PROSTATE CANCER

CURRENT CLINICAL ONCOLOGY

Breast Cancer
B.J. Kennedy, M.D., *Editor*

Late Effects of Treatment for Childhood Cancer
Daniel M. Green, M.D., and Giulio J. D'Angio, M.D., *Editors*

Prostate Cancer
Nancy A. Dawson, M.D., and Nicholas J. Vogelzang, M.D.,
Editors

Lung Cancer
Bruce E. Johnson, M.D., and David H. Johnson, M.D., *Editors*

PROSTATE CANCER

Editors

Nancy A. Dawson, M.D.
Walter Reed Army Medical Center
Washington, DC

Nicholas J. Vogelzang, M.D.
The University of Chicago Medical Center
The Pritzker School of Medicine
Chicago, Illinois

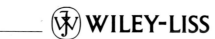 **WILEY-LISS**

A JOHN WILEY & SONS, INC., PUBLICATION
New York • Chichester • Brisbane • Toronto • Singapore

Address All Inquiries to the Publisher
Wiley-Liss, Inc., 605 Third Avenue, New York, NY 10158-0012

Copyright © 1994 Wiley-Liss, Inc.

Printed in the United States of America

While the authors, editors, and publisher believe that drug selection and dosage and the specification and usage of equipment and devices, as set forth in this book, are in accord with current recommendations and practice at the time of publication, they accept no legal responsibility for any errors or omissions, and make no warranty, express or implied, with respect to material contained herein. In view of ongoing research, equipment modifications, changes in governmental regulations and the constant flow of information relating to drug therapy, drug reactions, and the use of equipment and devices, the reader is urged to review and evaluate the information provided in the package insert or instructions for each drug, piece of equipment, or device for, among other things, any changes in the instructions or indication of dosage or usage and for added warnings and precautions.

Library of Congress Cataloging-in-Publication Data

Prostate cancer / editors, Nancy A. Dawson, Nicholas J. Vogelzang.
      p.   cm. — (Current clinical oncology series)
    Includes index.
    ISBN 0-471-58834-2
    1. Prostate—Cancer. I. Dawson, Nancy A. II. Vogelzang,
Nicholas. III. Series: Current clinical oncology.
    [DNLM: 1. Prostatic Neoplasms. WJ 752 P9662 1994]
    RC280.P7P742 1994
    616.99'463—dc20
    DNLM/DLC
    for Library of Congress   93-44295

The text of this book is printed on acid-free paper.

Contents

Contributors

Frederick R. Ahmann, M.D.
Section of Hematology/Oncology, Tucson
VA Medical Center, Tucson, AZ 85723
[215]

Peter C. Albertsen, M.D.
Division of Urology, University of
Connecticut Health Center, Farmington,
CT 06032 **[185]**

Gerald L. Andriole, M.D.
Division of Urologic Surgery, Washington
University School of Medicine, St. Louis,
MO 63110 **[95]**

Gregory T. Bales, M.D.
Department of Surgery, The University of
Chicago The Pritzker School of Medicine,
Chicago, IL 60637 **[65]**

Michael J. Barry, M.D.
Division of Urology, University of
Connecticut Health Center, Farmington,
CT 06032 **[185]**

Otis W. Brawley, M.D.
Division of Cancer Prevention and
Control, National Cancer Institute,
Bethesda, MD 20892 **[47]**

Peter R. Carroll, M.D.
Department of Urology, University of
California School of Medicine, San
Francisco, CA 94143 **[175]**

Michael L. Cher, M.D.
Department of Urology, University of
California School of Medicine, San
Francisco, CA 94143 **[175]**

Bruce L. Dalkin, M.D.
Section of Hematology/Oncology, Tucson
VA Medical Center, Tucson, AZ 85723
[215]

Nancy A. Dawson, M.D.
Hematology-Oncology Service, Walter
Reed Army Medical Center, Washington,
DC 20307 **[235]**

Jaya Gaddipati, Ph.D.
Department of Surgery, USUHS,
Bethesda, MD 20814 **[19]**

Glenn S. Gerber, M.D.
Department of Surgery, The University of
Chicago The Pritzker School of Medicine,
Chicago, IL 60637 **[65]**

Ruth D. Goldberg, M.B.B.Ch.
4501 Park Glen Road, #124, Saint Louis
Park, MN 55416 **[113]**

Gregory S. Grose, M.D.
Department of Urology, University of
Wisconsin Medical School, Madison, WI
53792 **[197]**

Joseph V. Gulfo, M.D.
CYTOGEN, 600 College Road East,
Princeton, NJ 08540 **[77]**

David W. Keetch, M.D.
Division of Urologic Surgery, Washington
University School of Medicine, St. Louis,
MO 63141 **[95]**

The page number in brackets is the opening page number of the contributor's article.

Thomas E. Kingston, M.D.
Division of Urology, Brown University
School of Medicine, Providence, RI 02912
[165]

Ken Kobayashi, M.D.
Section of Hematology/Oncology, The
University of Chicago The Pritzker
School of Medicine, Chicago, IL 60637
[235]

Barnett S. Kramer, M.D., M.P.H.
Division of Cancer Prevention and
Control, National Cancer Institute,
Bethesda, MD 20892 [47]

David G. McLeod, M.D., J.D.
Urology Service, Walter Reed Army
Medical Center, Washington, DC 20307
[1]

Edward M. Messing, M.D.
Department of Urology, University of
Wisconsin Medical School, Madison, WI
53792 [197]

Judd W. Moul, M.D.
Department of Surgery, USUHS,
Bethesda, MD 20814 [19]

Daniel B. Rukstalis, M.D.
Department of Surgery, The University of
Chicago The Pritzker School of Medicine,
Chicago, IL 60637 [151]

Kenneth J. Russell, M.D.
Department of Radiation Oncology,
University of Washington Medical
Center, Seattle, WA 98195 [133]

Katsuto Shinohara, M.D.
Department of Urology, University of
California School of Medicine, San
Francisco, CA 94143 [175]

Edward B. Silberstein, M.D.
Radioisotope Laboratory, University of
Cincinnati Medical Center, Cincinnati,
OH 45267 [261]

Eric J. Small, M.D.
Division of Medical Oncology, University
of Calfornia School of Medicine, San
Francisco, CA 94143 [175]

Shiv Srivastava, Ph.D.
Department of Surgery, USUHS,
Bethesda, MD 20814 [19]

Barry S. Stein, M.D.
Division of Urology, Brown University
School of Medicine, Providence, RI 02903
[165]

Francis H. Straus II, M.D.
Department of Pathology, The University
of Chicago Hospitals, Chicago, IL 60637
[113]

Nicholas J. Vogelzang, M.D.
Section of Hematology/Oncology, The
University of Chicago The Pritzker
School of Medicine, Chicago, IL 60637
[235]

John H. Wasson, M.D.
Division of Urology, University of
Connecticut Medical Center, Farmington,
CT 06032 [185]

Foreword

This volume on prostate cancer in the *Current Clinical Oncology* series is most timely. Prostate cancer is the most common malignancy in men in this country and is likely to grow in frequency with the aging of our population. During the past few years there have been some significant developments in our ability to screen for earlier detection of prostate cancer, and new agents for the treatment of this malignancy based on our understanding of its hormonal dependence. Recently a national trial was begun to determine if prostate cancer can be prevented.

Some of these developments have raised new questions for our consideration that are being subjected to the test of clinical trials. One important example is the opportunity for detecting prostate cancer earlier through the use of prostate-specific antigen (PSA) and the diagnostic imaging technique—transrectal ultrasound (TRUS). There has not yet been definitive demonstration that these techniques for earlier detection will have a significant impact on survival. Furthermore, their availability raises new issues concerning the proper treatment of localized prostate cancer, and even if in some individuals treatment is needed at all. A challenge is presented to further understand the biology of prostate cancer in order to define more clearly which tumors in older men will have a relatively benign indolent course, and which, if left untreated, will have a greater propensity for growth and metastasis.

Currently there is controversy about which is the most appropriate curative approach to localized cancer—surgery or radiation therapy. Here the consideration is not only which is most likely to be curative, but also which will result in the least long-term complications affecting the quality of life of the patient who has been cured.

The availability of new agents for hormonal manipulation presents opportunities for the palliative treatment of those individuals who already have metastatic disease. Ongoing clinical trials will provide information concerning the best regimens and certainly opportunities for testing newer agents as they become available. The availability of an agent finesteride, which was introduced to alleviate benign prostatic hypertrophy, raises the possibility of its use in the prevention or delay in clinical onset of prostate cancer in high-risk men.

There is still much to be learned about the biology of prostate cancer and the identification of specific risk factors. We have learned a great deal about risk factors for other cancers that have led to opportunities for preventive strategies. Hopefully, further studies of the epidemiology of this cancer and its biology at a molecular level will lead to information of value in the design for approaches to prevention in the future.

Alvin M. Mauer, M.D.
John E. Ultmann, M.D.

Preface

Prostate cancer is the most common nonskin malignancy in men in the United States. The American Cancer Society (ACS) estimated that 165,000 new cases were diagnosed in 1993, accounting for 25% of all cancer cases in men. Overall, it is the third most common malignancy, only exceeded by breast cancer (182,000 new cases) and lung cancer (170,000 new cases). With the rapidly increasing incidence of the disease, due in part to prostate-specific antigen (PSA) screening and the ease of transrectal prostate biopsies, it is widely believed that there will be over 200,000 new cases of prostate cancer by the year 2000. At present, prostate cancer is the second leading cause of cancer mortality, with only lung cancer killing more American males. An estimated 35,000 men will die of prostate cancer in 1993.

Despite its prevalence, only in the last decade has public awareness surged and prostate cancer research funding significantly risen. Prostate Cancer Awareness Week has facilitated large-scale prostate cancer screening and dissemination of medical information. The stigma of having prostate cancer has been significantly mitigated as numerous public figures have shared their experiences as prostate cancer survivors. Chapters of Us Too, a prostate cancer support group, are forming in every state in the country. Patient Advocates for Advanced Cancer Treatment (PAACT) has focused predominantly on promoting prostate cancer care, communication, and legislation to prevent discrimination against cancer patients and to expand research. Funding of prostate cancer research, especially directed at cancer screening and cancer prevention, has significantly increased. These funds are federal (NIH), voluntary (ACS), and pharmaceutical.

In this atmosphere of heightened awareness and accelerated research efforts, it becomes apparent that there are far more controversies in prostate cancer research than there are answers. Prostate cancer screening is increasing the detection of early-stage disease, but its impact on disease-specific mortality is unproven. Recent analyses suggest that therapies directed at localized cancer result in relatively little gain in years of life expectancy for most patients. If this is true, then how can our strained health care system either afford or justify mass screening?

Nonetheless, there are exciting new diagnostic and therapeutic techniques and treatment modalities. Radical prostatectomy and external beam radiation, the two standard approaches to localized disease, can be complicated by impotence, incontinence, and radiation-induced cystitis or enteritis. Cryosurgery, which uses subzero temperatures to destroy diseased tissue, and laser therapy, which induces tumor necrosis with light energy transformed into heat, both show promise in the control of localized prostate cancer with decreased morbidity. The use of neoadjuvant hormonal therapy to decrease tumor size preoperatively and potentially "downstage" locally advanced disease is also a promising area under active investigation.

In the arena of metastatic disease, a novel new therapeutic agent, suramin, has shown significant activity in hormone-refractory prostate cancer. The use of new beta-emitting, bone-seeking radiopharmaceuticals, which include strontium-89, samarium-153 EDTMP, and rhenium-186 diphosphonate, can significantly reduce pain and improve mobility and quality of life in the majority of terminal patients with symptomatic bone metastases.

It is the focus of this book to concentrate on these and other new advances in prostate cancer and the current status of the most crucial controversial issues.

Nancy A. Dawson, M.D.
Nicholas J. Vogelzang, M.D.

Prostate Cancer: Past, Present, and Future

David G. McLeod, M.D., J.D.

HISTORY OF THE TREATMENT OF PROSTATE CANCER

Prior to 1900 the diagnoses of diseases of the prostate were inexact and were often lumped together under hyperplasia of the prostate. Thus any cause of urinary obstruction, benign prostatic hyperplasia (BPH), prostatic carcinoma (PCa), bladder calculi, prostatitis, and/or ureteral strictures were not always differentiated. Usually a prostate condition was discovered due to the resulting condition, i.e., urinary obstruction. In 1855, Gross wrote that prostatic cancer ("scirrhus") was a rare disease.[1] Although he stated that he had not treated a case, he felt that the recommended treatment was rest, diet, anodynes, and occasional application of leeches to the perineum. During the 19th and early 20th century, while prostate cancer was felt to be uncommon, it is certain that many cases attributed to BPH and other conditions were in reality cancer of the prostate.

In 1817 Langstaff was the first to describe a case of cancer of the prostate.[2] Wadd in that same year presented a case of urinary obstruction in a patient with "fungus haematodes" in which he felt that the obstruction was secondary to prostatic cancer.[3] Attention began to be directed toward PCa as a disease entity when in 1844 Tanchon reviewed 8,289 cases and found five cases of the disease and 10 years later Thompson reported on 29 cases.[4,5] The 20th-century interest in the disease can be attributed in part to the work of Albarran and Hallé.[6] These authors examined 100 specimens of supposed BPH and found 14 cases of PCa, which they called "epithelioma adenoide," and reported their work in 1900.

Lydston in his textbook *The Surgical Diseases of the Genito-Urinary Tract*, published in 1899, stated some conclusions regarding PCa that when closely examined bear some occasional similarities to a description of the disease in today's terms.[7] An excerpt follows:

> Malignant disease of the prostate is rare, yet it is probably more frequent than ordinarily supposed, being often erroneously diagnosed. Histologically, malignant disease of the prostate occurs in two forms, viz.: sarcoma and carcinoma. It is found at the two extremes of life, being exceptional between the ages of ten and fifty years. It is occasionally found in very young children. In something over 85 per cent. of cases the malignant affection assumes the form of carcinoma, the remainder being of a sarcomatous character. Sarcoma is the form that is most likely to be met with in young patients.

Cancer of the prostate occurs clinically in three forms, viz.:(1) primary; (2) as an infection secondary to malignant disease of contiguous organs; (3) by infection via the blood. The form most often seen is secondary to malignant disease of the penis, testes, bladder, or kidneys. As Guyon has shown, primary prostatic cancer has but little tendency to invade the bladder, but speedily involves the lymphatics, especially of the pelvis. This latter clinical fact suggested to Guyon the term prostato-pelvic cancer. The disease may be at first circumscribed. It is usually, however, diffuse. The capsule of the gland may alone be affected, at least primarily. Eventually extensive pelvic invasion occurs, with involvement of the seminal vesicles, base of the bladder and sometimes its mucous membrane, the rectum, and urethra. Mixed infection and suppuration may eventually develop.

SYMPTOMS.—Frequent and painful micturition with hematuria—and, ulceration of the prostate exists, more or less purulent discharge—constitute the main symptomatic features. Pain is likely to be most severe at night, and is often referred to the region of the rectum. As the pelvic tissues become extensively involved, pressure irritation and resulting pain in one or both sciatic nerves is likely to develop. Intrapelvic pressure also may produce more or less obstruction of the iliac veins, with resistant edema of the limbs. Marked cachexia comes on at a comparatively early period. A fatal result is inevitable.

DIAGNOSIS.—In the differential diagnosis tuberculosis and prostatic hypertrophy only are worthy of consideration. A hard, nodular enlargement of the prostate with cachexia, pronounced symptoms referable to the vesical neck, and extreme pain suggestive of pelvic involvement, taken in connection with enlargement of the pelvic lymphatic glands and those of Scarpa's triangle, warrant a diagnosis of cancer. When cancer exists elsewhere in the body, and especially if it has invaded organs contiguous to or correlated with the prostate, the diagnosis is a very simple matter.

TREATMENT.—Treatment must necessarily be palliative. All radical attempts at surgical relief have thus far failed of their object. The author believes that early suprapubic section and the establishment of a permanent artificial urethra is the principal surgical indication. Great relief of some of the most annoying symptoms of the disease and prolongation of life are likely to result from the rest and relief from mechanic irrigation thus secured.

Although the perineum had been the site used to approach the prostate and bladder, particularly for attempts to remove bladder calculi; it was Bilroth who, in 1867, first performed perineal prostatectomy for carcinoma of the prostate.

The introduction of surgery for carcinoma of the prostate in the United States began in 1904 when Young, with Halsted as his assistant, performed the first radical perineal prostatectomy at Johns Hopkins. He reported on this case and three others in 1905.[8] From 1904 to 1927 Young performed perineal prostatectomy on 24 patients. Jewett later reported on 222 cases starting with Young's initial case in 1904 and including all cases through May 1948.[9] It is interesting that he reported a failure to diagnose cancer on microscopic examination in 24 of the cases, while in another eight the pathology reports were missing—experiences that, although uncommon, still occur. Jewett felt that the surgical technique of a radical perineal prostatectomy was relatively simple, with the mortality at the time being approximately 3%. Also, he felt that in properly selected cases the five-year disease-free survival rate was 51%, while the 10-year rate was 29%. He implored physicians not to wait for the appearance of metastatic disease before making the diagnosis of PCa, and he advocated that radical perineal prostatectomy was the procedure of choice for early cancer.

Opinions differed in the early and middle 20th century, as they do today, on the most effective treatment of PCa. There were several factors which sparked controversy during the years following Young's introduction to radical prostatectomy in this country. Culp and Meyer stated that there were innumerable "conscientious objectors" to perineal prostatectomy.[10] As they pointed out, many urologic surgeons were never comfortable with the procedure. When Millin published his experiences with the retropubic approach for benign disease in 1947, which led to the modern-day retropubic approach for localized cancer of the prostate, many surgeons felt that it too was a difficult operation to master, and there was no rush to embrace the latter procedure.[11] The early proponents of surgery had other factors with which to contend. Staging was inexact, there were frequently improperly selected patients, and indeed in some instances surgery was carried out by poorly qualified surgeons. Timing of appropriate surgery was obviously important; this fact, plus the inability to discern PCa in a potential curable stage, along with the prevailing view that if it could be detected clinically it probably was already incurable, all added to the controversy as to the most efficacious form of treatment.

Irradiation therapy competed with surgery during the first half of the 20th century in this group of patients. In 1911 Pasteau reported on the first radiotherapeutic approach to the treatment of PCa by using radium inserted through a ureteral catheter.[12] However, as with the surgical approach, most patients were not cured due to the extent of their disease. It was not until 1930 when Attwater reported on orthovoltage as a means of obtaining better control of the tumor that radiotherapy began to be viewed as a viable treatment modality.[13] Next in the development of irradiation therapy was Flock's interstitial therapy with radioactive gold ^{198}Au seeds.[14] He compared 1,193 patients treated by various modalities to 430 treated with ^{198}Au placed transrectally or transperineally, with the five-year survival in the two groups being 33% and 47%, respectively. The interest in brachytherapy waned, at least temporarily, with the advent of megavoltage external beam irradiation therapy in the mid-1950s. Cancerocidal doses could now be delivered to deep tissues without exceeding the radiation tolerance to other tissues and the skin. This had been a major drawback to the use of orthovoltage therapy. Irradiation therapy, combined with the prevailing view that few patients were candidates for radical surgery, along with the continuing perception that radical surgery was extremely difficult, pushed radiotherapy, as the treatment of choice for localized prostate cancer, at least for a period of time. As refinements of both techniques—surgery and irradiation—improved, controversy began to be generated over which was the better modality, an ongoing debate today. During the 1960s, interstitial implantation of encapsulated radioactive sources enjoyed a revival of interest due primarily to investigators at Memorial Sloan-Kettering Cancer Center. Their use of isotopes included ^{222}radon, ^{192}iridium, and ^{125}iodine, but most of the work carried out at Memorial in the 1970s was primarily with ^{125}iodine due to this isotope's ability to maintain a high radiation dose throughout the prostate while at the same time reducing the radiation exposure to personnel performing the implantation[15] (see also Chapter 8).

With the advent of transrectal ultrasonography (TRUS), more accurate placement of the radioactive implant is now possible. Although brachytherapy has enjoyed a resurgence lately with other isotopes such as ^{109}Pd, external beam irradiation has been at the forefront of definitive treatment from the viewpoint of most radiotherapists. Led by the early work of Bagshaw, Badhraja, and others, external beam irradiation has been, and remains, a viable alternative therapy for localized disease[16,17] (see also Chapter 8). Attempts have been made to achieve greater local control by combining external irradiation plus brachytherapy, and at Stanford Bagshaw added localized hyperthermia.[18]

In the past several years retropubic radical prostatectomy has become a surgical procedure that is now employed more than ever. The renewed interest in this technique and its wide employment in the treatment of localized disease is due primarily to its refinement and to a better understanding of the anatomical dissection. The seminal work of Walsh and his associates at Johns Hopkins University focused attention on the procedure, resulting in a more meticulous dissection that resulted in less blood loss and a higher incidence of preservation of potency.[19] Recently with laparoscopic pelvic node dissection, perineal prostatectomy, although never completely abandoned, is being used by a growing number of urologic surgeons (see also Chapter 9).

Although White in 1895 had performed castration on 111 men with symptoms of BPH, noting that they had responded well, it is fairly certain that some of his patients' symptoms were from cancer of the prostate and their improvement was due to androgen withdrawal.[20] However, it was the work of Charles Huggins and his student Clarence Hodges that ushered in the modern era of research on prostate cancer. These two investigators discovered the androgen dependency of PCa in 1941.[21] Prostate cancer was affected by endocrine therapy, either orchiectomy or the oral synthetic diethylstilbestrol estrogen (DES), and hormonal therapy competed as a form of therapy with this population of patients. Their work was based in part on the knowledge of biochemistry of the disease, knowledge that was based on the work of Gutman and Gutman, who had shown in the mid-1930s that PCa and its metastases secreted greater than normal levels of the enzyme acid phosphatase.[22] There was an initial period of optimism that endocrine therapy would be the answer to the treatment, or at least a portion

of the treatment for all patients with the disease (see also Chapter 14).

Prostate cancer is ubiquitous, as has been described in several autopsy series. From 1939 to 1941, independent autopsy series found its incidence to range from 14 to 46%.[23–26] In most cases the cancers seen at autopsy were small, contained within the prostate, were incidental to the patients' death, and but for the fact that an autopsy was performed would not have been diagnosed. The concept of "indolence" of the disease was introduced. In other words, carcinoma of the prostate was a disease one might likely die with but not a disease that would usually cause one's demise. However, some patients have tumors that are so malignant that metastases occur before any local symptoms do. At the other extreme are the indolent tumors that remain so throughout a patient's life. The mechanism(s) by which the body controls the development of this disease is unknown. The reasons for this indolent or dormant disease on the one hand and the rapid dissemination of disease on the other are still the quest of investigations. Franks elaborated on latency versus active prostate cancer without considering stage or grade of the tumor and made the observation that in men over the age of 80, while clinical cases became less frequent, latent cases were very common.[27] He also stated that there was no reliable method of distinguishing latent from aggressive carcinomas.

It was 1925 when Broders published his paper introducing tumor grading as a means of differentiating latent tumors from their more aggressive counterparts.[28] Since then, grading has been the pathologist's attempt to prognosticate the behavior of prostate cancer, and the problems are myriad.[29] In 1979 the National Prostate Cancer Detection Project (NPCDP) recommended the Gleason system. This system recognizes a primary and a secondary pattern and, in each, five different patterns.[30]

There is extensive literature on the subject, many in favor of the system, others against it, and two excellent reviews.[31,32] The major problem with the system is its reproducibility. Even in Gleason's hands the reproducibility was only 80%. Dissatisfaction with the Gleason system has lead to proposals for other compilations (see also Chapter 7).

Since 1979 five different systems have been proposed. The simplest of these is the one proposed by Dhom.[33] He grouped PCa with less than 10% of tissue involved by tumor as group I, those with more than 10% as group II, and those with 100% tumor as group III. This is the most easily reproducible system.

The World Health Organization (WHO) grading system takes into account the degree of nuclear anaplasia (nuclear grades) and the pattern of glandular differentiation (histologic grades).[34] Nuclear anaplasia is defined as variation of nuclear size, shape, chromatin distribution, and the character of nucleoli. Such variation could be slight (nuclear Grade I), moderate (nuclear Grade II), and marked nuclear anaplasia (nuclear Grade III).

A number of modifications of the WHO system have been proposed. Gaeta et al. take into account differentiation or nuclear anaplasia and base the final grade on the worst of the two.[35] Brawn et al. use a grading system based on differentiation alone.[36] Irrespective of the system used, all grading systems recognize the good tumors and the bad tumors. There is some disagreement in the intermediate group, but the major problems with all grading systems are that most tumors fall in the intermediate grade and none is applicable to individual patients.

In 1969, in a detailed autopsy study of 45 men with prostatic cancer, McNeal advanced the hypothesis that the malignant potential of prostate cancer was related to tumor size, and tumors less than 1 cm³ in volume have little potential for dissemination.[37] Added to the above observations is the fact that in 1900 life expectancy for a man was 47 years, around 1950 it had increased to 67 years, and at present it is 76. Whereas in 1950 there were 16 million men over age 50, today there are approximately 28 million in this category. In 1994 it is estimated that there will be 200,000 men diagnosed with prostate cancer and 38,000 will die of the disease.

TNM STAGING SYSTEM

Numerous systems of staging prostatic carcinoma have been devised but here also agreement has precluded any universal acceptance. The staging system most commonly used in the United States is the one introduced by Whitmore and later modified by both he and Jewett.[38] Using this staging system, PCa has been classified into four clinical categories, A through D. Recently there has been considerable enthusiasm for worldwide use of the Tumor–Nodes–Metastases (TNM) system. The various staging systems are described in Table 1.

As mentioned previously, no one stage system satisfies all aspects of clinical practice. With continuing refinements in diagnostic modalities we shall continue to see modifications and refinements in staging and grading of these lesions. The TNM system (Table 1) is the most accurate staging system to date, and there is increasing pressure to use it in staging PCa.

Stage A (T_1)

These are tumors that are not detectable on digital rectal exam (DRE) but are usually found on subsequent examination of prostatic tissue removed during a transurethral resection of the prostate (TURP). There is no clinical evidence of spread outside the prostate. This stage is subdivided into A_1 (T_{1a}) disease, i.e., well-differentiated cancer in less than 5% of the resected tissue, and A_2 (T_{1b}) disease, i.e., any cancer other

TABLE 1. Adenocarcinoma of the Prostate: Clinical Staging Systems

Description	Modified Whitmore	Modified Jewett	TNM (1992)[a]
Clinically localized disease			
Incidental TURP	A	A	T_1
• Focal, low-grade	A_1	A_1	T_{1a}
• Diffuse, high-grade	A_2	A_2	T_{1b}
Diagnosed on TRUS Guided Biopsy— prompted by elevated PSA only	—	—	T_{1c}
Clinically Detected			
• Palpable tumor 1 lobe	$B_1(\leq 2cm)$	$B_{1N}(\geq 1cm)$	$T_{2a}(<\frac{1}{2}$ lobe$)$ $T_{2b}(>\frac{1}{2}$ lobe but <1 lobe$)$
	$B_2(>2cm)$		
• Palpable tumor both lobes	B_3	B_2	T_{2c} (both lobes)
• Palpable beyond capsule	C	C	T_{3-4}
• Extending to lateral sulcus	C_1	—	T_3(unilat.) T_3(bilat.)
• Extending to base of sem. vesicle(s)	C_2	—	T_3
• Beyond base of sem. vesicle(s)	C_3	—	—
• Invades sphincter, bladder neck, or rectum	—	—	T_4
• Invades levator muscles or pelvic side wall	—	—	T_4
Metastatic disease	D	D	$T_{1-4}N_{1-3}M_0$
• Pelvic lymph nodes only	D_1	D_1	$T_{1-4}N_1M_0$
• Bones, lung, etc.	D_2	D_2	$T_{1-4}N_{1-3}M_1$ (bone)
• Lung, liver, brain	—	—	$T_{1-4}N_{1-3}M_{1c}$
• Elevated acid phos. only	D_0	D_0	—
• Hormonally refractory	\multicolumn{3}{Commonly referred to as D_3}	

[a]Manual for Staging of Cancer, 4th ed, American Joint Committee on Cancer, 1992.

than well-differentiated and/or cancer in more than 5% of the resected tissue. Men with A_1 disease have a better prognosis than those with A_2 disease, and several studies have shown that patients with a small focus of well-differentiated tumor do as well as the age-matched control population.[39-42] However, some investigators have advocated a re-TURP to ensure that the amount of tumor removed was indeed a small focus and not just the "tip" of more diffuse and therefore more aggressive disease.[43] Historically approximately 10–15% of patients undergoing TURP for BPH have exhibited PCa; however, at the present time stage A (T_{1a} and T_{1b}) disease is being diagnosed less often due to the use

of prostate-specific antigen (PSA), which is usually drawn during routine evaluation prior to TURP. Prostate-specific antigen is a 34-kd protein that is specific to the prostatic epithelium. Its use for diagnosis and staging is undergoing extensive investigations (see also Chapter 6), but it is the rare patient who undergoes treatment for BPH today who has not had a PSA drawn along with a DRE. If one or both of these studies are abnormal, then TRUS is usually employed. The occasional case of prostatic cancer is still being found when either a PSA was not drawn prior to surgery or else the prostate was benign feeling and of such a size that PCa was not suspected, even in the face of a mildly elevated PSA.

In our practice the rate of detection of stage A (T_{1a} and T_{1b}) disease has fallen from 10% to 2% since we have been drawing a PSA on all patients prior to TURP. In patients treated by other surgical modalities, e.g., laser therapy, where no tissue is removed, the possibility of overlooking PCa is always present. However, in patients with an abnormal PSA and/or DRE and subsequent investigation by TRUS with a possible biopsy, the amount of overlooked PCa is now very small. In addition to those patients who have no tissue removed because of alternate surgical procedures, the chance to overlook PCa is also present in those patients who are having their BPH treated with medical therapy.

Stage B_0 (T_{1c})

This proposed classification recently has emerged due to increasing diagnostic abilities, which have in turn led to PCa being diagnosed more frequently. In men with "normal" glands on DRE and in whom PSA values are elevated, the latter will frequently prompt a TRUS examination. Strictly speaking, if the prostate is normal on TRUS and an empirical sextant biopsy reveals PCa, the patient is said to have T_{1C} disease. However, when an abnormal area is seen on TRUS, and biopsy reveals PCa, most urologists consider this lesion also to be stage T_{1C} although these lesions are more appropriately be T_{2a} or T_{2b}.

Stage B (T_2)

This stage of PCa refers to those tumors that are palpable on DRE and felt to be confined solely to the prostate. This stage has been subdivided into B_1, B_2, and B_3 disease or T_{2a}, T_{2b}, and T_{2c} disease. A lesion that is a palpable tumor confined to one lobe and is less than 2 cm in size is classified as B_1, while a greater than 2 cm lesion is B_2. In solitary lesions confined to one lobe that are less than 1 cm in diameter, another subclassification has occasionally been used: B_{1N}. The TNM system distinguishes T_{2a} ($<1/2$ of a lobe involved) and T_{2b} ($>1/2$ of a lobe involved). In those lesions that involve both lobes on rectal examination, stage B_3 or T_{2c} is used. Although still useful in the clinical setting, reproducibility in discerning prostate lesions from one examiner to another has been difficult and is, in reality, often impossible. In other words, one examiner's B_1 lesion might, in the estimation of another, be a B_2 lesion. Digital rectal examination is useful but its limitations, although recognized for some time, are being further accentuated in the past several years as a result of TRUS and the increasing use of PSA values. Prostatic-specific antigen is clearly reproducible and is much more reliable than DRE. Nevertheless the two tests are complementary and should be used together.

The true B lesion should be amenable to radical prostatectomy, but should not irradiation therapy also be curable? To try and settle this controversy the National Prostate Cancer Project in the mid-1980s attempted a clinical trial. In those patients with clinical A_2 or B disease and who would agree to a randomization between the two treatment regimens, a pelvic node dissection was carried out. Randomization was performed prior to surgery, and if the nodes were negative, the patient proceeded immediately to a radical prostatectomy or, depending on the randomization, surgery was terminated and the patient received irradiation after recovering from his surgery. Initially patients were to receive their randomization at the time of surgery when the pelvic nodes were found to be negative. In an attempt to accrue more patients it was pointed out to the statisticians that patients needed to be randomized preoperatively, that is, prior to surgery, knowing that the occasional patient would turn out to be ineligible if his nodes were positive. Nevertheless, this study had to be abandoned after several years when the accrual was only eight patients. Another more recent attempt by the Southwestern Oncology Group (SWOG) was also abandoned due to lack of accrual. Although it would be ideal to settle the issue of irradiation versus surgery it is doubtful if the question can ever be answered.

Stage C (T_3 and T_4)

This stage consists of those cancers that clinically have spread outside the prostate but have not metastasized. Again, clinical determination by DRE is very subjective and upon pathological examination up to 50% of the prostate specimens, which were felt to have the cancers contained within them, are found to have disease either to the inked margin, into the periprostatic tissue, or into the seminal vesicles. Stage C disease has been subdivided into C_1, C_2, and C_3 (T_{3a}, T_{3b}, and T_{3c}). Classically these tumors have been treated with external beam irradiation. Lymph node involvement has been found to be present in approximately 50% of patients, upstaging them to stage D_1 (pelvic node positive). Initially lymphangiography was utilized to ascertain pelvic nodal involvement. It has been abandoned since obturator and hypogastric nodes are infrequently visualized. In addition, when the visualized nodes were biopsied the false-negative rate was high; the procedure was tedious, time-consuming, and not without morbidity, e.g., pneumonitis. Pelvic computerized tomography (CT) scanning and more recently laparoscopic node dissection have antiquated this diagnostic modality.

Side effects are usually minimal when irradiation is used for either B or C lesions (see Chapter 8). With modern techniques they consist of mild diarrhea, rectal urgency, dysuria, and frequency. In general most patients tolerate radiation therapy well, and if they have any of the aforementioned symptoms conservative therapy usually results in abatement of their complaints.

Very few patients develop rectal or urinary incontinence. The most serious side effects seen today are in those patients who develop small-capacity bladders and/or frequent, sometimes life-threatening hematuria months to years following therapy. These complications are frequently aggravated by recurrent local disease, and on rare occasions patients must have a urinary diversion because of them. There have been no prospective randomized studies comparing irradiation to surgery, and the natural history of the disease allows some patients in all series to do well. Furthermore, all retrospective analyses suffer from lack of control, occasional concomitant endocrine therapy, and variable follow-up. Thus the debate between physicians who prefer surgical or irradiation management techniques for stage C (T_3) is likely to continue unabated.

Stage D ($T_{1-4}N_{1-3}$)

This group of patients has also been divided into several subsets. Patients with disease in only pelvic lymph nodes are classified as D_1 disease (see also Chapter 13). Staging lymphadenectomy at the time of radical prostatectomy has been found to be positive in as many as 20% of patients in the Mayo Clinic series.[44] Their experience suggested better results with radical prostatectomy and endocrine therapy when compared to therapy with endocrine therapy alone. Survival was apparently better in those patients who had diploid tumors. Irradiation therapy alone was not found to be efficacious and radical prostatectomy alone, although superior to irradiation, did not seem to control metastatic spread in their patients.

TREATMENT TO DATE

In 1978 the National Prostate Cancer Project (NPCP) completed two protocols that evaluated adjuvant systemic therapy following surgery (Protocol 900) or radiation (Protocol 1,000).[45] All patients had a staging pelvic lymphadenectomy. Patients were randomized to receive estramustine phosphate 600 mg/m² orally daily for two years, cyclophosphamide 1 gm/m² intravenously every three weeks, or observation. It is interesting that the progression-free survival and overall survival were greater in Protocol 900 (surgery) as compared to those patients in Protocol 1,000, regardless of the adjuvant therapy. This is not too surprising as, in general, the patients in the surgically treated group had a lower pathologic stage. Lymph node involvement was seen in 49% of those patients in Protocol 900 and in 63% in Protocol 1,000. In the patients in the irradiation-treated group there was a greater progression-free survival for all patients, including those with limited and extensive nodal disease, who received estramustine phosphate.

In those patients with bony metastases and/or distant nodal or soft tissue spread (D-2) it is important to remember that endocrine treatment of PCa is palliative in nature. Three studies of early hormonal treatment demonstrated prolonged life in patients with metastatic prostate cancer. Vest and Frazier compared 71 patients who had bilateral orchiectomy with a similar group of patients who were not treated.[46] The untreated patients in their series were patients who were followed prior to the discovery of hormonal manipulation, and this group of patients did not live as long as the subsequently treated ones. Nesbitt and Plumb reported on a series of 795 patients selected from an era before the advent of hormonal treatment of metastatic disease.[47] They compared this group to a later cohort of 75 patients treated by bilateral orchiectomy and estrogens and found the latter group's overall survival rate to be better. Then in yet another early study of this question by Nesbitt and Baum, the survival rate of the untreated patients in

the Nesbitt and Plumb series was compared with that for 263 patients treated by hormonal therapy (i.e., orchiectomy or estrogens).[48] The conclusion gleaned from these three series was that patients with metastatic cancer should be treated at the time of diagnosis. These studies are criticized because comparisons were made in groups of patients in different eras of medical treatment. It is impossible to determine the impact of antibiotic therapy and refinement of surgical procedures (e.g., transurethral prostatectomy) on the later groups of patients who were also treated by hormonal therapy. These individualized and uncontrolled studies do not pass the stringent controls imperative in modern clinical trials.

In 1967, the first randomized study was undertaken by the Veterans Administration Cooperative Urological Research Group (VACURG).[49] This study accrued a total of 1,093 patients with clinical stage C or D disease. Patients received one of the following: (1) placebo, (2) orchiectomy, (3) 5 mg daily of DES, or (4) 5 mg of DES and orchiectomy. At the time of progression each group was crossed over to a different treatment arm. The study thus allowed for the placebo group to be treated by hormone therapy at the time of progression. However, within one year the majority of patients had endocrine treatment initiated. Basically two conclusions can be drawn from this series: (1) the delayed therapy in the control group did not show an increase in time to death compared to other groups; (2) there was a higher incidence of cardiovascular morbidity and mortality in the DES-treated groups. In the DES groups there were fewer cancer deaths but this observation may be due to the number of patients who died from cardiovascular causes before they could die from PCa. Although the findings of the first VACURG study were apparently at odds with those of the three earlier studies, in reality the question of hormonal therapy versus no hormonal therapy could not be answered ethically or scientifically.

Due to the increase in cardiovascular deaths attributable to estrogen therapy, the next VACURG study focused primarily on lowering the estrogen dosage.[50] Patients were randomized to receive placebo or one of three daily DES dosages; 0.2, 1.0, or 5.0 mg. This study demonstrated that there was a slight survival advantage among patients who received 1.0 mg of DES daily. Also it was found that orchiectomy was equal to DES therapy. The combination of orchiectomy and DES did not offer an advantage over either therapy alone. These results seem to imply that there was a difference in survival in patients treated early with hormonal therapy. Once again this study suffered from design flaws, such as the lack of statistical analysis and the fact that placebo-treated patients were not crossed over to receive hormonal therapy. Additionally there was a median follow-up of only one year. A reexamination of these data found the mean length of survival for all patients to be approximately 30 months. This study therefore complemented the first VACURG study. In summary, these often-quoted and early studies favor hormonal therapy over no hormonal therapy, while the two controlled VACURG studies appeared to show no difference in early versus later hormonal therapy.

Bilateral orchiectomy has been, and is, considered the standard by which all forms of hormonal therapy are measured. Psychological aspects of orchiectomy are frequently cited, and in a recent study in which patients were offered either an orchiectomy or the luteinizing hormone-releasing hormone (LHRH) agonist goserlin (Zoladex), 70% of patients chose the latter.[51] Nevertheless, orchiectomy has much to offer a patient when cost, ease of procedure, immediate control of testosterone production, and compliance are all considered. It is important to remember that patients usually do not know the difference between orchiectomy and emasculation. When the physician explains to the patient that the scrotum remains and the penis is intact, most, though not all, will accept the procedure. It is my preference to make a small incision in each hemiscrotum to effect the bilateral orchiectomy. One incision in the median raphe will suffice, incisions can be carried out in the same amount of time, but I am spared the explanation of how I removed both testes through one incision. With a single incision I have not infrequently had to reassure the patient repeatedly that I had indeed removed both testes because invariably it seems that one spermatic cord is longer that the other, and the patient feels that he has one testicle remaining.

The operation of subcapsular orchiectomy is used by some urologists. Although I cannot quantify this statement, I have heard the operation advocated by a small but growing number of urologists. This renewed interest in this procedure may be attributed to a growing interest in this type of operation as an alternative option between "total" orchiectomy and a medical castration. Side effects of orchiectomy are usually impotence and occasional hot flashes.

The oral administration of estrogen, usually DES, inhibits luteinizing hormone (LH) production from the anterior pituitary. With this stimulation "blocked," the Leydig cells of the testes cease producing testosterone; however, it may take one to two weeks to achieve castrate levels. A daily dose of 3 mg of DES is felt to be required to block the diurnal production of testosterone. DES administered in daily doses of less than 3 mg does not consistently block the diurnal production of testosterone. As a method of hormonal treatment, DES has fallen into disfavor with the advent of LHRH agonists, due to the former's potential side effects. Although the cost of DES is negligible, the potential side effects are not. Cardiovascular problems (e.g., thrombophlebitis and peripheral edema) are serious and can be life-threatening. Gynecomastia is a major concern also, but after careful exclusion of a positive cardiovascular history and with an informed consent, if the decision is made to use DES, breast irradiation therapy for one to three days prior to initiation of treatment is recommended. As mentioned, the cardiovascular risks make the use of this drug questionable. Its use is somewhat antiquated, and I personally have not prescribed this therapy in several years; however, DES may still have a very limited role in the treatment of the occasional patient who refuses orchiectomy and will not allow medical castration by injection, albeit this type of patient is a rare entity.

In 1971, Schally et al. isolated the naturally occurring LHRH and later synthesized the compound.[52] The identification of this decapeptide has led to a new class of drugs for the treatment of advanced prostate cancer. The synthetic analogs of naturally occurring LHRH are approximately 100 times more potent than naturally occurring LHRH. These compounds cause a paradoxical desensitization of the pituitary, with sustained administration of LHRH parenterally. However, during initial treatment with an LHRH analog there is an initial increase in LH, with a resultant increase in testosterone. This increase of testosterone can cause worsening of symptoms of "flare" during the initial three to four days of treatment. The possibility of flare makes this drug contraindicated in patients with severe verbal metastases and in patients with acute ureteral obstruction. If it is necessary that these patients or those who are very symptomatic from bone pain be treated with an LHRH analog, initial simultaneous administration of an antiandrogen can prevent flare.[53] In these types of patients, orchiectomy, in my opinion, is the initial treatment of choice.

The efficacy of LHRH was demonstrated in a randomized prospective clinical trial in previously untreated patients with metastatic disease (stage D2).[54] Patients received either a 1 mg daily subcutaneous dose of leuprolide acetate (Lupron) or 3 mg orally of DES. When the data on the objective response to the DES and the leuprolide arms of the study were reviewed, there was no difference between the two treatment populations. In addition, there was no difference between the two arms in improvement of bony pain, performance status, and median time to progression. The survival statistics were also similar; however, there was a difference in side effects. Although patients who received leuprolide had a higher incidence of hot flashes, the incidence of serious cardiovascular complications and gynecomastia was significantly higher in the DES-treated group.

Following this study, leuprolide acetate was the first LHRH analog to be approved for use in the United States by the Food and Drug Administration (FDA). Initially the drug was given in a self-administered daily subcutaneous leuprolide dose of 1 mg. Subsequently, in early 1989 a monthly depot formulation of leuprolide became available. In this formulation a monthly intramuscular injection of 7.5 mg is administered and maintains therapeutic levels for up to five weeks. It is recommended that leuprolide be given on a monthly basis, although during the fifth week following injection, the drug continues to provide a concentration that achieves a castrate level. These extra days are enough to provide the patient a clinical window if he cannot keep his appointment at exactly four-week intervals.

About the same time that leuprolide became available in depot form, another analog, goserelin (Zoladex) became available. In this type of compound, a pellet is implanted subcutaneously via a 14-gauge needle. This 3.60-mg pellet has a constant release of drug over a one-month period.

This compound does not have the several "extra days" that leuprolide allows and should be given every 28 days for a total of 13 dosages per year. Makers of both drugs are actively carrying out research to develop a three-month depot preparation.

Buserelin (Suprefact) is an LHRH analog used extensively in Europe in depot form. Although a daily subcutaneous preparation was investigated in a large clinical trial in the United States, a decision was made not to seek FDA approval. There is one other LHRH analog used in the United States: nafarelin acetate (Synarel). This compound is administered intranasally twice daily, alternating nasal passages with inhalation. Nafarelin acetate is indicated for use solely in patients with endometrioses.

Regardless of the method of hormonal treatment (orchiectomy, DES, or LHRH agonist), the median time to progression and the median time for survival are 12 to 18 months and 24 to 30 months, respectively.

At the present time there are two overriding questions concerning treatment of metastatic prostate cancer, and both are presently under investigation. The first question is one of early versus delayed hormone therapy, and the second is whether combined androgen blockade is superior to treatment by monohormonal therapy.

Labrie et al. advanced the concept that improvement in time progression and also in survival could be made in patients by simultaneously excluding both testicular and adrenal androgens, the latter being blocked by the use of antiandrogen.[55] This observation was greeted with a great deal of skepticism by the urologic community as a whole and numerous clinical trials testing his hypothesis have been carried out (see also Chapter 14).

In 1989 the results of the National Cancer Institute (NCI) Intergroup study 0036 were published by Crawford et al.[56] They used daily injections of leuprolide in comparison with leuprolide plus flutamide in a prospective randomized study of 603 patients with previously untreated metastatic prostate cancer. There was a significant difference in favor of maximal androgen suppression for both time to progression and overall survival. Median time to progression was 16.5 months and median duration of survival was 35.6 months for the combination arm versus 13.9 and 28.3 months in the leuprolide arm. Most striking was the fact that patients with minimal disease and good performance who were on the combination showed marked advantage over those patients in the monotherapy arm.

Although not all studies have shown the same results, as data from the other studies mature there definitely appears to be an advantage for total androgen blockade (Table 2).

Although approximately 80% of patients respond to palliative hormonal therapy initially, these patients ultimately relapse. Numerous phase II and phase III clinical trials using single-agent and combination chemotherapy in the treatment of hormone-resistant prostate cancer failed to demonstrate any clear advantage for any single agent or group of agents. The apparent resistance to chemotherapeutic drugs by prostatic carcinoma is possibly due to the tumor's slow doubling time and the difficulty with quantifying extent of the lesions initially and during treatment. Since most patients' disease is marked by osteoblastic bone involvement, and it is only the rare patient who has bidimensional disease, present methods to evaluate therapy are problematic. Of note is the difficulty in trying to quantify positive bone scans.

One drug that has been used extensively in Europe, and to a lesser extent in the United States, is estramustine phosphate (Emcyt). This drug has a dual mechanism of action in that it has significant clinical estrogenic effects as well as cytotoxic properties. It has been shown that

TABLE 2. Results of Various Clinical Trials Utilizing Total Androgen Blockade (TAB) in the Treatment of Patients with Metastatic Disease

Study	n	Design	Progression-Free Survival	Overall Survival	Cancer-Specific Survival	Comments
NCI[56]	603	LHRH + placebo vs LHRH + flutamide	2.6 mo advantage ($P = .039$)	7.3 mo advantage ($P = .035$)	Parameter not evaluated	Largest study comparing TAB to medical castration
Janknegt[61]	423	Orchiectomy + placebo vs orchiectomy + nilutamide	4.3 mo advantage ($P = .005$)	3.1 mo advantage; no significant difference	7.0 mo advantage ($P = .071$); approaching significance	Benefits of TAB could not be from flare suppression
EORTC 30853[62]	327	Orchiectomy vs LHRH + flutamide	5.9 mo advantage ($P = .002$)	7.3 mo advantage ($P = .02$)	15.1 mo advantage ($P = .007$)	Compliments NCI trial data
Canadian Anadron Study Group[63]	189	Orchiectomy + placebo vs orchiectomy + nilutamide	No significant difference	6.0 mo advantage ($P = .046$)	7.0 mo advantage ($P = .048$)	Benefits of TAB could not be from flare suppression
DAPROCA[64]	262	Orchiectomy vs LHRH + flutamide	No significant difference	No significant difference	Median survival just reached	Insufficient statistical power to detect differences in survival; data not mature

estramustine exerts antimicrotubule effects on cells and is cytotoxic in cells capable of dividing.[57] The use of estramustine phosphate in the United States has been limited to oral administration, whereas in Europe it is frequently given intravenously. The NPCP studied the drug extensively in comparative trials.[58] Although response criteria are open to debate, there were those occasional patients who have had subjective improvement while taking the drug. Adverse effects were gastrointestinal complaints and cardiovascular complications. At present, there is some renewed interest in using this drug in combination with vinblastine in clinical trials.

Diethylstilbestrol diphosphate (Stilphostrol) has been used for refractory patients either orally or in intravenous loading doses followed by oral administration. Although there are numerous anecdotal reports about the efficacy of DES diphosphate, this compound has never been tested in a controlled clinical setting.

Numerous clinical trials by the NPCP tested chemotherapy in numerous single-agent or combination studies. The same agents have been used with standard hormonal therapy in newly diagnosed metastatic prostatic cancer patients. A partial list of agents includes 5-fluorouracil (5-FU), mithramycin, mitomycin (Mitomycin-C), melphalan, prednimustine, and vincristine, to name the most common chemotherapeutic drugs. Raghavan concisely summarized chemotherapy for metastatic prostate cancer.[59] As he pointed out, when therapeutic agents have been used, their response has been largely stabilization of disease and only rarely has clinical objective improvement been documented. Again the same problems with the lack of measurable disease, age of patients, presence of comorbid medical conditions, and the variable natural history of the disease have clouded results. To date there is no evidence that chemotherapy prolongs survival.

FUTURE DIRECTIONS IN THE TREATMENT OF PROSTATE CANCER

It is ironic that the use of PSA, a test that makes it possible to diagnose more cases of PCa at an earlier stage, is also at the same time generating such controversy. Opponents of screening are pointing out that the test does not meet the criteria of an adequate screening program. But it must be remembered that screening and early detection are not necessarily the same. The natural history of prostatic cancer is variable and the histologic incidence is greater than the clinical significance, but when a patient is in the office of a physician the latter is forced to think in terms of early detection. At a time when we are diagnosing more PCa as a result of PSA testing, it is well to remember that an estimated 20% of patients will have elevated PSAs secondary to BPH. Also, at the same time, more cancers could be detected if the PSA level were lowered to the 2 ng/ml, but would this be advantageous? Nevertheless, PSA is the most clinically useful tumor marker to date for the diagnosis of PCa. As more work is done on this marker one would hope the controversy will abate and we shall be able to better diagnose and treat patients with this disease. As Osterling has recently shown, PSA concentration is directly correlated with patient age. This finding is primarily due to increasing prostatic volume seen with advancing age.[60]

Certain risk factors allow identification of high-risk individuals, for whom screening programs are most efficient. For prostate cancer, age is clearly the most important factor; less than 1% of cases are detected in men younger than 50 and only 16% are detected in men 50–64. The second important risk factor is family history: a single first-degree relative with prostate cancer imparts an increased risk that is approximately double the baseline risk. Third, race is an important factor.

Black men are at increased risk for prostate cancer, the magnitude of increased risk perhaps as high as 50%.

The NCI should, by the time of this publication, have instituted its screening trial where men will be randomized to yearly DRE and PSA versus no testing. Whether or not this study is feasible with the public awareness of PSA testing remains to be seen. Another study soon to be launched is a cancer prevention trial where the 5-alpha reductase inhibitor finesteride will be used in a randomized double-blind placebo controlled study in an attempt to determine the drug's efficacy as a cancer prevention agent (see also Chapter 3). The results of these studies will take years and will require time, money, and a lot of effort in order to achieve meaningful results. Two other studies to address screening are also underway, the American Cancer Society National Prostate Cancer Detection Project and a European effort, both of which are involved in screening for PCa.

Also, there is an NIH-sponsored study that is presently in the planning stage, whereby patients with clinical stage B disease will be randomized to radical prostatectomy or watchful waiting. Initially irradiation was to be a third arm in the study. Although irradiation has been dropped at this time, this valuable study will, in the author's opinion, be a very difficult one to complete.

With more patients being operated upon and positive margins being seen in approximately 50% of specimens, the question of adjunctive irradiation is also of paramount importance. In an attempt to answer the question of the value of irradiation for positive margins, SWOG and the Eastern Cooperative Oncology Group (ECOG) have been involved in a trial where patients with positive margins following surgical extirpation for cancer are randomized to receive either irradiation or only observation. This study, started before PSA values were being used, has been accruing patients slowly and there is some concern whether the accrual goal will be reached. With the large numbers of patients with positive margins, other studies are in the formative stage, e.g., adjunctive therapy with an antiandrogen.

Another area of increasing interest is the role of neoadjuvant hormonal manipulation in the treatment of localized prostatic cancer. The basis for this approach is to eliminate androgen-dependent tumor cells, leaving the residual hormonally unresponsive cells to be eliminated by surgical removal (see also Chapter 11). The Radiation Therapy Oncology Group (RTOG) has been evaluating this downstaging, or more appropriately downsizing, of the prostate prior to definitive irradiation. Results of these group studies are still being evaluated.

As mentioned before, chemotherapy has not in general proved to be very effective in the treatment of hormonal refractory disease. It is important to remember that due to the advanced median age of these patients and their frequently comprised medical conditions, adequate cytotoxic doses of chemotherapy have frequently not been administered. In the future, with the development of bone marrow progenitor cell growth factors such as granulocyte colony-stimulating factor (G-CSF), granulocyte-macrophage CSF (GM-CSF), and interleukin-3 (IL-3), it is possible that more therapeutic doses of chemotherapeutic agents can be given with decreased toxicity.

In addition, there are several promising new agents now undergoing phase II trials. Suramin, an antiparasitic compound that inhibits certain growth factors, is undergoing clinical testing (see also Chapter 15). Another new drug that has recently become available for use in this disease is taxol. This compound has been isolated from the Pacific yew and has been found to bind to cellular microtubules. To date it has been found to be effective against several prostatic cancer cell lines.

It may now be possible to monitor some patients with PSA when they are initially treated with chemotherapeutic agents. If the PSA is reduced, perhaps these patients would then become candidates for combination hormonal and chemotherapeutic trials. If this hypothesis is correct, the side effects from chemotherapy may be justified in patients in whom there is a reduction in their PSA values initially. Trials involving suramin with and without TAB are being conducted under the auspices of the NCI, and meetings are being held to formulate the trials with the cooperative groups.

Finally there is the issue of perineal cryotherapy in the treatment of localized disease. The approach of investigators using this technique has focused on those patients who have rising PSAs and positive prostate biopsies, following definitive irradiation for stage B and C lesions. The technique is also being used in several institutions for patients with stage B lesions who would otherwise have undergone radical prostatectomy, or in some instances irradiation therapy (see also Chapter 10). Although cryoablation had been used in the past, advocates of the technique feel that by using TRUS, optimal perineal placement of the cryoprobes can be performed utilizing real-time imaging. Whether or not the use of real-time placement will prove to be a viable treatment option for cryoablation or for brachytherapy remains to be seen.

In conclusion, the diagnosis and treatment options for patients with prostatic carcinoma are rapidly changing. Funding is increasing and opportunities abound for individual institutions and cooperative groups to participate in meaningful urologic research.

REFERENCES

1. Gross SD: A practical treatise on the diseases, injuries and malformations of the urinary bladder, prostate gland and urethra. Philadelphia: Blanchard, Lee, 2nd ed, pp 716–717, 1855.

2. Langstaff, cited by Herbst RH and Polskey HJ: Prostatic malignancy. In: Ballenger EG, Fontz WA, Hamer HG, Lewis B (eds): History of Urology. Baltimore: Williams & Wilkins Co., vol 2, chap 6, p 187, 1933.

3. Wadd W: Cases of Diseased Bladder and Testicle. London: Smith and Day, 1817.

4. Tanchon LB: Recherches sur le die cancer, Gaz. d. hop., 1984, v. 313. Cited by Herbst RH and Polkey HJ: Prostatic malignancy. In: Ballenger EG, Fontz WA, Hamer HG, Lewis B (eds): History of Urology. Baltimore: Williams & Wilkins Co., vol 2, chap 6, p 187, 1933.

5. Thompson H: The Enlarged Prostate, Its Pathology and Treatment. London: J & A Churchill, Ltd., p 212, 1858.

6. Albarran J, Hallé N: Hypertrophie et neoplasies épitheliales de la prostate. Ann des Mag Genitourin 18:113, 225, 1900.

7. Lydston GF: In: Surgical Diseases of the Genito-Urinary Tract Venereal and Sexual Diseases. Philadelphia: F.A. Davis, p 168, 1899.

8. Young HH: The early diagnosis and radical cure of carcinoma of the prostate. Being a study of 40 cases and presentation of a radical operation which was carried out in 4 cases. Johns Hopkins Hosp Bull 16:315–321, 1905.

9. Jewett HJ: Radical perineal prostatectomy for cancer of the prostate: an analysis of 190 cases. J Urol 61:277–280, 1949.

10. Culp OS, Meyer JJ: Radical prostatectomy in the treatment of prostatic cancer. CA 32:1113–1118, 1973.

11. Millin T: Retropubic Urinary Surgery. London: Livingstone, 1947.

12. Pasteau O: Traitment du cancer de la prostate par la radium. Review des Maladies du la Nutrition, pp 363–398, 1911.

13. Attwater HL: Malignant diseases of prostate and bladder. Postgrad Med J 6:6–17, 1930.

14. Flocks RH, Kerr HD, Elkins HB, et al.: Treatment of carcinoma of the prostate by interstitial radiation with radioactive gold (AU 198): a preliminary report. J Urol 68:510–522, 1952.

15. Whitmore WH Jr, Hilaris B, Grabstad H: Retropubic implantation of iodine-125 in the treatment of prostatic cancer. J Urol 108:918–920, 1972.

16. Bagshaw MA, Kaplan HS: Radical external radiotherapy of localized prostatic carcinoma. Presented at Tenth International Congress Radiology, Montreal, Canada, September 15–18, 1962.

17. Badhraja SN, Anderson JC: An assessment of the value of radiotherapy in the management of carcinoma of the prostate. Br J Urol 36:535–540, 1964.

18. Bagshaw MA, Prionas SD, Goffinet DR, et al.: External beam irradiation combined with the use of 192-iridium implants and radiofrequency-induced hyperthermia in the treatment of prostatic carcinoma. In: Smith PH, Pavone-Macaluso M (eds): EORTC Genitourinary Group monograph 10: Urological oncology: Reconstructive surgery, organ conservation and function restoration. New York: Wiley-Liss, pp 276–279, 1991.

19. Walsh PC, Lapor H, Eggleston JC: Radical prostatectomy with preservation of sexual function: anatomical and pathological considerations. Prostate 4:473–485, 1983.

20. White TJ: The results of double castration in hypertrophy of the prostate. Am Surg 22:1, 1945.

21. Huggins C, Hodges CV: Studies of prostatic cancer: 1. Effect of castration, estrogen, and androgen injections on serum phosphatases in metastatic carcinoma of the prostate. Cancer Res 1:293–297, 1941.

22. Gutman EB, Sproul EE, Gutman AB: Significance of increased phosphatase activity of bone at the site of osteoblastic metastases secondary to carcinoma of the prostate gland. Am J Cancer 28:485–495, 1936.

23. Rich AR: On frequency of occurrence of occult carcinoma of prostate. J Urol 33:215–233, 1935.

24. Moore RA: Morphology of small prostatic carcinoma. J Urol 33:224–234, 1935.

25. Kahler JE: Carcinoma of prostate gland: Pathologic study. J Urol 41:557–574, 1939.

26. Baron E, Angrist A: Incidence of occult adenocarcinoma of prostate after 50 years of age. Arch Pathol 32:787–793, 1941.

27. Franks LM: Latent carcinoma of prostate. J Pathol Bacterial 68:603–616, 1954.

28. Broder AC: The grading of carcinoma. Minn Med 8:726–730, 1925.

29. Mostofi FK, Sesterhenn IA, Davis CJ Jr: Problems in pathologic diagnosis of prostatic carcinoma. Semin Oncol 3:161–169, 1976.

30. Gleason DF: Classification of prostatic carcinomas. Cancer Chemother Rep 50:125–128, 1966.

31. Grayhack JT, Assimos DG: Prognostic significance of tumor grade and stage in patients with carcinoma of the prostate. Prostate 4:13–33, 1983.

32. Mostofi FK: Grading of prostatic carcinoma: current status. In: Bruce A, Trachtenberg J (eds): Adenocarcinoma of the Prostate. New York: Springer-Verlag, pp 29–46, 1987.

33. Dhom G: Classification and grading of prostatic carcinoma. Recent Results Cancer Res 60:14–26, 1977.

34. Mostofi FK: Grading of prostatic carcinoma. Cancer Chemother Rep 59:111–117, 1975.

35. Gaeta JF, Asirwatham JE, Miller G, et al.: Histologic grading of primary prostatic cancer: A new approach to an old problem. J Urol 123:689–693, 1980.

36. Brawn PN, Ayala AA, Eschenbach AC, et al.: Histologic grading study of prostatic adenocarcinoma: development of a new system and comparison with other methods. Cancer 49:113–120, 1982.

37. McNeal JE: Origin and development of carcinoma in the prostate. Cancer 23:24–34, 1969.

38. Whitmore WF Jr: Natural history and staging of prostate cancer. In: Urologic Clinics of North America. Philadelphia: W.B. Saunders Co., 11:2, pp 205–220, 1984.

39. Hanash KA, Utz DC, Cook EN, et al.: Carcinoma of the prostate: a 15-year follow-up. J Urol 107:450–453, 1972.

40. Correa RJ, Anderson RG, Gibbons RP, et al.: Latent carcinoma of the prostate—why the controversy. J Urol 111:644–646, 1974.

41. Barnes RW, Ninan CA: Carcinoma of the prostate: biopsy and conservative therapy. J Urol 108:897–900, 1982.

42. Khalifa NM, Jarman WD: A study of 48 cases incidental carcinoma of the prostate followed 10 years or longer. J Urol 116:329–331, 1976.

43. McMillen SM, Wettlaufer JN: The role of repeat transurethral biopsy in stage A carcinoma of the prostate. J Urol 116:759–760, 1976.

44. Zincke H, Bergstralh EJ, Larson-Keller JL, et al.: Stage D1 prostate cancer treated by radical prostatectomy and adjuvant hormonal treatment. Cancer (Suppl) 70:311–323, 1992.

45. Schmidt JD, Gibbons RP, Murphy GP, Bartolucci A: Adjuvant therapy for localized prostate disease. Cancer (Suppl) 71:3, 1005–1018, 1993.

46. Vest SA, Frazier TH: Survival following castration for prostate cancer. J Urol 56:97–111, 1946.

47. Nesbitt RM, Plumb RT: Prostatic carcinoma: a follow-up of 795 patients treated prior to the endocrine and a comparison of survival rates between these and patients treated by endocrine therapy. Surgery 20:263–272, 1946.

48. Nesbitt RM, Baum WC: Endocrine control of prostatic carcinoma: clinical and statistical survey of 1818 cases. JAMA 143:1317–1320, 1950.

49. Veterans Administration Cooperative Urological Research Group (VACURG): Treatment and survival of patients with cancer of the prostate. Surg Gynecol Obstet 124:1401, 1967.

50. Bailar JC III, Byar DP, VACURG: Estrogen treatment for cancer of the prostate: early results with three doses of diethylstilbestrol and placebo. Cancer 26:257, 1970.

51. Soloway MS, Chodak G, Vogelzang NJ, et al.: Zoladex versus orchiectomy in treatment of advanced prostate cancer: a randomized trial. Urology 37:46–51, 1991.

52. Schally AV, Arimura A, Coy DA: Recent approaches to fertility control based on derivatives of LHRH. In: Murson PL, Glover E, Diezfalusy E, et al. (eds): Vitamins and Hormones. San Diego: Academic Press, pp 257–323, 1980.

53. Kuhn JM, Billebaud T, Navnatil H, et al.: Prevention of the transient adverse effects of a gonadotropin-releasing hormone analogue (buserelin) in metastatic prostate carcinoma by administration of an antiandrogen (nilutamide). N Engl J Med 321:413–418, 1989.

54. The Leuprolide Study Group: Leuprolide vs diethylstilbestrol for metastatic prostate cancer. N Engl J Med 311:1281–1286, 1984.

55. Labrie F, Dupont A, Lacourciere Y, et al.: Combined treatment with flutamide in association with medical and surgical castration. J Urol 135 (Suppl):203A, 1985.

56. Crawford DA, Eisenberger MA, McLeod DG, et al.: A controlled trial of leuprolide with and without flutamide in prostatic carcinoma. N Engl J Med 321:419–424, 1989.

57. Sterns ME, Tew KD: Antimicrotubule effects of estramustine, an antiprostatic tumor drug. Cancer Res 45:3891–3894, 1985.

58. Schmidt JD, Scott WW, Gibbons R, et al.: Chemotherapy programs of the National Prostatic Cancer Project (NPCP). Cancer 45:1937–1946, 1980.

59. Raghavan D: Non-hormone chemotherapy for prostate cancer: principles of treatment and application to the testing of new drugs. Semin Oncol 15:371–389, 1988.

60. Osterling JE, Jacobsen SJ, Chute CG, Guess NA, et al.: Serum prostate-specific antigen in a community based population of healthy men. JAMA 270:7, 860–864, 1993.

61. Janknegt RA, Abbou CC, Bartoletti R, et al.: Orchiectomy and nilutamide or placebo as treatment of metastatic prostate cancer in a multinational double-blind randomized trial. J Urol 149:77–83, 1993.

62. Denis LJ, Whelan P, Carneiro de Moura JL, et al.: Goserelin acetate and flutamide versus bilateral orchiectomy: a phase III EORTC 30853 trial. Urology, in press.

63. The Canadian Anadron Study Group: Total androgen ablation in the treatment of metastatic prostate cancer. Semin Urol 8:159–165, 1990.

64. Iversen P, Christensen MG, Friis E, et al.: A phase III trial of Zoladex and flutamide versus orchiectomy in the treatment of patients with advanced carcinoma of the prostate. Cancer 66 (Suppl):1058–1066, 1990.

Molecular Biology of Prostate Cancer: Oncogenes and Tumor Suppressor Genes

Judd W. Moul, M.D., **Jaya Gaddipati,** Ph.D, and **Shiv Srivastava,** Ph.D.

INTRODUCTION

Advances in molecular biology over the last decade have occurred at breakneck speed. For the practicing clinician, this rapid accumulation of knowledge has made it difficult to keep abreast. Although genetic damage has been postulated since the turn of the century to lie at the heart of tumorigenesis, molecular biologic techniques developed since the 1970s have allowed identification of specific genes implicated in causing cancer. These specific genes fall into two categories: cancer-causing genes, called oncogenes, and tumor-suppressor genes or antioncogenes.

HISTORY AND BACKGROUND

The notion that cancer may be attributed to discrete genetic elements was first supported experimentally in 1911 when Rous reported that a sarcoma in chickens could be induced by cell-free filtrates.[1] Interestingly, Rous later decried the role of genetic mutations in the genesis of cancer.[2]

Decades later, reverse transcriptase and retroviruses were discovered and a unique gene v-*src* was found to be responsible for Rous sarcoma.[3,4] Many other viral oncogenes were discovered and genes of similar structure were found in many higher species, including humans. It was then deduced that these viral DNA sequences originated in the eukaryotic organisms and represented genes that code for cellular proteins important in cell growth controls. These normal gene sequences were termed proto-oncogenes and the altered counterparts were termed oncogenes. By the mid-1970s, the concept of "cancer genes," i.e., oncogenes, as predicted by Huebner and Todaro in 1969, had been given a good deal of experimental support.[5]

Oncogenes function in a dominant manner; the presence of the altered gene is tumorigenic even in the presence of one normal allele. The concept that tumor-suppressor genes exist and whose *absence* may induce the neoplastic state also developed in the 1970s.[6] Tumor suppressor genes have also been termed antioncogenes or recessive oncogenes and they function in a recessive manner. Each gene has matching copies on the paired chromosomes that are termed alleles. If one copy

The opinions and assertions contained herein are the private views of the authors and should not be construed as reflecting the views of the Department of Defense or the United States Army.

of the gene is already missing or otherwise defunctionalized because of an inherited defect, then a loss of the sole remaining copy of the gene results in complete absent expression of that gene's product. The complete loss of function of certain genes can lead to the neoplastic state and so the concept of tumor-suppressor genes. The loss of both alleles of a gene was termed the "two-hit" hypothesis by Knudson in 1971 and explained the epidemiology of retinoblastoma (RB), which was later found to be due to the loss of the RB suppressor gene.[7,8]

ONCOGENES: INTRODUCTION AND DEFINITION

As of early 1991, over 60 oncogenes have been identified as being implicated in contributing to the neoplastic state.[9] The normal sequence coding for a cellular protein is called a proto-oncogene and the altered version, an oncogene. Proto-oncogenes participate in normal cell growth and proliferation, encoding for a variety of proteins that may function as growth factors, growth factor receptors, regulators of DNA synthesis, regulators of RNA transcription, modifiers of protein function by phosphorylation, and many other cellular components. It is easy to understand how alterations of these critical genes can subvert cellular mechanisms to cause aberrant growth and contribute to neoplastic transformation. The alteration that converts a proto-oncogene to an oncogene can take several forms. There may be a mutation (base substitution) in the gene sequence. The prototype of this mechanism is the *ras* oncogene. Single base substitutions (point mutations) at characteristic areas of the gene sequence convert the *ras* gene to an oncogene. This gene has been widely studied in a variety of human tumors, including urologic neoplasms[10,11] (see further discussion below). A second mechanism occurs when there are extra copies of a normal DNA sequence gene which con-

verts the proto-oncogene to an oncogene. The prototypes for this mechanism, called amplification, include *N-myc* in neuroblastoma and *c-erb-B-2* (also called *HER*-2 or *neu*) in breast cancer. Extra gene copy number correlates with adverse outcomes in both these cancers. A third mechanism for conversion occurs when the oncogene is moved or translocated to a different place on the same chromosome or to a different chromosome. In this scenario, the normal sequence of the gene comes under control of different upstream promoters or regulators. The inappropriate or overexpression of such a gene may be oncogenic. Alternatively, a portion of the gene is translocated and this portion may fuse with a different gene sequence at the new location to create a new hybrid gene, which is an oncogene. This is termed translocational rearrangement. The prototype example of translocation/rearrangement is the *c-abl* proto-oncogene in leukemia. In chronic myelogenous leukemia (CML), translocation between chromosomes 9 and 22 results in the Philadelphia chromosome. We now know that a portion of the *c-abl* gene transfers from chromosome 9 to the breakpoint cluster region (bcr) of chromosome 22, creating a fusion gene, bcr-*abl*, which is oncogenic.[12] Translocations/rearrangements are also important in the pathogenesis of other leukemias and lymphomas, particularly in Burkitt lymphoma, in which the *c-myc* proto-oncogene is moved from chromosome 8 to 14.[12]

ONCOGENES IN PROSTATE CANCER

Despite the fact that prostate cancer is the most common cancer in men and the second leading cause of male cancer deaths in the United States, amazingly little is known concerning the molecular mechanisms involved in prostate tumorigenesis [13–20]. Research regarding oncogenes in prostate cancer has been limited and fragmentary and no oncogene has been correlated conclusively with the initiation or progression of prostate cancer.[21] Considering the importance of this cancer as a public health problem, it is disturbing that more molecular genetic data are not yet available.[22,23] Also, considering the clinical dilemma that not all histological prostate cancer will progress or interfere with the life span of the host, molecular markers of progression are urgently needed.[23,24] Although over 60 oncogenes have been currently identified, very few have been studied in prostate cancer. In this section we review the oncogenes that have received some study in prostate cancer: *ras*, *myc*, *c-erb-B-2*, and some of the growth factor oncogenes. There are a plethora of biologic markers that have received at least some study in prostate cancer, including morphometric markers such as nucleolar organizer regions, proliferation markers, neuroendocrine markers, cytoplasmic proteins, cytokeratins, lectins, mucins, stromal factors, blood group antigens, and even cell culture characteristics.[25] In addition, growth factors have recently received attention in prostate cancer and are reviewed elsewhere.[26,27] This chapter focuses on oncogenes and tumor-suppressor genes.

Of the oncogenes, members of the *ras* gene family, e.g., Harvey (H)-, Kirsten (K)-, and Neuroblastoma (N)-*ras*, have been most widely studied in prostate cancer.[21] The current understanding of how *ras* p21 functions is described in Figure 1. Viola et al. were among the first to report enhanced expression of p21 protein, the *ras* gene product in fresh prostate tissue utilizing a broadly reactive monoclonal antibody.[28] With increased Gleason grade, there was increased p21 expression and the authors postulated that *ras* expression would be a clinically useful prognostic marker. Sumiya et al. have also found a similar correlation between histological differentiation and *ras* p21 protein expression; however, in no cases was this protein

considered to be overexpressed.[29] Unfortunately, these initial antibodies were found to be nonspecific in later work[30] and further study with formalin-fixed and paraffin-embedded tissues disclosed no differences in p21 expression in various grades/stages of prostate cancer.[31] In another study examining a primary and bony metastasis from the same patient, the p21 protein was detected in most metastatic cells but only in 20% of the primary tumor.[32] It was postulated that metastases originated from the *ras* expressing subpopulation. *ras* oncoproteins have also been detected in the urine of prostate cancer patients, but this has not been pursued further and the clinical relevance is unknown.[33] The prostatic cell lines PC-3 and DU 145 do not overexpress *ras* proteins.[34] At the mRNA level, studies of c-H-*ras* mRNA have revealed increases as prostate tumors progress from androgen-dependent low-grade tumors to high-grade androgen-independent tumors.[35,36] On the other hand, there appears to be no correlation with tumor progression and mRNA expression for either K-*ras* or N-*ras* oncogenes.[35,36] Further work in human prostate tissue samples is necessary to clarify these discrepancies. Antibodies specific for H-, K-, and N-*ras* p21 proteins need to be used to study both fresh and archival specimens. Specifically, there is a need to determine, at both the mRNA and protein level, which, if any, of the *ras* family of oncogenes is overexpressed in this neoplasm and if any *ras* protein will be a clinically useful marker.[24]

Regarding mutations in the *ras* genes, which have been so commonly seen in other human tumors,[10,11] these appear to be infrequent in human prostate cancer.[34,37-42] (Table 1). It has been demonstrated that transfection of the mutated v-H-*ras* oncogene into a tumorigenic nonmetastatic Dunning rat prostatic cancer cell line results in the acquisition of metastatic ability,[43] decreased expression of fi-

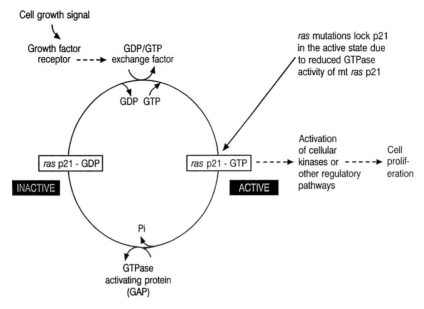

Fig. 1. *ras* p21 protein binds guanine nucleotides and possesses intrinsic GTPase activity. The GTP bound form of the *ras* protein represents the biochemically "active" form, whereas the GDP bound form represents the "inactive" or "downregulated" form. The conversion of the *ras* p21 between the "active" and "inactive" states is achieved by its interaction with other proteins. GTPase activating protein (GAP) activates *ras* p21 GTPase to convert the *ras* p21-GTP form (active) into *ras* p21-GDP form (inactive). The activation of the *ras* p21-GDP form is brought about by proteins that dissociate GDP from the *ras* p21 or exchange GTP for GDP on *ras* p21. A cell growth signal brings about the conversion of inactive *ras* p21 into its active form, which then interacts with downstream targets, leading to accumulation of second messengers that in turn activate cellular protein kinases. The downstream functions of *ras* p21, not yet well understood, finally bring about cell proliferation. The mutant *ras* p21 associated with diverse tumors exhibits severly reduced GTPase activity and therefore the active form of *ras* p21 is increased, favoring cell proliferation.

bronectin,[44] and increased cellular motility[45] if H-*ras* p21 is overexpressed. At least concerning mutations activating *ras*, these animal findings do not seem to translate to human prostate cancer.

Peehl, Wehner, and Stamey were the first to study *ras* mutations in prostate cancer, finding one of eight cases with a K-*ras* activation by the 3T3 transfection assay.[37] No amplification of K-*ras*, H-*ras*, or N-*ras* was detected. The one case with apparent K-*ras* activation was a large Gleason 5/5 tumor and the authors postulated that the *ras* mutation was a late event in prostate cancer progression. More recently, the

polymerase chain reaction (PCR)/oligo-nucleotide hybridization assay has been used to survey for *ras* mutations in prostate cancer. Carter, Epstein, and Isaacs studied radical prostatectomy cases for *ras* mutations and in their cohort DNA was extracted from fresh-frozen samples.[38] One of their 24 cases exhibited an H-*ras* mutation at codon 61, although this was from a rare atypical primary ductal carcinoma. All of their cases were clinically localized. Gumerlock et al. studied 19 localized and metastatic prostate cancers for *ras* mutations, finding only one case with an H-*ras* 61 mutation.[39] Ten of these cases

TABLE 1. ras Mutations in Human Prostate Cancer

Author	Reference	Type of Tissue/Assay	No. of Cases Studied	No. with Mutation	Mutation Rate (%)	ras Codon
Peehl et al.	37	Fresh tumor DNA 3TC transfection	8	1	12.5	c-Ki-ras
Carter et al.	38	Frozen tumors (radical prostatectomy) PCR/OLIGO	24	1	4	c-Ha-ras-61 Position 2, A to G
		Cell lines: PC-82, TSU-PR1, LNCaP, PC-3, DU 145	5	1 (TSU-PR1)	20	C-Ha-ras-12 Position 2, G to T
Gumerlock et al.	39	Frozen and archival tumors (stage B D, Gleason 3–10) PCR/OLIGO	19	1	5	c-Ha-ras-61 Position 2, A to T, G or C
		Cell lines: LNCaP, PC-3, DU 145	3	0	0	
Konishi et al.	40	Frozen and archival (incidental autopsy tumors—Japanese) PCR/OLIGO	23	6	26	c-Ki-ras-12 (4) Position 2, G to T (1) Position 2, G to A (1) Position 2, G to A, G to T
Moul et al.	41	Archival tumors (radical prostatectomy, stage B–C—American) PCR/OLIGO	24	0	0	—
Pergolizzi et al.	34	K, N-ras 12, 13: Fresh metastatic	9	1	11	c-Ki-ras-12
		Fresh primary	2	0	0	
		Archival	5	0	0	
		Cell lines	13	3 (DU 145, LNCaP, PC-3)	23	c-Ki-ras-12
Anwar et al.	42	Archival tumors Japanese clinical cases A–D	68	16	24	c-Ha-ras-61 (11) Position 2, A to T N-ras-12 (4) Position 1, G to A c-Ki-ras-61 (2) Position 1, C to A

were archival and nine were fresh tissue for which the investigators used RNA-PCR analysis. The one mutation was from RNA analysis of a stage C, Gleason 7, diploid tumor.

Our own laboratory has also not found H-, K-, or N-*ras* codon 12, 13, or 61 mutations in a cohort of 24 clinically localized prostate cancers.[47] Another recent study has found N- or K-*ras* codon 12 or 13 mutations in 1 of 9 metastatic fresh prostatic specimens, 0/2 primary tumors (fresh), and 0/5 archival specimens.[34]

These four studies[34,38,39,41] confirm the infrequency of *ras* mutations (3/83—3.6%) in prostate cancer patients from the United States. *ras* mutation analysis of human prostate cancer cell lines has also been performed. Carter et al. studied five lines (PC-82, TSU-PR1, LNCaP, PC-3, DU 145) with the TSU-PR1 line having an H-*ras* 12 mutation.[38] This was a G-to-T transversion at position 2 resulting in a glycine to valine amino acid substitution. Gumerlock et al. studied three lines (LNCaP, PC-3, DU 145) without detecting a mutation.[39] As Carter et al. have noted, it is unclear whether cell line mutations were present in vivo or occurred during in vitro passage of the line.[38] In contrast Pergolizzi et al. reported that 3 of 13 prostate cell lines (DU 145, LNCaP, PC-3) contained K-*ras* codon 12 mutations.[34] In reviewing this paper, however, the mutation signals on the Southern blot hybridization corresponding to these alleged mutations are quite weak. Overall, the cell line studies support the rarity of *ras* mutations in prostatic cancer.

In contrast to the work noted above, Konishi et al. have found 6/23 (25%) K-*ras* 12 mutations in a cohort of Japanese latent autopsy prostate tumors.[40] Four of these mutations were position 2, G-to-T, one was position 2, G-to-A, and one case had two mutations, position 2, G-to-A and G-to-T. These authors speculate that there may be a difference between latent and clinically evident cancers or there may be

racial differences. Alternatively, when working with PCR, the possibility of cross-contamination must always be considered.[46] In addition, the possibility of false positives resulting from the nonspecific binding of the mutation-specific probe must also be considered when using oligonucleotide mismatch assay. Konishi et al. did confirm results with direct sequencing in two of their cases.[40] Similarly, Anwar et al. have also recently reported a 24% mutation rate in Japanese clinical prostate cancers.[42] Eleven of the 16 (69%) mutations detected were restricted to codon 61 of H-*ras* and 8 of these 11 (73%) were in stage D patients. Similarly of the 4 N-*ras* 12 and 2 K-*ras* 61 mutations, 3 were stage D and two were stage C. Clearly, this study is unlike the others[38–41] in having a majority of stage D cases.

To summarize the data on *ras* mutations, there has been a very low incidence detected in cases from the United States, whereas, in cases from Japan, both incidental and advanced clinical, about one-fourth appear to harbor *ras* mutations. From our own work and experience with these assays,[41,47,48] the potential for false-positive results, especially because of the sensitivity of PCR and subjectiveness of the oligonucleotide assay, must be considered. Conversely, prostate cancer in this Japanese cohort may indeed harbor *ras* mutations, especially in the advanced-disease cases, which have been underrepresented in the U.S. studies.

The *myc* family of oncogenes, in particular *c-myc*, has also received attention regarding a possible role in prostate cancer.[21] A number of studies showed that *c-myc* messenger RNA was elevated in prostate cancers compared to BPH and normal tissues and that there tended to be enhanced expression with higher grade tumors.[49–53] As Peehl notes, the heterogeneous nature of the prostate complicates the interpretation of data obtained from the RNA studies, which were of homogenized tissue extracts of epithelium and stroma of benign areas admixed with neoplastic areas.[21] One study has localized the c-myc expression to the epithelium of one BPH specimen by in situ hybridization.[54] More recently, eight prostate carcinomas and four BPH specimens were examined for c-myc expression via in situ expression of mRNA.[55] Two well-differentiated carcinomas expressed c-myc but similar levels were seen in adjacent nonmalignant BPH. One of the four BPH samples expressed c-myc. Based on these findings, these investigators suggested that myc expression is not common in prostate cancers. Although c-myc amplification has been seen in some prostate cancer cell lines,[56,57] it does not appear that the c-myc gene is amplified in human tumors.[37,51] Based on this RNA overexpression in some tumors, it is surprising that no one has examined myc in a larger cohort as a potential clinical marker of stage or outcome. Most recently, c-myc mRNA has been found to be regulated by androgen in LNCaP cells.[58] Further work is obviously necessary.

Despite these unresolved issues regarding ras and myc in human prostate cancers, interesting experimental study has been done in animal models. In a mouse prostate model, vH-ras alone (only in high concentrations) induced dysplasia, and myc overexpression alone induced hyperplastic lesions.[59] Together, ras plus myc induced predominantly malignant carcinomas. The study concluded that single oncogenes can induce phenotypes resembling distinct premalignant stages of tumorigenesis, whereas the activation of multiple oncogenes and/or inactivation of tumor-suppressor genes is likely carcinogenic in the prostate.[60]

c-erbB-2, neu, and HER-2 are all names for the same gene that was initially identified in 1981 from a rat neuroglioblastoma.[61] The c-erbB-2/neu/HER-2 (hereafter c-erbB-2) was independently identified in human tumor tissue by two groups in 1985.[62,63] The c-erbB-2 gene, located at chromosome 17q21, codes for a protein that is similar, but not identical to, the epidermal growth factor receptor. The most common mechanism of c-erbB-2 activation in human neoplasms is genomic DNA amplification, which almost always results in overproduction of c-erbB-2 mRNA and protein.[62–65] Amplification of c-erbB-2 has been found in a significant number of cell lines derived from human adenocarcinomas, but rarely in cancer cell lines of other origin.[65] Similarly, analysis of tumor tissue itself has generally revealed amplification in adenocarcinomas only.[66] Amplification of the c-erbB-2 oncogene has been most extensively studied in breast carcinoma, with most studies correlating c-erbB-2 amplification/overexpression to poorer prognosis.[67,68] Approximately 20% of breast cancers exhibit c-erbB-2 activations, mostly by DNA amplification, and breast carcinomas with c-erbB-2 amplification contain 2 to 40 times more c-erbB-2 mRNA than found in normal tissues.[69] In addition to amplification, c-erbB-2 activation in breast and other neoplasms may occur by overproduction of c-erbB-2 mRNA and protein without DNA amplification or by protein overproduction alone.[70] The c-erbB-2 oncogene has also been implicated in ovarian, gastric, and bladder neoplasms but does not appear to be involved in pulmonary, hematological, sarcomatous, or renal tumors.[75]

Study of the c-erbB-2 gene in human prostate cancer has been confounded by conflicting results (Table 2). Initial studies showed no amplification of the c-erbB-2 gene, no increased RNA species of c-erbB-2, and no protein expression by immunohistochemistry.[71,72] In contrast, Sikes and Chung transfected the rat neu point mutationally activated gene into a rat ventral prostate epithelial cell line, NbE-1.4, which is normally nontumorigenic.[73] When multicopy transfection resulted in overexpression of the activated neu, the

TABLE 2. c-erbB-2 in Human Prostate Cancer

Author	Reference	No. of Cases	Methods	c-erbB-2 DNA amp[a]	c-erbB-2 mRNA exp[a]	c-erbB-2 Protein exp[a]
McCann et al.	71	23 Ca	IHC—archival 21N pAB	—	—	0/23
Klotz et al.	72	13 Ca, 3 BPH	DNA, RNA, slot blot, DNA probe	0/13, 0/3	0/13, 0/3	
Natali et al.	76	7 Ca, 5 NL	IHC—archival & fresh MAb4D5	—	—	2/7 (29%), 0/5
Zhau et al.	74	25 Ca, 3 cell lines	Western blot—fresh & IHC	—	—	13/25 (52%), LNCap > PC-3 > DU 145
Sadasivon et al.	77	25 Ca, 15 BPH	IHC—fresh tissue, MAb TA 1	—	—	7/25 (28%), 0/15
Natoli et al.	78	51 Ca	IHC—archival—MAb	—	—	7/51 (14%)
Grob et al.	79	14 Ca, 7 BPH, 5 NL	IHC—archival—MAb & radioimmunoassay and Western blot	—	—	12/14 (86%), 1/7 (14%), 0/5
Ware et al.	80	24 Ca, 34 BPH, 10 Ca, 8 Ca, 11 BPH	IHC—archival—pAB-60 (Triton); MAb-1 (Triton); fresh-frozen MAb-1 (Triton)	—	—	17/24 (71%), 21/34 (62%), 0/10, 7/8 (88%), 11/11 (100%)
Mellon et al.	81	29 Ca, 34 BPH	IHC—fresh—MAb NCL-CB11 (Novocastra Labs, GB)	—	—	6/29 (21%), 6/34 (18%)
Zhau et al.	75	16 Ca, 15 Ca, 8 BPH, 8 NL, 10 Ca, 3 cell lines	Western blot; IHC—archival—MAb-3 (Oncogene Science Inc.); 2-IHC, 6 Western; 2-IHC, 5-IHC, 3 Western; fresh-frozen-Southern; fresh-Southern	0/10, 0/3	Androgen dependent	11/16 (69%), 12/15 (80%), 0/8, 0/8
Visakorpi et al.	82	147 Ca, 17 BPH, 2 NL	IHC—archival—MAb-1 (Triton)	—	—	0/147, 0/17, 0/2
Kuhn et al.	84	53 Ca, 9 BPH, 18 Ca, (pos. IHC)	IHC—archival—pAB-1 (Triton); Differential PCR	0/18	—	18/53 (34%), 0/9

[a]amp, amplification; exp, expression.
Ca, carcinoma; BPH, benign prostatic hyperplasia; NL, normal; IHC, immunohistochemistry; pAB, polyclonal antibody; MAb, monoclonal antibody; PCR, polymerase chain reaction.

cell line acquired a tumorigenic phenotype. Low-level expression of the *neu* gene, however, did not result in tumor formation. This group also found that the LNCaP cell line demonstrated predominantly cytoplasmic c-*erb*B-2 oncoprotein expression, whereas the PC-3 line showed membranous expression.[74] Furthermore, 13 of 25 (52%) prostate cancer samples contained detectable levels of the c-*erb*B-2 oncoprotein by Western blot analysis and with histochemical staining. These investigators' most recent work found 11 of 16 (69%) prostate cancers exhibited overexpression of c-*erb*B-2 protein via Western analysis, 12 of 15 (80%) by immunohistochemistry, but 0 of 10 cases and no cell lines had gene amplification.[75] The c-*erb*B-2 messenger RNA was positively regulated by androgen similar to PSA expression.[75]

A number of investigators have also studied prostate cancer via immunohistochemistry for c-*erb*B-2 oncoprotein expression.[75–85] Natali et al. studied seven prostate cancers and five cases of BPH as part of a large survey of a variety of human tissues, finding 2 of the 7 (29%) undifferentiated prostate cancers demonstrating c-*erb*B-2 oncoprotein expression.[76] As opposed to intense membranous staining for c-*erb*B-2 in many breast cancers, the staining in the prostate and various other neoplasms was characterized as heterogeneous and weak plasma membrane staining.[76] Sadasivan et al. found 7 of 25 prostate cancers had expression of c-*erb*B-2 via immunohistochemistry using a monoclonal antibody (TA-1) in fresh samples and concluded that c-*erb*B-2 expression correlated to higher grade and high S-phase and aneuploidy on flow cytometry.[77] In a later report from this same group, 19 of 25 prostate cancers (76%) but no BPH cases (0/15) show c-*erb*B-2 overexpression, which was generally confirmed with two monoclonal antibodies (TA-1 and 3B5). Furthermore, overexpression was correlated with more

advanced stage (6 of 7 stage C and D showed 2+ and 3+ staining) and higher Gleason score. Natoli et al. studied c-*erb*B-2 and epidermal growth factor receptor (EGFR) oncoprotein in 51 prostate cancers, finding 7 (14%) with c-*erb*B-2 expression and 18/51 (35%) with EGFR expression.[78] Grob et al. performed immunohistochemical analysis on 14 prostate carcinomas, seven cases of BPH, and five normal prostates using a monoclonal antibody for c-*erb*B-2 in archival tissue, finding 12 (86%) carcinomas, one BPH, and no normals demonstrating c-*erb*B-2 expression.[79] These authors also performed differential PCR assay and found certain cases with DNA amplification of c-*erb*B-2.

Ware and associates found the monoclonal antibody mAB-1 (Triton Diagnostic, Alameda, CA) did not react on archival tissues; however, the pAB-60 (Triton) yielded positive staining in 17/24 prostate cancers.[80] Benign areas of six of these cases exhibited c-*erb*B-2 staining and 12 of 13 BPH cases also stained positively, with most of the staining occurring in the cytoplasm; however, exposure to the antibody at 4°C decreased staining on benign tissues. Mellon et al., using a monoclonal antibody, NCL-CB11 (Novocastrs Labs, UK), found 6 of 29 (21%) prostate cancers and 6 of 34 (18%) BPH cases exhibited epithelial expression.[81] No significant relationship was observed between tumor stage or grade and the expression of c-*erb*B-2.[81] Most recently, Visakorpi et al.[82] found similar results to Ware et al.[80] in that mAB-1 did not react in archival prostate cancers. Our laboratory has examined 53 clinically localized archival prostate cancers obtained from radical prostatectomy utilizing a polyclonal antibody pAB-1 (Triton), finding 18 (34%) with expression of the oncoprotein.[84] No association was found between c-*erb*B-2 expression and grade or pathologic stage (B vs. C), however, there was trend toward higher recurrence rates in patients who expressed the oncoprotein. Using a PCR assay, we did not find DNA amplification of c-erbB-2 in those cases expressing the protein.[84] Most recently, Fox et al. examined epidermal growth factor receptor, c-erbB-2, P53, and c-myc protein expression by immunohistochemistry in 45 stage A1 prostate cancer patients.[85] Only c-erbB-2 was significantly related to survival ($P = 0.008$) and c-erbB-2 expression conferred a 4.6-fold increased risk of dying of prostate cancer.

A subset of human prostate cancers appears to express the c-erbB-2 oncoprotein in immunohistochemistry assays. The variety of both polyclonal and monoclonal antibodies, the use of fresh versus archival tissues, and variations in technique and interpretation of positive staining has undoubtedly resulted in different expression rates. Much more work is necessary with regard to the importance of the c-erbB-2 gene in prostate cancer. We currently do not believe that the observed oncoprotein expression is due to gene amplification, based on our differential PCR data and work by others.[72,75] However, it is unknown if the oncoprotein expression is due to overexpression at the mRNA level or strictly at the protein level. More study is obviously needed to clarify this diversity of results with various monoclonal and polyclonal antibodies, to determine the exact nature of this gene's expression in prostatic carcinoma and in light of this gene's importance in breast cancer, to further define any possible prognostic utility for the c-erbB-2 oncogene.

The proto-oncogene c-sis has also been studied in prostate cancer.[50,52,86–88] The protein product of c-sis is identical to the B-chain of platelet-derived growth factor (PDGF). Expression of sis has been seen in PC-3, DU 145, and PC-82 cell lines.[86,87] c-sis may play a role in the growth of prostate tissue by androgens as well as its repression by corticosteroids.[50,88] c-sis has also been studied in prostate tissues by using RNA dot blots; sis was elevated in poorly differentiated carcinomas.[50] c-sis protein-derived peptides were detectable in the urine of prostate cancer patients, but this work has not been pursued.[33] Most recently immunohistochemical analysis of the PDGF alpha and B-chains (c-sis protein) was performed on prostate tissues.[89] The antibody for the B-chain (c-sis) did not react in any of the tissues; however, the B-chain receptor antibody did stain BPH and some of the carcinomas. Further work is necessary to define the role, if any, of c-sis in prostate cancer.

The c-fos oncogene encodes a protein that is postulated to act at a central position in intracellular signal transduction by initiating the regulation of gene expression in response to external signals and is therefore considered a "master switch."[90] c-fos seems to play a role in transformation by other oncogenes and plays a pivotal role in the regulation of transcription.[90] Little work has been done regarding c-fos in prostate cancer. There may be a relationship between androgen receptor content and c-fos expression in prostate cancer.[50,86,91] Androgen deprivation has been shown to reduce c-fos expression by 90% in some cell lines.[86] No amplification of the c-fos gene has been seen in prostate cancer.[26]

Preliminary work has recently been reported for the oncogenes Bcl-2 and c-kit in prostate cancer.[92,93] Bcl-2 is the only known proto-oncogene that functions in a manner to circumvent normal endogenous programmed cell death mechanisms. It has now been shown that Bcl-2 protein is undetectable in a majority of androgen-dependent prostate cancers, whereas a vast majority of hormone refractory cases exhibited diffuse high expression.[92] The authors feel that Bcl-2 is involved in the progression from androgen dependence to independence and that this oncogene deserves further study.[92] c-kit encodes for a membrane receptor of the tyrosine kinase family and its ligand is the stem cell factor

(SCF). In a recent immunohistochemical study *c-kit* protein was detected in 5/22 carcinomas and the ligand in 8/22 cases.[93] The implications of these results are not yet known and further work is necessary.

Undoubtedly, more proto-oncogenes will be identified as potentially playing a role in prostate cancer. Even with the oncogenes studied to date, little clinical correlation has been done. More work is necessary to determine if any of these gene expressions can function as clinically useful tumor markers. For prostate cancer, molecular markers to distinguish clinically insignificant from important neoplasms are necessary.

TUMOR SUPPRESSOR GENES: INTRODUCTION AND DEFINITION

As previously noted, oncogenes act in a dominant fashion. Despite a normal counterpart allele, the oncogene can transform cells. To quote Nobel laureate J.M. Bishop, "Evil overrides good."[9] In contrast, when both alleles of a tumor-suppressor gene (TSG) are lost, inactivated, or damaged, the gene protein product is absent or attenuated. This protein product was necessary to suppress susceptibility to the neoplastic state. The absence, either functional or complete, then contributes to oncogenesis. The two most famous tumor-suppressor genes to date are the RB gene, or retinoblastoma gene,[94–98] discovered as the cause of retinoblastoma and the p53 gene[97–100] implicated in a number of neoplasms, as well as in genetic predisposition of Li-Fraumeni syndrome families to diverse neoplasms.[101–103] The WT gene in Wilms tumor, DCC and FAP in colon carcinoma, NF in neurofibromatosis, and MEN in tumors of the multiple endocrine neoplasia syndrome are other recently identified tumor-suppressor genes.[97,98] Cytogenetic studies of other tumors have suggested many other consistent regions of genetic loss which will undoubtedly

lead to discovery of other suppressor genes.

The retinoblastoma gene, or RB, was the first identified tumor-suppressor gene. This gene's existence was predicted based on the inheritance of retinoblastoma in the "two-hit" hypothesis of Knudson.[7] The first "hit" inactivates one allele and this would generally occur in the germ line, thereby transmitting this alteration to all body cells. The second "hit" occurs in a somatic cell to the only remaining normal allele, thereby eliminating normal expression of the gene. The RB gene has been found to be located on chromosome 13 at 13q14 and the RB gene transcript is ~4.7 kilobases (kb) in length.[104–106] This ~4.7 kb RB gene transcript codes for a 110 kilodalton (PP110) nuclear phosphoprotein which interacts with cell cycle related proteins.[12,97] The RB gene product functions to suppress cell division by preventing cells in G1 phase from entering S-phase.[95,97] Retinoblastoma patients also develop other neoplasms, and the RB gene has been implicated in these and other cancers.[14,97]

Although initially felt to be an oncogene, p53 is now considered to be a tumor-suppressor gene.[107] The p53 gene, like RB, is a nuclear phosphoprotein that is postulated to arrest cells in G1. For cellular growth to occur, cells must enter the S-phase and p53 cell growth arrest functions must be inactivated.[107] The p53 protein has been recently implicated in the regulation of genes induced by agents which damage DNA.[108]

The current understanding of p53 alterations in tumors and diverse functions of p53 is summarized in Figure 2. Recent reports also suggest the function of p53 in programmed cell death, or apoptosis.[109,110] The p53 gene has been mapped to the short arm of chromosome 17 at 17p13. This short arm of chromosome 17 is a commonly deleted area of many human tumors and recent studies have shown that the remaining p53 allele frequently harbors

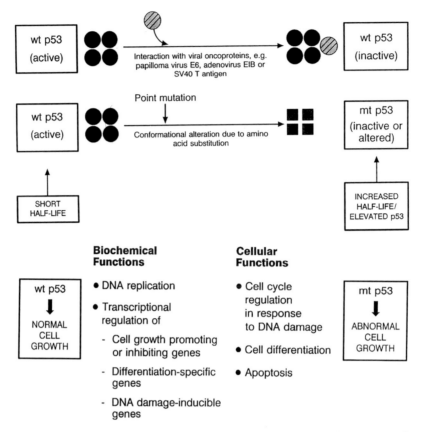

Fig. 2. The tumor-suppressor gene p53 is the most frequently altered gene yet analyzed in human tumors. Various biochemical and cellular functions have been described for the p53 protein. The interaction of wild type (wt) p53 with DNA viral oncoproteins, SV 40 T antigen and E1B, inactivates its normal functions, e.g., DNA binding and transcription transactivation. Interaction of p53 with human papilloma virus E6 results in its degradation. p53 mutations associated with human tumors give rise to the mutant p53 proteins, which lack sequence-specific DNA binding or transcriptional transactivation function. A number of mutant p53 proteins exhibit increased half-life, thereby giving the appearance of increased p53 protein upon immunohistochemical analysis of tumors. wt p53 (normal) appears to play a critical role in control of cell cycle events. Cells containing wt p53 exhibit G1 and G2 arrest upon exposure to irradiation, whereas cells lacking wt p53 or containing mutant (mt) p53 do not arrest in G1. The functions of wt p53 also include regulation of apoptosis, which has been shown to be altered in cells lacking wt p53.

point mutations.[99,100] By this process, the normal p53 protein product is lost from tumor cells and can contribute to oncogenesis in diverse neoplasms. Like RB, germ-line mutations in p53 gene have also been described in rare cancer-prone families with Li-Fraumeni syndrome.[101–103]

TUMOR-SUPPRESSOR GENES IN PROSTATE CANCER

The studies of TSGs in prostate cancer are just beginning to emerge. Analysis of nonrandom loss of the genetic material, as well as the alterations of known TSGs such as RB and p53, are being currently evaluated in prostate cancer. Studies utilizing different cytogenetic and molecular approaches reviewed here comprise the current strategies to identify and analyze prostate cancer-specific alterations in TSGs.

The observations on the association of consistent chromosomal alterations such as deletions during the traditional karyotypic analysis of tumor cells, e.g., in retinoblastoma, Wilms' tumor, neurofibromatosis, familial colon cancer, Von Hippel-Lindau syndrome, have provided the early clues for the localization and eventual identification of the respective TSGs for these cancers[97, 98]. However, the karyotype analyses in prostate cancer have been limited due to the problems encountered in the culturing of the prostate cancer cells. A survey[111] of available cytogenetic data in prostate adenocarcinomas has revealed the loss of chromosome 1, 2, 5, and Y and the gain of chromosomes 7, 14, 20, and 22. These authors[111] also reported the rearrangements involving chromosome arms 2p, 7q, and 10q and suggest that multiple hot spots might be of relevance in the genesis of prostate cancer. The cytogenetic analysis of 62 primary prostatic adenocarcinomas by Micale et al.[112] revealed normal male diploid karyotype in 87% of all the cells analyzed and the coexistence of clonally aberrant, nonclonally aberrant, and normal diploid cells. This report also described nonrandom chromosome alteration including gain of chromosome 7 and loss of Y chromosome. A possible relationship between the amount of constitutive heterochromatin on chromosomes 1 and 16 and susceptibility to an early development of prostate cancer has also been reported. These authors reported loss of 7q, 8p, and 10q as common aberrations in 13 of the 15 tumor specimens exhibiting clonal karyotypic abnormalities.[113] A comprehensive summary of the chromosomal abnormalities in prostate cancer can be found in an excellent recent review by Sandberg.[114]

A recent study utilizing in situ hybridizations with chromosome-specific DNA probes has shown the losses of chromosomes 7, 16, and Y in prostate cancer specimens.[115] Using similar techniques, another report[116] has suggested that numerical chromosome alterations in prostate cancer coincide with aggressive tumor behavior. Recent analysis of cytogenetic aberrations in prostate cancer by use of the complementary methods, e.g., PCR amplification of nucleotide repeat polymorphic loci and fluorescence in situ hybridization (FISH) using centromere-specific probe, showed a higher frequency of chromosomes 8p, 10q, and Y alterations in one or more cancer foci per patient.[117] Furthermore, another group utilizing FISH and chromosome 7-specific probe has suggested that trisomy 7 may be a common feature associated with local and metastatic progression of human prostate cancer.[118] Although cytogenetic analyses have suggested chromosomal alterations in prostate cancer, a comprehensive analysis involving more specimens is needed to better define the association of specific chromosomal alterations. It is expected that the introduction of these new techniques of in situ hybridization utilizing DNA probes for specific chromosomal loci on fresh, as well as archival, tissue sections will provide better understanding of cytogenetic alterations in prostate neoplasms. These techniques should also be useful in distinguishing early versus late genetic alterations in prostatic neoplasms.

Molecular analysis of alleles on a specific chromosome locus due to restriction fragment length polymorphisms (RFLPs) and tumor-associated loss of heterozygosity (LOH) has yielded a wealth of information that has led to the identification of neoplasm-specific TSGs.[97, 98] Tumor-suppressor genes involved in the genesis of retinoblastomas,[104–106] Wilms' tumor,[119–121] neurofibromatosis,[122–125] colon cancer,[126–130] and Von Hippel-Lindau disease[131] have already been identified and cloned, and several of these TSGs are already being utilized in the clinical setting. A review of the literature reveals that search for allelic losses in prostate cancer is also receiving more attention.

Carter et al.[132] examined 28 prostate cancer specimens for LOH at 11 different chromosome arms, including 3p, 7q, 9q, 10p, 10q, 11p, 13q, 16p, 16q, 17p, and 18q. Thirteen of 24 clinically localized tumors and 4 of 4 metastatic tumors exhibited LOH on at least one chromosome. The highest frequency of chromosomal losses were seen on 16q and 10q and these sites may contain the loci for TSGs important in prostate tumorigenesis. Another study[133] of alleotyping of prostate carcinoma revealed a high frequency of allelic deletions on chromosome 8, 10, and 16. A comprehensive analysis of 18 cases showed that 65% had deletions on 8p with minimally deleted region between the *PLAT* locus and p ter. Allelic deletions of the long arm of chromosome 16 were found in 56% informative cases and a relatively small percentage of specimens also exhibited a complex pattern of deletions on chromosome 10. Kunimi et al.[134] have also reported frequent allelic losses on chromosomes 16q, 8p, 18q, 10p, and 10q in 18 cases of prostatic adenocarcinoma. Taken together, these reports suggest the frequent involvement of TSGs located on chromosomes 8p, 10q, and 16q in prostate oncogenesis.

Recent observations[135] on decreased expression of E-Cadherin, a cell adhesion protein, in high-grade prostate tumors, along with the earlier reports[132,133] of frequent deletions of the region of chromosome 16q, where E-Cadherin gene is located, are very exciting new findings. In fact, an earlier study has already shown an association of decreased E-Cadherin expression with the invasive phenotype of rat prostate cancer cells.[136] Taken together, these reports[135,136] suggest that E-Cadherin may function as a suppressor of invasive phenotype associated with prostate

cancer. Thus E-Cadherin may represent a first characterized TSG, frequently altered in prostate cancer. Further studies to evaluate the utility of E-Cadherin in staging of prostate cancer is of paramount clinical significance. A recent report also suggests that loss of the expression of proteins, e.g., α-catenin, with which E-Cadherin interacts to mediate cell adhesion, may also be responsible for invasive phenotype of prostate cancer cell lines even when E-Cadherin is expressed normally.[137]

In search of genetic alterations that could serve as markers for the extent of clinical disease in prostate cancer, Macoska et al.[138] have reported the LOH on two loci on the chromosome 17p: p53 and D17S5 in a lymph node metastasis sample. D17S5 locus on chromosome 17p, probably harboring a new suppressor gene distinct from p53, has been recently shown to be a site of hypermethylation in 80–90% of prostate cancer specimens analyzed.[139] Recent studies of LOH from microdissected prostate tumor specimens utilizing RFLP on Southern blots or utilizing a new technique based on PCR amplification of short tandem repeats further emphasize that allelic losses on 8p, 16q, and 10q loci are frequent events in prostate tumorigenesis.[140,141] It is rather obvious that future studies will focus on the cloning and characterization of the TSGs on these chromosome loci.

The most stringent test for a gene to qualify as TSG is its ability to suppress the tumorigenic phenotype of a tumor or cells derived from a tumor. The TSG is either introduced into tumor cells as a cloned cDNA in an appropriate expression vector or an individual chromosome-harboring candidate TSG is introduced into tumor cells by microcell transfer technique. Both these approaches are being utilized for the analysis of TSGs in prostate cancer. The RB and p53 tumor-suppressor activities have already been tested in prostate cancer cell lines. The introduction of a retroviral vector containing wt RB cDNA into a prostate cancer cell line DU 145 resulted in an approximately 15-fold reduction in the tumorigenicity of the transfectants in nude mice as compared to the parental cell line without wt RB cDNA.[142] Additionally, the small tumors that developed in nude mice lacked exogenous wt RB. These results, therefore, have convincingly shown that RB gene can suppress the tumorigenic phenotype of this prostate cancer cell line. Cytomegalovirus promoter-enhancer mediated expression of the wt p53 cDNA in prostate cancer cell lines TSU-PR-1 and PC-3 severely inhibited the growth of these cells as evidenced by reduced level of thymidine incorporation into DNA.[143] This study suggested a functional role for the wt p53 gene in suppressing prostatic tumorigenesis. Since the growth inhibitory effects of RB and p53 are not specific to prostate cancer cell lines, the protein encoded by RB and p53 probably represents key proteins involved in negative cell growth controls for diverse cell types. However, inactivation of p53 and RB genes in prostate tumorigenesis may still play an important role in the tumorigenesis, like several other tumor types.[97–100]

To identify possible suppressor genes specific to prostate cells, Peehl et al.[144] created somatic cell hybrids by fusing normal prostate cells with malignant HeLa cells. The normal phenotype was dominant in these hybrids; however, one hybrid clone was found to be tumorigenic, possibly due to the loss of a putative TSG. Further characterization of prostate-specific TSG from this approach is still awaited.

Similar assays, utilizing transfer of specific chromosomes into tumor cells to inhibit their growth, are also underway to identify prostate-specific TSGs. Introduction of chromosome 11 into a highly metastatic rat prostate cell line by microcell-mediated chromosome transfer resulted in the suppression of the metastatic ability without any effect on the tumorigenicity.[145] The region on chromosome 11 capable of suppressing metastatic phenotype was localized between 11p11.2–13 but not including Wilms' tumor-1 locus.[146] Microcell transfer of human chromosome 17 into human prostate cancer cell line TSU resulted in the loss of tumorigenicity of this line in nude mice.[147] These authors suggested that the suppression of tumorigenicity may be due to p53 activity or due to another suppressor on chromosome 17. Future molecular characterizations will undoubtedly include identification of metastatic suppressor genes on chromosomes 11 and 17. Although frequent losses of chromosome 8p have been reported in prostate cancer, the introduction of this chromosome thus far has not shown any inhibitory effect on prostate cancer cells.[140] Further studies are needed to understand the significance of these observations. A combination of functional assays, as well as physical mapping of genes by LOH assays, appears to be the current strategy for the identification of prostate cancer-specific TSGs.

Although RB gene alterations were originally described in inherited as well as sporadic retinoblastomas, somatic mutations of RB genes are present in diverse tumors.[97,98] Initial study of RB gene in prostate cancer cell lines revealed the presence of abnormal RB protein in a prostate cancer cell line: DU 145, due to a point mutation in the splice junction site which resulted in the mutated RB protein lacking 35 amino acids encoded by exon 21.[148] Analysis of seven primary prostate carcinomas further revealed the absence or reduced expression of RB protein in two specimens. The prostate carcinoma specimen lacking RB protein had a 103 bp deletion containing the transcriptional start site.[148] The allelic losses of RB have also been reported recently in 11 out of 47 tumors analyzed by PCR of highly polymorphic variable number tandem repeat (VNTR) in the intron 20 of the RB gene.[149] However, a recent report analyzing RB gene in seven prostate tumor specimens did not detect any exon 21 alterations or deletions in the promoter region.[150] The preceding reports therefore suggest that RB gene is altered in 10–20% of the specimens analyzed. A more comprehensive analysis of RB is needed in tumor specimens and this may be achieved better with the availability of better antibodies suited for the immunodetection of RB protein in paraffin sections or RB transcript analysis by in situ PCR on tumor tissue sections.

Like RB, somatic mutations of p53 gene have been reported in diverse neoplasms, and in fact p53 mutations represent the most common genetic alterations in human cancers analyzed to date.[100–107] With the exception of Li-Fraumeni syndrome and a very small fraction of other neoplasms,[101–103] most of the p53 alterations represent late somatic alterations in the process of tumorigenesis.[100,107] Prostate cancer specimens are being extensively evaluated for p53 by the analysis of increased p53 protein level in tumor sections, as several mutations in p53 gene are known to stabilize p53 gene product.[107] Additionally, the relatively smaller size of the p53 gene as opposed to RB makes it pliable to mutational analysis by single strand conformational polymorphism (SSCP) and DNA sequencing of the PCR-derived DNA fragments. Various recent reports of p53 alterations[143,151–159] in prostate cancer specimens are summarized in Table 3. The majority of studies with tumors describe p53 alterations in 6–20% of specimens tested. However, two reports[156,159] have described p53 alterations in 60–80% of specimens analyzed. p53 mutations have also been reported at a higher frequency in prostate tumor-derived cell lines.[143,153] It is observed that p53 mutations might associate with higher grade tumors and alterations of p53 are not common in BPH (Table 3). A very interesting recent study has described p53 mutations in 11 of 56 specimens analyzed.[158] Further

analysis showed that 9 of the 11 tumors with p53 mutations were derived from the hormone refractory patients.[158] In fact, an earlier report on p53 mutations in prostate tumor cell lines[143] reported that cell lines LNCaP and PC-82, which require the presence of hormone to elicit tumorigenicity in nude mouse, did not exhibit p53 mutations. From these recent observations, it also appears the p53 mutations may be more relevant in the late stage and/or hormone-refactory prostate neoplasms. Recent studies from our laboratory have shown that a high fraction of hormone refractory prostate cancer specimens (20 of 26) harbor p53 alterations as judged by immunostaining and SSCP (unpublished). Further studies in this regard will undoubtedly provide better insights into association of p53 mutation and prostate tumor staging.

In a recent study aimed toward understanding the molecular basis of androgen withdrawal-induced apoptosis in the rat prostate gland, elevated p53 expression along with other cell cycle-related genes has been observed in castrated rats.[160] Thus it appears that p53 may also play an important role in apoptosis resulting from androgen withdrawal. Future studies on these lines might also shed light on how alterations of p53 expression during apoptosis contribute toward hormonal response of the prostate gland. As we previously discussed, studies have recently shown that introduction of an activated *ras* gene into reconstituted prostate causes mild hyperplasia, whereas a combination of *ras* and *myc* oncogenes lead to the development of carcinomas.[59] It was quite surprising, therefore, to note from these studies that p53 mutations were found in the reconstituted organs containing *ras* alone, whereas wt p53 (no p53 mutations) was detected in carcinomas containing *ras* and *myc*. It was even more unexpected to find that these carcinomas exhibited elevated expression of the wt p53.[161] The ramifica-

TABLE 3. p53 Alterations in Prostate Cancer

Author	Reference	Type of Tissue/ Cell Line	Type of Assay	No. of Cases Studied	No. of Cases with p53 Alteration	Frequency of p53 Alteration (%)
Isaacs et al.	143	Cell lines: TSU, PC-3, DU 145, LNCaP, PC-82	Mutational analysis between exons 5–9 by DNA sequencing	5	3	60
Rubin et al.	151	Primary tumors Cell lines: DU 145, PC-3	DNA, RNA protein	2 2	1 1	50 50
Effert et al.	152,153	Cell lines: 1 LN, DU-pRO, DU 145	Mutational analysis by SSGP; DNA sequencing	3	3	100
Mellon et al.	154	Primary tumors Metastatic tumors Locally advanced prostate tumors BPH	p53 Immunostaining	10 2 29 34	1 1 5 0	10 50 17 0
Soini et al.	155	Tumor specimens	p53 Immunostaining	34	2	6
Veldhuizen et al.	156	Tumor specimens	p53 Immunostaining	33	26	79
Bookstein et al.	157	Tumor specimens	Immunostaining; SSCP; and DNA sequencing	150	18; More alterations in stage C & D	12
Hamdy et al.	158	Primary tumor specimens	Immunostaining	56	11	20
		Subset of hormone refractory tumors	Immunostaining	11	9	80
de Vere White et al.	159	Prostate carcinoma BPH	RNA/PCR expression	51 13	31 4	61 38

tions of these observations are not clear at this point, but they do suggest that alterations of p53 by mechanisms other than point mutations might also contribute toward tumor development.

In addition to p53 and RB, there are also a few recent reports of the analysis of other candidate TSGs in human prostate cancer. The candidate TSG at chromosome locus 18q21·3 called DCC (deleted in colon carcinoma)[162] exhibited allelic losses in 3 of 16 (19%) BPH specimens and 9 of 25 (38%) carcinomas.[163] Another recent report has shown reduced expression of DCC in 86% of prostate tumor specimens analyzed.[164] The decreased expression of the members of the nm23 gene family (nm23 H-1 and nm23 H-2) has been reported as a measure of metastatic potential.[165] The analysis of nm23 H-2 gene expression by RNA/PCR revealed that its expression decreased significantly as the stage of the prostate carcinoma advanced.[166] In contrast to breast cancer, where nm23-H1 gene is important, alterations of nm23-H2 expression appear to be more relevant in prostate cancer.

The search for TSGs has been very productive in familial cancer syndromes where loss of specific gene(s) is associated with the presence of characteristic neoplasms in certain cancer-prone families.[97,98] The current sophisticated cloning and sequencing methodologies have been largely responsible for the identification of a TSG after the approximate position of that TSG is mapped on a particular chromosome. Using these approaches TSGs involved in the genesis of hereditary retinoblastoma,[104–106] Wilms' tumor,[119–121] neurofibromatosis,[122–125] colon cancer,[126–130] and Von Hippel-Lindau disease[131] have already been identified. It also appears that the TSG which is involved in a specific type of familial cancer is also involved in the genesis of the same type of cancer in sporadic situations. While a germ-line defect would be present in a TSG in hereditary cancers, sporadic cancers of the same type would result from somatic alterations in the same TSG with much later onset. Thus, if there is evidence of a familial clustering for a specific neoplasm, identification of neoplasm-specific genes can be best approached by characterization of these genes in affected individuals belonging to these families.

Early evidence for familial aggregation for prostate cancer was shown by Woolf[167] from the study of first degree relatives of 228 white males who died from carcinoma of the prostate. An approximate threefold increase in the deaths of male relatives due to prostate cancer was observed. Another study[168] of 150 prostate cancers diagnosed before the age of 62 showed fourfold increased risk in the brothers of probands compared to the controls who were brothers-in-law of the probands. Furthermore, the analysis of families of 2,821 probands found that prostate cancer has a higher familiality than colon and breast carcinomas.[169] In another study, the pedigree of 691 prostate cancer patients and 640 spouses who served as controls were analyzed.[170] Men with first degree relatives affected were at twice the risk of developing prostate cancer.

This familial clustering of prostate cancer could be due to two factors: the first and potentially most important one is that there is an inherited genetic risk factor, while the second is that there is an environmental carcinogen leading to exposure of related family members.[171] Recently 691 families with prostate cancer incidence were investigated to assess the role of genetic factors in prostate cancer development.[172] The probands in this study were grouped according to age at the onset of prostate cancer (<53 years, 53–65 years, and >65 years) and were analyzed for the cumulative prostate cancer risk for probands' first degree relatives in these age groups. These estimates showed that the relatives of probands with a younger age had a higher risk of developing prostate cancer as compared to relatives of older probands and also suggested a stronger familial clustering among those with earlier onset of disease.

Segregation analysis of prostate cancer in these families was performed to understand the inheritance pattern and familial aggregation. The autosomal dominant model provided a good fit with the distribution data of prostate cancer in these families. Genotype-specific penetrance estimates for an autosomal dominant model indicated 88% penetrance in both homozygous dominant and heterozygous carriers by age 85, whereas for recessive noncarriers it was only 5% by age 85. As prostate cancer occurrence in U.S. Caucasian men before age 55 accounts for 2% of cases,[173] the total number of cancers due to inherited factors is small. It can be concluded that a small fraction of prostate cancers occurs due to a Mendelian autosomal dominant gene with high penetrance. Molecular genetic characterization of this subset of prostate neoplasms might provide information on prostate neoplasm-specific gene(s). Recent reviews dealing with the studies of the oncogenes and tumor-suppressor genes in prostate cancer are also recommended for additional reading.[14–21,174,175]

SUMMARY

Over the last few years, a growing list of genes have been discovered that are implicated in causing or helping to cause human cancer. These genes fall into two categories: oncogenes whose presence allows or stimulates neoplastic transformation and tumor-suppressor genes whose absence allows neoplastic transformation. Recent studies are addressing the role of oncogenes and tumor-suppressor genes in prostate cancer while cytogenetic analyses have shown chromosomal abnormalities at 7q, 8p, 10q, 16q, and 18q loci. Analyses using molecular probes have confirmed frequent loss of heterozygosity on 8p, 10q,

and 16q loci. Loss of expression of the E-Cadherin gene which is located on chromosome 16q has also been reported in prostate cancers. The well-studied tumor-suppressor genes RB and p53 are being extensively evaluated. Families at high risk for prostate cancer are being utilized for identification of candidate tumor-suppressor genes. Oncogene studies have shown a low incidence of ras oncogene activation; however, the c-erbB-2 oncogene may be overexpressed at the protein level in some tumors. Thus alterations of oncogenes, tumor-suppressor genes, and possibly other novel genes are beginning to define prostate neoplasms at the molecular genetic level, some of which may be early events while others may be later events in prostate tumorigenesis. Future work should uncover specific genetic alterations in prostate cancer and will apply these findings to the discovery of clinically relevant new tumor markers and as targets for new therapies.

ACKNOWLEDGMENTS

Supported by the Center for Prostate Disease Research, a program of the Henry M. Jackson Foundation for the Advancement of Military Medicine, Rockville, MD.

REFERENCES

1. Rous P: A sarcoma of the fowl transmissible by an agent separable from the tumor cells. J Urol Med 13:397, 1901.
2. Varmus H: A historical review of oncogenes. In: Weinberg RA (ed): Oncogenes and the Molecular Origins of Cancer. New York: Cold Spring Harbor Labortory Press, pp 3–44, 1989.
3. Baltimore D: RNA-dependent DNA polymerase in virons of RNA tumor viruses. Nature 226:1209, 1970.
4. Martin GS: Rous sarcoma virus: A function required for the maintenance of the transformed state. Nature 227:1021, 1970.
5. Huebner RJ, Todaro GJ: Oncogenes of RNA tumor viruses as determinants of cancer. Proc Natl Acad Sci 64:1087, 1969.

6. Comings DE: A general theory of carcinogenesis. Proc Natl Acad Sci 70:3324, 1973.

7. Knudson AG: Mutation and cancer: Statistical study of retinoblastoma. Proc Natl Acad Sci 68:820, 1971.

8. Dryja TP, Rapaport JM, Joyce JM, Petersen RA: Molecular detection of deletions involving band q14 of chromosome 13 in retinoblastomas. Proc Natl Acad Sci 83:7319, 1986.

9. Bishop JM: Molecular themes in oncogenesis. Cell 64:235–248, 1991.

10. Bos JL: *ras* oncogenes in human cancer: A review. Cancer Res 49:4682–4689, 1989.

11. Barbacid M: *ras* oncogenes: Their role in neoplasia. Eur J Clin Invest 20:225–235, 1990.

12. Fishleder AJ: Oncogenes and cancer: Clinical applications. Cleveland Clin J Med 57:721–726, 1990.

13. Thompson TC: Growth factors and oncogenes in prostate cancer. Cancer Cells 2:345–354, 1990.

14. Schalken JA, Bussemakers MJG, Debruyne FMJ: Oncogene expression in prostate cancer. Oncogenes 7:97–105, 1990.

15. Gelmann EP: Oncogenes and growth factors in prostate cancer. Journal NIH Res 3:62–64, 1991.

16. Schalken JA: Biological progress in prostate cancer. Current Opin Urol 1:8–10, 1991.

17. Isaacs WB, Carter BS: Genetic changes associated with prostate cancer in humans. Cancer Surveys 11:15–23, 1991.

18. Ichikawa T, Ichikawa Y, Isaacs JT: Genetic factors and metastatic potential of prostate cancer. Cancer Surveys 11:35–41, 1991.

19. Schalken JA: Molecular methods for predicting the metastatic potential of prostate cancer. Cancer Surveys 11:43–53, 1991.

20. Stearns ME, McGarvey T: Prostate cancer: therapeutic, diagnostic, and basic studies. Lab Invest 67:540–552, 1992.

21. Peehl DM: Oncogenes in prostate cancer: an update. Cancer 71:1159–1164, 1993.

22. Viola MV: Genetic changes in prostate carcinoma cells. Cancer Invest 11:92–93, 1993.

23. Chiarodo A: Prosstate cancer working group: National Cancer Institute roundtable on prostate cancer: future research directions. Cancer Res 51:2498–2505, 1991.

24. Rinker-Schaeffer CW, Isaacs WB, Isaacs JT: Molecular and cellular markers for metastic prostate cancer. Cancer Metast Rev 12:3–10, 1993.

25. Bostwick DG, Montironi R, Nagle R, et al.: Current and proposed biologic markers in prostate cancer. J Cell Biochem (Suppl) 16H:65–67, 1992.

26. Habib FK, Chisholm GD: The role of growth factors in the human prostate. Scand J Urol Nephrol (Suppl) 126:53–58, 1991.

27. Davies P, Eaton CL: Regulation of prostate growth. J Endocrin 131:5–17, 1991.

28. Viola MV, Fromowitz F, Oravez S, et al.: Expression of *RAS* oncogene p21 in prostate cancer. N Engl J Med 314:133–137, 1986.

29. Sumiya H, Masai M, Akimotot S, Yatani K, Shimazaki J: Histochemical examination of the expression of *RAS* p21 protein and R-1881-Binding protein in human prostatic cancers. Eur J Cancer 26:786–789, 1990.

30. Sanowitz WS, Paull G, Hamilton SR: Reported binding of monoclonal antibody RAP-S to formalin fixed tissue sections is not indicative of *ras* p21 expression. Hum Pathol 19:127–132, 1988.

31. Varma VA, Austin GE, O'Connell AC: Antibodies to *ras* oncogene p21 proteins lack immunohistochemical specficity for neoplatic epithelium in human prostate tissue. Arch Pathol Lab Med 113:16–19, 1989.

32. Fan K: Heterogeneous subpopulations of human prostatic adenocarcinoma cells: potential usefulness of p21 protein as a predictor for bone metastasis. J Urol 139:318–322, 1988.

33. Niman HL, Thompson AMH, Yu A, Markman M, Willems JJ, Herwig KR, Habib NA, Wood CB, Houghten RA, Lerner RA: Antipeptide antibodies detect oncogene-related proteins in urine. Proc Natl Acad Sci 82:7924–7928, 1985.

34. Pergolizzi RG, Kreis W, Rottach C, Susin M, Broome JD: Mutational status of codons 12 and 13 of the N and K *ras* genes in tissue and cell lines derived from primary and metastatic prostate carcinomas. Cancer Invest 11:25–32, 1993.

35. Cooke DB, Quarmby VE, Petrusz P, Mickey DD, Der CJ, Isaacs JT, French FS: Expression of ras proto-oncogenes in the Dunning R-3327 rat prostatic adenocarcinoma system. Prostate 13:273–287, 1988.

36. Bussemakers MJG, Isaacs JT, Debruyne FMJ, Van de Ven WJM, Schalken JA: Oncogene expression in prostate cancer. World J Urol 9:58–63, 1991.

37. Peehl DM, Wehner N, Stamey TA: Activated Ki-*ras* oncogene in human prostatic adenocarcinoma. Prostate 10:281–289, 1987.

38. Carter BS, Epstein JI, Isaacs WB: *ras* gene mutations in human prostate cancer. Cancer Res 50:6830–6832, 1990.

39. Gumerlock PH, Poonmallee UR, Meyers FJ, de Vere White RW: Activated *ras* alleles in human carcinoma of the prostate are rare. Cancer Res 51:1632–1637, 1991.

40. Konishi N, Enomoto T, Buzard G, Ohshima M, Ward JM, Rice JM: K-*ras* activation and *ras* p21 expression in latent prostatic carcinomas in Japanese men. Cancer 69:2293–2299, 1992.

41. Moul JW, Lance RS, Friedrichs PA, Theune SM, Chang EH: Infrequent *ras* oncogene mutations in human prostate cancer. Prostate 20:327–338, 1992.

42. Anwar K, Nakakuki K, Shiraishi T, Naiki H, Yatani R, Inwua M: Presence of *ras* oncogene mutations and human papillomavirus DNA in human prostate carcinomas. Cancer Res 52:5991–5996, 1992.

43. Treiger B, Isaacs JT: Expression of a transfected v-Harvey-*ras* oncogene in a Dunning rat prostate adenocarcinoma and the development of high metastatic ability. J Urol 140:1580–1586, 1988.

44. Schalken JA, Ebeling SB, Isaacs JT, Treiger B, Bussemakers MJG, de Jong MEM, Van de Ven WJM: Down modulation of fibronectin messenger RNA in metastasizing rat prostatic cancer cells revealed by differential hybridization analysis. Cancer Res 48:2042–2046, 1988.

45. Partin AW, Isaacs JT, Treiger B, Coffey DS: Early cell motility changes associated with an increase in metastatic ability in rat prostate cancer cells transfected with v-Harvey-*ras* oncogene. Cancer Res 48:6050–6053, 1988.

46. Kwok S, Higuchi R: Avoiding false positives with PCR. Nature 339:237–238, 1989.

47. Moul JW, Theune SM, Chang EH: Detection of RAS mutations in archival testicular germ cell tumors by polymerase chain reaction and oligonucleotide hybridization. Genes Chromosomes Cancer 5:109–118, 1992.

48. Moul JW, Bishoff JT, Theune SM, Chang EH: Absent *ras* gene mutations in human adrenal cortical neoplasms and pheochromocytomas. J Urol 149:1389–1394, 1993.

49. Fleming WH, Hamel A, MacDonald R, et al.: Expression of the c-*myc* protooncogene in human prostatic carcinoma in benign prostatic hyperplasia. Cancer Res 46:1535–1538, 1986.

50. Phillips MEA, Ferro MA, Smith PJB, Davies P: Intranuclear androgen receptor deployment and protoncogene expression in human diseased prostate. Urol Int 42:115–119, 1987.

51. Buttyan R, Sawczuk IS, Benson MC, Siegal JD, Olsson CA: Enhanced expression of the c-*myc* proto-oncogene in high-grade human prostate cancer. Prostate 11:327–337, 1987.

52. Cooke DB, Quarmby VE, Mickey DD, Isaacs JT, French FS: Oncogene expression in prostate cancer: Dunning R3327 rat dorsal prostatic adenocarcinoma system. Prostate 13:263–272, 1988.

53. Eaton CL, Davies P, Phillips MEA: Growth factor involvement and oncogene expression in prostatic tumors. J Steroid Biochem 30:341–345, 1988.

54. Matusik RJ, Fleming WH, Hamel A, Westenbrink TG, Hrabarchuk B, MacDonald R, Ramsey E, Gartner JG, Pettigrew NM, Johnston B, Alam TG, Dodd JG: Expression of the c-myc proto-oncogene in prostatic tissue. Prog Clin Biol Res 239:91–112, 1987.

55. Funa K, Nordgren H, Nilsson S: *In-situ* expression of mRNA for proto-oncogenes in benign prostatic hyperplasia and in prostatic carcinoma. Scand J Urol Nephorol 25:95–100, 1991.

56. Fukumoto M, Shevrin DH, Roninson IB: Analysis of gene amplification in human tumor cell lines. Proc Natl Acad Sci 85:6846–6850, 1988.

57. Nag A, Smith RG: Amplification, rearrangement, and elevated expression of c-myc in the human prostatic carcinoma cell line LNCaP. Prostate 15:115–122, 1989.

58. Wolf DA, Kohlhuber F, Schulz P, Fittler F, Eick D: Transcriptional down-regulation of c-*myc* in human prostate carcinoma cells by the synthetic androgen mibolerone. Br J Cancer 65:376–382, 1992.

59. Thompson TC, Southgate J, Kitchener G, Land H: Multistage carcinogenesis induced by *ras* and *myc* oncogenes in a reconstituted organ. Cell 56:917–930, 1989.

60. Carter HB, Piantadosi S, Isaacs JT: Clinical evidence for and implications of the multistep development of prostate cancer. J Urol 143:742–746, 1990.

61. Shih C, Padhy LC, Murray M, et al.: transforming genes of carcinomas and neuroblastomas introduced into mouse fibroblasts. Nature 290:261, 1981.

62. Semba K, Kamata N, Toyoshima K, et al.: A V-erb related proto-oncogene, c-erb-B-2 is distinct from the c-*erb*B-1 epidermal growth factor receptor gene and is amplified in a hu-

man salivary gland adenocarcinoma. Proc Natl Acad Sci 82:6497, 1985.

63. King CR, Kruas MH, Aaronson SA: Amplification of a novel c-erbB related gene in a human mammary carcinoma. Science 229:974, 1985.

64. Fukushige SI, Matsubara KI, Yoshida M, et al.: Localization of a novel c-erbB related gene, c-erbB-2, on human chromosome 17 and its amplification in a gastric cancer cell line. Mol Cell Biol 6:955, 1986.

65. Maguire HC, Greene MI: The neu (c-erbB-2) oncogene. Sem Oncol 16:148, 1989.

66. Yokota J, Toyoshima K, Sugimura T, et al.: Amplification of c-erbB-2 oncogene in human adenocarcinomas in vivo. Lancet 1:765, 1986.

67. Slamon DJ, Clark GM, Wong SG, et al.: Human breast cancer: Correlation of relapse and survival with amplification of the erbB-2neu oncogene. Science 235:177, 1987.

68. Slamon DJ, Godolphin W, Jones LA, et al.: Studies of HER-2/neu proto-oncogene in human breast and ovarian cancer. Science 244:707, 1989.

69. Singleton TP, Strickler JG: Clinical and pathologic significance of the c-erbB-2 (HER-2/neu) oncogene. Pathol Ann 27(p1):165–190, 1992.

70. Hynes NE, Gerber HA, Saurer S, Groner B: Over-expression of the c-erbB-2 protein in human breast tumor cell lines. J Cell Biochem 39:167, 1989.

71. McCann A, Dervan PA, Johnston PA, et al.: c-erbB-2 oncoprotein expression in primary human tumors. Cancer 65:88, 1990.

72. Klotz LH, Auger M, Andrulis I, Srigley J: Molecular analysis of neu, sis, c-myc, fos, and P53 oncogenes in benign prostatic hypertrophy and prostatic carcinoma. J Urol 143:401A, 1990.

73. Sikes RA, Chung LWK: Acquisition of a tumorigenic phenotype by a rat ventral prostate epithelial cell line expressing a transfected activated neu oncogene. Cancer Res 52:3174–3181, 1992.

74. Zhau HE, Wan D, Chung LK, Li W, Hsich J, Ro J, Chung LWK: Expression of the HER-2/neu proto-oncogene in human prostate cancer. J Urol 145:348A, 1991 (abstr).

75. Zhau HE, Wan DS, Zhou J, Miller GJ, Von Eschenbach AC: Expression of c-erbB-2/neu proto-oncogene in human prostatic cancer tissues and cell lines. Mol Carc 5:320–327, 1992.

76. Natali PG, Nicotra MR, Bigotti A, et al.: Expression of the P185 encoded by HER-2 oncogene in normal and transformed human tissues. Int J Cancer 45:457–461, 1990.

77. Sadasivan R, Morgan R, Jennings S, et al.: Over-expression of HER-2/neu may be an indicator of poor prognosis in prostate cancer: Proc Am Assoc Cancer Res 32:166, 1991 (abstr).

78. Natoli C, Angelucci D, Tinari N, et al.: Epidermal growth factor receptors, HER-2/neu, and ploidy in prostate cancer. Proc Am Assoc Cancer Res 32:166, 1991 (abstr).

79. Grob MB, Schellhammer PF, Wright GL, et al.: Expression of the c-erbB2 oncogene in human prostatic carcinoma. J Urol 145:294A, 1991.

80. Ware JL, Maygarden SJ, Koontz WW, Strom SC: Immunohistochemical detection of c-erbB-2 protein in human benign and neoplastic prostate. Hum Pathol 22:254, 1991.

81. Mellon K, Thompson S, Charlton RG, et al.: P53, c-erb-B2 and the epidermal growth factor receptor in the benign and malignant prostate. J Urol 147:496–499, 1992.

82. Visakorpi T, Kallioniemi OP, Koivula T, Harvey J, Isola J: Expression of epidermal growth factor recptor and ERBB2 (Her-2/neu) oncoprotein in prostatic carcinomas. Mod Pathol 5:643–648, 1992.

83. Sadasivan R, Morgan R, Jennings S, Austenfeld M, Van Veldhuizen P, Stephens R, Noble M: Over expression of NER-2/neu may be an indicator of poor prognosis in prostate cancer. J Urol 150:126–131, 1993.

84. Kuhn EJ, Kurnot RA, Sesterhenn IA, Chang EH, Moul JW: Expression of the c-erbB-2 (HER-2/neu) oncoprotein in human prostatic carcinoma. J Urol 150:1427–1433, 1993.

85. Fox SB, Persad RA, Collins CC, Royds J, Silcocks SB: EGFR, c-erbB-2, P53 and c-myc expression in stage A1 prostate adenocarcinoma: prognostic determinants? J Urol 149:331A, 1993 (abstr 475).

86. Rijnders AWM, van der Korput JAGM, van Steenbrugge GJ, Romijn JC, Trapman J: Expression of cellular oncogenes in human prostatic carcinoma cell lines. Biochem Biophys Res Comm 132:548–554, 1985.

87. Sitaras NM, Sariban E, Bravo M, Panatazis P, Antoniades HN: Constitutive production of platelet-derived growth factor-like proteins by human prostate carcinoma cell lines. Cancer Res 48:1930–1935, 1988.

88. Smith RG, Nag A: Regulation of c-sis expression in tumors of the male reproductive tract. Prog Clin Biol Res 239:113–122, 1987.

89. Fudge K, Wang CY, Stearns ME: Immunocytochemical analysis of PDGF A/B chain and PDGF alpha and Beta receptor expression in BPH and Gleason graded human prostate adenocarcinomas. Proc Am Assoc Cancer Res 34:193 (1151), 1993.

90. Lucibello FC, Muller R: Transcription factor encoding oncogenes. Rev Physiol Biochem Pharmacol 119:225–257, 1992.

91. Davies P, Eaton CL, France TD, Phillips ME: Growth factor receptors and oncogene expression in prostate cells. Am J Clin Oncol 11 (Suppl 2):1–7, 1988.

92. McDonnell TJ, Troncoso P, Brisbay SM, Logothetis CJ, Chung LK, Hsieh JT, Tu SM, Campbell ML: BCL-2 expression in androgen-independent prostate carcinoma. J Urol 149:221A (29), 1993.

93. Simak R, Cohen D, Fair WR, Scher H, Birkett NC, Melamed J, Reuter V, Cordon-Cardo C: Expression of c-kit and kit-ligand in human prostate cancer tissues. Proc Am Assoc Cancer Res 34:256 (1525), 1993.

94. Seemayer TA, Cavenee WK: Biology of disease: molecular mechanisms of oncogenesis. Lab Invest 60:585–599, 1989.

95. Benedict WF, Xu HJ, Takahashi R: The retinoblastoma gene: its role in human malignancies. Cancer Invest 8:535–540, 1990.

96. Hunter T: Cooperation between oncogenes. Cell 64:249–270, 1991.

97. Weinberg RA: Tumor suppressor genes. Science 254:1138–1146, 1991.

98. Marshall CJ: Tumor suppressor genes. Cell 64:313–326, 1991.

99. Nigro J, Baker SJ, Preisinger AC, et al.: Mutations in the p53 gene occur in diverse human tumor types. Nature 342:705–708, 1989.

100. Hollstein M, Sidransky D, Vogelstein B, Harris: p53 mutations in human cancers. Science 253:49–53, 1991.

101. Malkin D, Li FP, Strong LC, Fraumeni J Jr, Nelson CE, Kim DH, Kassel J, Gryka MA, Bischoff FZ, Tainsky MA, Friend SH: Germ line p53 mutations in a familial syndrome of breast cancer, sarcomas and other neoplasms. Science 250:1233–1238, 1990.

102. Srivastava S, Zou Z, Pirollo K, Blattner W, Chang EH: Germ-line transmission of a mutated p53 gene in a cancer-prone family with Li-Fraumeni syndrome. Nature 348:747–749, 1990.

103. Frebourg T, Friend SH: Cancer risks from germ-line p53 mutations. J Clin Invest 90:1637–1641, 1992.

104. Friend SH, Bernards R, Rogelj S, Weinberg RA, Rapaport JM, Albert DM, et al.: A human DNA segment with properties of the gene that predisposes to retinoblastoma and osteosarcoma. Nature 323:643–646, 1986.

105. Lee WH, Bookstein R, Hong F, Young LJ, Shew JY, Lee EYHP: Human retinoblastoma susceptibility gene: cloning, identification, and sequence. Science 235:1394–1399, 1987.

106. Fung YKT, Murphree AL, T'Ang A, Qian J, Hinrichs SH, Benedict WF: Structural evidence for the authenicity of the human retinoblastoma gene. Science 236:1657–1661, 1987.

107. Levine AJ, Momand J, Finlay CA: The p53 tumor suppressor gene. Nature 351:453–456, 1991.

108. Kastan MB, Zhan Q, El-Deiry WS, Carrier F, Jacks T, Walsh WV, Plunkett BS, Vogelstein B, Fornance AJ Jr: A mammalian cell cycle checkpoint pathway utilizing p53 and GADD45 is defective in ataxia-telangiectasia. Cell 71:587–597, 1992.

109. Lowe SW, Schmitt EM, Smith SW, Osborne BA, Jacks T: p53 is required for radiation induced apoptosis in mouse thymocytes. Nature 362:847–849, 1993.

110. Clarke AR, Purdie CA, Harrison DJ, Morris RG, Bird OC, Hooper ML, Wyllie AH: Thymocyte apoptosis induced by p53-dependent and independent pathways: Nature 302:849–852, 1993.

111. Brothman AR, Peehl DM, Patel AM, McNeal JE: Frequency and pattern of karyotypic abnormalities in human prostate cancer. Cancer Res 50:3795–3803, 1990.

112. Micale MA, Mohamed A, Sakr W, Powell IJ, Wolman SR: Cytogenetics of primary prostatic adenocarcinoma. Clonality and chromosome instability. Cancer Genet Cytogenet 61:165–173, 1992.

113. Lundgren R: Cytogenetic studies of prostatic cancer. Scand J Urol Nephrol (Suppl) 136:1–35, 1991.

114. Sandberg AA: Chromosomal abnormalities and related events in prostate cancer. Hum Pathol 23:368–380, 1992.

115. Van Dekken H, Kerstens HM, Tersteeg TA, Verhofstad AA, Vooijs GP: Histological pre-

servation after *in situ* hybridization to archival solid tumor sections allows discrimination of cells bearing numerical chromosome changes. J Pathol 168:317–324, 1992.

116. Henke RP, Kruger E, Ayhan N, Hubner D, Hammerer P: Numerical chromosomal aberrations in prostate cancer: correlation with morphology and cell kinetics. Virchows Arch A Pathol Anat Histopathol 422:61–66, 1993.

117. Macoska JA, Wolman SR, Micale MR, Sakr WA: Analysis of molecular genetic and cytogenetic aberrations in prostate cancer. Proc Am Assoc Cancer Res 34:254 (1513), 1993.

118. Bandyk MG, Zhao LC, Leland WK, Troncoso P, Liang JC: Trisomy 7: A potential cytogenetic marker of human prostate cancer progression. Proc Am Assoc Cancer Res 34:210 (1254), 1993.

119. Call KM, Glaser T, Ito CY, Buckler AJ, et al.: Isolation and characterization of a zinc finger polypeptide gene at the human chromosome 11 Wilms' tumours locus. Cell 60:509–520, 1990.

120. Gessler M, Poustka A, Cavenee W, Neve RL, et al.: Homozygous deletion in Wilms tumours of a zinc-finger gene identified by chromosome jumping. Nature 343:774–778, 1990.

121. Rose EA, Glaser T, Jones C, Smith CL, et al.: Complete physical map of the WAGR region of 11p13 localizes a candidate Wilms' tumor gene. Cell 60:495–508, 1990.

122. Cawthon RM, Weiss R, Xu G, Viskochil D, et al.: A major segment of the neurofibromatosis type 1 gene: cDNA sequence, genomic structure, and point mutations. Cell 62:193–201, 1990.

123. Viskochil D, Buchberg AM, Xu G, Cawthon RM, et al.: Deletions and a translocation interrupt a cloned gene at the neurofibromatosis type 1 locus. Cell 62:187–192, 1990.

124. Wallace MR, Marchuk DA, Anderson LB, Letcher R, et al.: Type 1 neurofibromatosis gene: identification of a large transcript disrupted in three NF1 patients. Science 249:181–186, 1990.

125. Xu G, O'Connell P, Viskochil D, Cawthon R, et al.: The neurofibromatosis type 1 gene encodes a protein related to GAP. Cell 62:599–608, 1990.

126. Joslyn G, Carlson M, Thliveris A, Albertsen H, et al.: Identification of deletion mutations and three new genes at the familial polyposis locus. Cell 66:601–613, 1991.

127. Groden J, Thliveris A, Samowitz W, Carlson M, et al.: Identification and characterization of the familial adenomatous polyposis coli gene. Cell 66:589–600, 1991.

128. Kinzler KW, Nilbert MC, Su LK, Vogelstein B, et al.: Identification of FAP locus genes from chromosome 5q21. Science 253:661–665, 1991.

129. Nishisho I, Nakamura Y, Miyoshi Y, Miki Y, et al.: Mutations of chromosome 5q21 genes in FAP and colorectal cancer patients. Science 253:665–669, 1991.

130. Peltomaki P, Aaltonen LA, Sistonen P, Pylkkanen L, et al.: Genetic mapping of a locus predisposing to human colorectal cancer. Science 260:810–812, 1993.

131. Latif F, Tory K, Gnarra J, Yao M, et al.: Identification of the von Hippel-Lindau disease tumor suppressor gene. Science 260:1317–1320, 1993.

132. Carter BS, Ewing CM, Ward WS, Treiger BF, et al.: Allelic loss of chromosomes 16q and 10q in human prostate cancer. Proc Natl Acad Sci 87:8751–8755, 1990.

133. Bergerheim USR, Kunimi K, Collins VP, Ekman P: Deletion mapping of chromosomes 8, 10 and 16 in human prostate carcinoma. Genes Chromosome Cancer 3:215–220, 1991.

134. Kunimi K, Uchibayashi T, Hisazumi H: Oncogene amplification and inactivation of tumor suppressor genes in urological malignant tumors—the application of restriction fragment length polymorphism analysis. Nippon Hinyokika Gakkai Zasshi, 82:1930–1938, 1991.

135. Umbas R, Schalken JA, Aalders TW, Carter B, et al.: Expression of cellular adhesion molecule E-cadherin is reduced or absent in high-grade prostate cancer. Cancer Res 52:5104–5109, 1992.

136. Bussemakers MJG, van Moorselaar RJA, Giroldi LA, Ichikawa T, et al.: Decreased expression of E-cadherin in the progression of rat prostatic cancer. Cancer Res 52:2916–2999, 1992.

137. Morton R, Ewing C, Nagafuchi A, Tsukita S: Expression of α-catenin in human prostate cancer cell lines. Proc Am Assoc Cancer Res 34:34 (198), 1993.

138. Macoska JA, Powell IJ, Sakr W, Lane MA: Loss of 17p chromosome region in a metastatic carcinoma of the prostate. J Urol 147:1142–1146, 1992.

139. Morton RA, Bova GS, Issacs WB: Hyper-methylation of chromosome 17p13·3 in human adenocarcinoma of the prostate. J Urol 149:376A (653), 1993.

140. Bova GS, Carter BS, Robinson J, Issacs WB: Tumor suppressor loci in human prostate cancer: high resolution search using Southern analysis and short tandem repeat polymorphism. J Urol 149:221A (30), 1993.

141. Macoska JA, Sakr W, Benson P, Pontes JE: Allelic loss at 8p, 10q and 16q in microdissected prostate tumors. J Urol 149:221A (31), 1993.

142. Bookstein R, Shew JY, Chen PL, Scully P, Lee WH: Suppression of tumorigenicity of human prostate carcinoma cells by replacing a mutated RB gene. Science 247:712–715, 1990.

143. Isaacs WB, Carter BS, Ewing CM: Wild-type p53 suppresses growth of human prostate cancer cells containing mutant p53 alleles. Cancer Res 51:4716–4720, 1991.

144. Peehl DM, Wong ST, McNeal JE, Stamey TA: Analysis of somatic cell hybrids derived from normal human prostatic epithelial cells fused with Hela cells. Prostate 17:123–126, 1990.

145. Ichikawa T, Ichikawa Y, Dong J, Hawkins AL: Localization of metastasis suppressor gene(s) for prostatic cancer to the short arm of human chromosome 11. Cancer Res 52:3486–3490, 1992.

146. Rinker-Schaeffer CW, Vukanonvic J, Issacs J: Identification and characterization of genes in metastatic progression of prostatic cancer cells. Proc Am Assoc Cancer Res 34:249 (1483), 1993.

147. Bova GS, Robinson JC, Isaacs WB: Chromosome 17 suppresses tumorgenicity of a human prostate cell line. Proc Am Assoc Cancer Res 34:540 (3222), 1993.

148. Bookstein R, Rio P, Madreperla SA, Hong F, et al.: Promoter deletion and loss of retinoblastoma gene expression in human prostate carcinoma. Proc Natl Acad Sci 87:7762–7766, 1990.

149. Brooks JD, Bova GS, Marshall FF, Isaacs WB: Allelic losses of retinoblatoma gene in primary renal and prostate cancers. J Urol 149:376A (652), 1993.

150. Sarkar FH, Sakr W, Li YW, Maloska J, et al.: Analysis of retinoblastoma (RB) gene deletion in human prostatic carcinoma. Prostate 21:145–152, 1992.

151. Rubin SJ, Hallahan DE, Ashman CR, Brachman DG, et al.: Two prostate carcinoma cell lines demonstrate abnormalities in tumor suppressor genes. J Surg Oncol 46:31–36, 1991.

152. Effert PJ, Neubauer A, Walther PJ, Liu ET: Alterations of the p53 gene are associated with the progression of a human prostate carcinoma. J Urol 147:789–793, 1992.

153. Effert PJ, McCoy RH, Walther PJ, Liu ET: p53 gene alterations in human prostate carcinoma. J Urol 150:257–261, 1993.

154. Mellon K, Thompson S, Charlton RG, Marsh C, et al.: ρ53 c-erb-2 and epidermal growth factor receptor in the benign and malignant prostate. J Urol 147:496–499, 1992.

155. Soini Y, Paakko P, Nuorva K, Kamel D, et al.: Comparative analysis of p53 protein immunoreactivity in prostatic, lung and breast carcinomas. Virchows Arch A Pathol Anat Histopathol 421:223–228, 1992.

156. Van Veldhuizen PJ, Sadasivan R, Garcia F, Austenfeld MS, Stephen RL: Mutant p53 expression in prostate carcinoma. Prostate 22:23–30, 1993.

157. Bookstein R, MacGrogan D, Sharkey F, Hilsenbeck SG, Aured DC: p53 mutations in human prostate cancer. Proc Am Assoc Cancer Res 34:537 (3205), 1993.

158. Hamdy CF, Thurrell W, Lawry J, Anderson JB, et al.: p53 mutant expression correlates with hormone sensitivity and prognosis in human prostatic adenocarcinoma. J Urol 149:377A (658), 1993.

159. de Vere White RW, Gumerlock PH, Chi SG, Meyers FJ: p53 tumor suppressor gene abnormalities are frequent in human prostate tissues. J Urol 149:376A (654), 1993.

160. Colombel M, Olsson C, Buttyan R: Hormone-regulated apoptosis results from reentry of differentiated prostate cells into defective cell cycle. Cancer Res 52:4313–4319, 1992.

161. Liu X, Park SH, Thompson TC, Lane DP: Ras-induced hyperplasia occurs with mutations of p53 but activated ras and myc together can induce carcinomas without p53 mutation. Cell 70:153–161, 1992.

162. Fearon ER, Cho KR, Nigro JM, Kerm SE, et al.: Identification of a chromosome 18q gene that is altered in colorectal cancers. Science 247:49–56, 1990.

163. Brewster SF, Harper S, Brown KF: Somatic alterations on chromosome 18q in human prostatic carcinoma implicate the DCC gene. J Urol 149:221A (32), 1993.

164. Gao X, Honn KV, Grignon D, Sakr W: Frequent loss of expression and loss of heterozygosity of the putative suppressor gene DCC in prostatic carcinoma. Cancer Res 53:2723–2727, 1993.

165. Golden A, Benedict M, Shearn A, Kimurs N, et al.: Nucleoside diphosphate kinases, nm23, and tumor metastasis: possible biochemical mechanisms. Cancer Treat Res 63:345–358, 1992.

166. Fishman JR, Gumerlock PH, Kim SY, Meyers FJ, de Vere White RW: Quantitation of nm23 expression in human prostate tissues. J Urol 149:374A (647), 1993.

167. Woolf CM: An investigation of the familial aspects of carcinoma of the prostate. Cancer 13:739–744, 1960.

168. Meikle AW, Smith JA, West DW: Familial factors affecting prostatic cancer risk and plasma sex steriod levels. Prostate 6:121–128, 1985.

169. Cannon L, Bishop DT, Skolnick M, Hunt S, et al.: Genetic epidemiology of prostate cancer in the Utah Mormon genealogy. Cancer Surveys 1:47–69, 1982.

170. Steinberg GS, Carter BS, Beaty TH, Childs B, Walsh PC: Family history and the risk of prostate cancer. Prostate 17:337–347, 1990.

171. Carter BS, Steinberg GD, Beaty TH, Childs B, Walsh PC: Familial risk factors for prostate cancer. Cancer Surveys, 11:5–13, 1991.

172. Carter BS, Beaty TH, Steinberg GD, Childs B, Walsh PC: Mendelian inheritance of familial prostate cancer. Proc Natl Acad Sci 89:3367–3371, 1992.

173. Devesa SS, Silverman DT, Young JL, Pollack ES, et al.: Cancer incidence and mortality trends among whites in the United States. J Natl Cancer Inst 79:701–770, 1987.

174. Linehan WM: Molecular genetics of tumor suppressor genes in prostate carcinoma: the challenge and promise ahead. J Urol 147:808–809, 1992.

175. Bookstein R, Allred DC: Recessive oncogenes. Cancer 71:1179–1186, 1993.

APPENDIX: DEFINITION OF TERMS

Allele: Because of the paired nature of chromosomes, each gene is present in two copies, each termed an allele.

Antioncogene (Tumor-Suppressor Gene): A gene whose protein products' *absence* contributes to tumor development/progression.

The gene normallly suppresses cellular growth and proliferation.

BCL-2: Proto-oncogene involved in prolonging programmed cell death (apoptosis). High expression has been seen in hormone refractory prostate cancer and has been implicated in pathogenesis of this phenotype.

Chromosome Translocation: The exchange of genes or portions of gene between different chromosomes. This is one mechanism for oncogene activation.

Codon: Refers to the position of a DNA 3-base coding message in the gene sequence. For example, in *ras* genes, the 12th, 13th, or 61st codon may be mutated, leading to oncogene activation.

DNA Probe: A short segment of DNA whose base sequence is specifically complementary to a particular gene segment. The probe can be used on a Southern blot, for example, to determine if a certain gene is present in a tumor DNA sample.

c-erbB-2 (also called HER-2 or neu): Oncogene that codes for a protein similar to the epidermal growth factor receptor. Clinically useful as prognostic marker in breast cancer where gene is amplified. May be involved in prostate cancer; studies currently in conflict.

c-fos: protein product of this oncogene forms part of the AP-1 transcription factor. *c-fos* involved in "master-switch" of transcription. In prostate, no amplification of *c-fos* but some may have overexpression. More work is needed.

c-kit: Proto-oncogene that encodes a cell surface tyrosine kinase growth factor receptor. The ligand of *c-kit* is the stem cell factor (SCF). The oncogene has recently been found to be expressed in a subset of prostate cancers but the implications are presently unknown.

c-sis: Proto-oncogene whose protein product is identical to the B-chain of the platelet derived growth factor (PDGF). Earlier work suggested that *c-sis* may be overexpressed in poorly differentiated prostate carcinoma, but little follow-up work has been done.

Gel Electrophoresis: Molecular biology laboratory technique in which DNA, RNA, or proteins are separated according to molecular weight, charge, and spatial characteristics in an electric field applied to a gel. Since DNA, for example, is negatively charged, it migrates toward the positively charged electrode.

Gene Amplification: Increased copy number per cell of an individual gene, usually a proto-oncogene. The c-*erb*B-2 and *N-myc* genes typically function as oncogenes in this manner.

Gene Expression: Refers to the gene of interest's rate of transcription to messenger RNA. For example, in prostate cancer study of mRNA from a tumor may show abundant mRNA species of the c-*erb*B-2 gene, indicating overexpression of the c-*erb*B-2 oncogene.

Heterozygosity: Two different forms of the same gene in a cell. For example, an oncogene is generally heterozygous; one allele may be mutated while the other copy remains normal. In addition, different forms of a gene may be normal variants. Variations in exact base sequence within DNA are common in the genome among the human population. These are called polymorphisms and are frequently responsible for the heterozygous state.

Loss of Heterozygosity (LOH): The heterozygous state of a particular locus on a specific chromosome as identified by restriction fragment length polymorphism and informative DNA probe helps to identify two copies of a gene on that locus. Generally, in normal cells two alleles of a candidate tumor-suppressor gene are detected, whereas in tumor cells one of the wild type (wt) alleles is lost and other allele is retained in the mutated form. Such an allelic loss in tumors as compared to normal cells is commonly referred to as the loss of heterozygosity, and this concept is the hallmark of the analysis of tumor-suppressor genes in human tumors. In prostate cancer there is a frequent loss of chromosomal loci 8p and 16q, as evidenced by LOH analysis.

Microcell Transfer: Microcells are cytoplasmic fragments that contain micronuclei composed of one or a few chromosomes. The fusion of a microcell population into target cell population results in the transfer of individual chromosomes into target cells. Thus, microcell transfer provides a way to transfer individual chromosomes from a donor cell to a recipient cell.

myc: Proto-oncogene family that includes *c-myc*, *N-myc*, *L-myc*, and *R-myc*. Encodes a nuclear associated DNA-binding proteins that affects DNA replication and transcription. Amplification of *N-myc* has been found to be of prognostic significance in neuroblastoma.

Northern Blot: Molecular biology techinque whereby RNA is transferred from a gel electrophoresis to a nylon membrane. The RNA is bound to the membrane and the membrane can be probed to determine RNA expression of various genes of interest.

Oncogenes: Cancer producing sequence of DNA; genes that have been implicated to contribute to the neoplastic state. An oncogene is a functionally or structurally aberrant form of its proto-oncogene. A proto-oncogene may become an oncogene via point mutation, amplification, translocation, and/or gene rearrangement.

PCR: Stands for "polymerase chain reaction." It is a technique to multiply genes or portions of genes in vitro if the sequence of the gene is known or partially known. Priming pieces of DNA called "primers" flank the region of gene of interest to be multiplied and a special heat stable enzyme called "taq-polymerase" creates DNA in the test tube. This technique has revolutionized molecular biology by allowing study of genes from very small or even degraded samples of tissue or tumor. For example, analysis for certain genes is possible from archival paraffin samples or from small quantities of cells.

Polymorphisms: Variations in exact base sequence of DNA making up the genome. These variations are normal and are common in human populations. Polymorphisms have been exploited in molecular genetics because these variations are inherited and polymorphisms near or within disease genes can be used in linkage genetic studies.

Proto-oncogenes: Genes that encode for a variety of proteins involved in normal cell growth and proliferation including growth factors, growth factor receptors, regulators of DNA synthesis, and modifiers of protein function by phosphorylation.

p53 Gene: Tumor-suppressor gene encodes a nuclear phosphoprotein, which arrests cell from entering S-phase of cell cycle. Recent observations also suggest that p53 protein is involved in the regulation of expression of the genes, induced during cell growth arrest triggered by DNA damaging agents, e.g., UV or ionizing radiations. Normal functions of p53 may also include regulation of apoptosis induced by ionizing radiation. Located on chromosome 17 (17p13), p53 is postulated to contribute to tumorigenesis of a diverse variety of cancers. Mutations have been commonly found in certain highly conserved regions of the gene in various human tumors.

ras: Family of genes that encode for similar cell membrane bound proteins that are involved in signal transduction. Three genes, *K-ras, N-ras,* and *H-ras* have been most widely studied in human tumors. The proto-oncogene becomes activated by point mutations, most commonly in specific codons of the gene sequence. The oncogenes have importance in colon and lung cancers but are uncommonly activated in prostatic neoplasms.

RB Gene: First discovered tumor-suppressor gene, which is a 4.7 kilobase gene located at chromosome 13q14. Encodes a 110,000 kilodalton nuclear phosphoprotein that suppresses the cell cycle. This gene is the cause of retinoblastomas and is involved in the pathogenesis of many other neoplasms.

Restriction Fragment Length Polymorphisms (RFLPs) in the Identification of TSGs: The changes in the specific recognition sequence of a restriction endonuclease due to the DNA polymorphism in one of the two alleles of a particular chromosome locus results in the generation of DNA fragments of different sizes representing different alleles. These DNA fragments can then be identified on a Southern blot utilizing an "informative DNA probe" derived from the same chromosome locus. This establishes heterozygosity for a particular locus which is usually found in normal, constitutional cells. The loss of one allele, usually of the one containing the wild form TSG, is termed a loss of heterozygosity (LOH) and is frequently associated with tumors. Thus the comparison of normal and tumor tissues from the same patient yields information on the frequent allelic loss or LOH in a specific neoplasm, which in turn is suggestive of the involvement of the TSG on that chromosome locus.

Single Strand Conformation Polymorphism (SSCP) Analysis of Point Mutations: This is a rapid method for the detection of changes in DNA sequences, including point mutations. The sequence of interest in the genomic DNA is PCR amplified and the two strands of the PCR-derived DNA are generated by denaturation. The resulting sample is run on polyacrylamide gel under nondenaturing condition. Single strand DNA exhibits a characteristic conformation and mobility on the gel. The mobility shift in comparison to control samples is detected on the gel due to conformational alterations caused by mutation(s).

Southern Blot: Molecular biology technique whereby DNA is transferred from a gel electrophoresis to a nylon or nitrocellulose membrane. The DNA can be fixed to these surfaces and further study with DNA probes can then detect, for example, the presence of an oncogene.

Transcription: Converting the DNA code into a complementary messenger RNA segment.

Translation: Converting a messenger RNA sequence into a protein product.

Wild-type Gene: Term used to describe the normal nonmutated, nonaltered gene or allele in the genome. A gene encoding a proto-oncogene would be considered to be a wild-type gene since it has not been altered.

3

The Epidemiology and Prevention of Prostate Cancer

Otis W. Brawley, M.D., and Barnett S. Kramer, M.D., M.P.H.

INTRODUCTION

The increasing incidence of prostate cancer has been attributed to improved medical surveillance, more precise medical technology, a greater awareness of the disease, or a true increase in prostate cancer. The precise contribution that each of these factors plays is unknown, but what is known is that latent or indolent prostate cancer is present in 50–70% of men by age 75. Is it possible that this increase in incidence is due solely to the ability of medical technology to detect latent or indolent prostate cancer?

This chapter reviews the controversial topic of latent or indolent prostate cancer, and reviews the risk factors that may cause promotion of latent cancer to clinically apparent cancer. Lastly, we review the ability of drugs to prevent prostate cancer or to block its progression.

EPIDEMIOLOGY

The Cancer Surveillance, Epidemiology, and End Results (SEER) Program of the National Cancer Institute provides the most complete information on cancer in the United States and documents the changing pattern of prostate cancer diagnosis.[1] SEER was begun in 1973; most recent data are available for 1990. Information is collected on all cases of cancer diagnosed in residents of nine areas of the United States. Approximately 10% of the American population lives in areas surveyed by SEER. Hospital pathology reports, discharge diagnoses, and death certificates are reviewed, as are records kept by physicians. The data are checked for accuracy and completeness in a routine quality-control program.[2]

SEER data demonstrates two important points: (1) that prostate cancer remains primarily a disease of older men; and (2) that African-American mortality from prostate cancer remains the highest in the world. In 1990, the age-adjusted incidence rate was 22.7 per 100,000 for men under the age of 65 and 884.1 per 100,000 for men aged 65 years and older. Figure 1 illustrates SEER data on age-specific prostate cancer incidence and mortality for African-Americans and white Americans from 1985 to 1990. During this period the median age at diagnosis of prostate cancer was 72, and median age at death was 77 years. The median age at diagnosis for African-Americans was 70 and median age at death was 75.

Figure 2 demonstrates the changes in prostate cancer incidence and mortality for black and white Americans from 1973 to 1990 in the SEER database. Age-adjusted incidence rates have increased an average

Prostate Cancer, pages 47–64 Published 1994 Wiley-Liss, Inc.

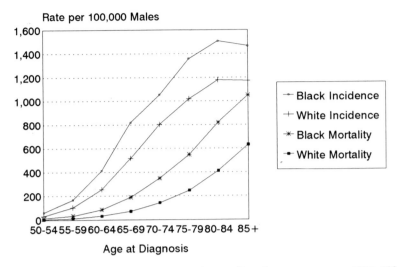

Fig. 1. U.S. age-specific incidence and mortality of prostate cancer, 1986–1990.

of 3.3% per year in the U.S. The rise is most rapid among whites. Prostate cancer mortality has also increased during the period, but the increase is not as dramatic as that of prostate cancer incidence. African-American prostate cancer mortality rates were twice those of white Americans throughout the period 1973 to 1990 and throughout all age groups. During the 1980s, the majority of men diagnosed with prostate cancer in the SEER registries had localized disease, although a disproportio-

nate number of black patients were diagnosed with distant disease (Table 1). Not surprisingly, those with low-stage disease had a distinct survival advantage when compared to advanced or distant disease. When compared to whites within the same stage, a lower proportion of black men survived five years (Table 2).

Throughout the 1980s, the age-adjusted prostate cancer incidence rate increase was 8% for black Americans and 30% for white Americans. Although the incidence rate

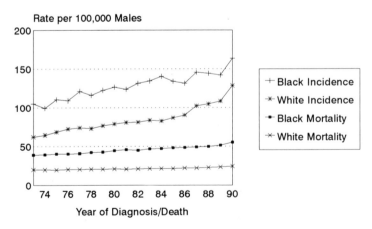

Fig. 2. U.S. incidence and mortality of prostate cancer, 1973–1990.

TABLE 1. Stage Distribution by Race[a]

	White Males (%) N = 34,371	Black Males (%) N = 4,174
Localized	59	52
Regional	15	12
Distant	17	26
Unstaged	9	10

[a]SEER patients diagnosed 1983–1987.

has been higher for black men, the ratio of black incidence to white incidence decreased from 1.6 in 1980 to 1.3 in 1990. The age-specific incidence ratio by race has been greatest among men in their early fifties. In the late 1980s, the age-specific incidence for black men age 50–54 was 61.7, and was 36.6 for white men (a black–white incidence ratio of 1.7).

The increase in diagnosed prostate cancers among white Americans as compared to African-Americans is reflected in changing lifetime risk estimates. These risk estimates are projections taking into account competing risk factors for death. In 1980, Seidman and colleagues, using incidence and population figures, estimated the lifetime risk of developing clinically significant prostate cancer to be 9.6% for an African-American man and 5.2% for a white American man. By 1985, the figures were 9.4% and 8.7%, respectively,[3] while by 1988–90 the figures increased to 11.3% and 13.3%. The lifetime risk of a white man dying of prostate cancer is 3.18%, while the calculated lifetime risk of an

TABLE 2. Five-Year Survival by Race[a]

	White Males	Black Males
All stages	77.2	63.1
Localized	91.6	85.3
Regional	81.7	68.3
Distant	28.7	21.7
Unstaged	69.9	53.1

[a]SEER patients diagnosed 1983–1987.

African-American man dying of prostate cancer is 3.96%.[4]

The recent dramatic increases in the white prostate cancer rates are likely an example of selection bias. A disproportionate number of middle and upper middle class Americans are undergoing prostate cancer screening. These socioeconomic groups are overwhelmingly white. In addition to screening, the increase in prostate cancer is associated with expanding availability and use of several diagnostic tools. The increasing number of transurethral resections of the prostate (TURPs) performed to treat benign prostatic hyperplasia (BPH) has been correlated with the rise in prostate cancer incidence rates.[5] Transrectal ultrasound and the spring-loaded transrectal biopsy "gun" technology have made diagnosis easier.[6] Serum prostate-specific antigen (PSA) became widely available in 1988. Much of the increase in diagnosed prostate cancers from the estimated 105,000 American cases in 1990 to the estimated 165,000 in 1993 can be attributed to screening with PSA.[7–9] Prostate cancer screening, and especially screening with PSA, is profoundly changing the incidence of diagnosed prostate cancer.

Prostate cancer is a disease with a high prevalence and variable biologic behavior. Most prostate cancers are indolent and of no threat to the patient; others are highly aggressive and lead to death. It has been estimated that 1 in 380 men with prostate cancer actually dies of it.[10] Autopsy data from a number of countries demonstrate a very high incidence of indolent prostate cancer in all populations. Greater than 30% of men over the age of 50 dying of causes other than prostate cancer have histologic evidence of prostate cancer.[11–36] These studies also demonstrate that the presence of histologic cancer increases with age. By age 75 approximately 50 to 70% of men have histologic evidence of prostate carcinoma at autopsy.

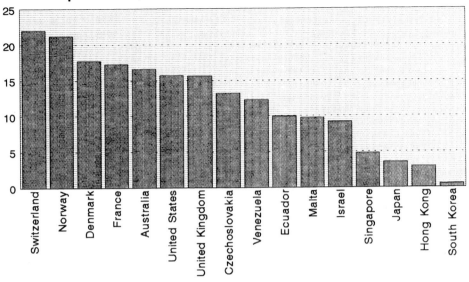

Fig. 3. Age-adjusted mortality rates of prostate cancer, 1986–1988.

The literature does not suggest a geographic or ethnic variability in the rate of latent carcinoma; indeed where carefully studied it appears the incidence of latent carcinoma is similar among countries and races even though there is a marked difference in prostate mortality (Fig. 3).[34] Recently Carter and colleagues have shown that the prevalence of histologic prostate cancer in Japan and the United States is similar even though the incidence of clinical prostate cancer and prostate cancer-specific mortality is markedly higher in Americans.[37] Sakr and colleagues have compared racial differences of latent prostate cancer among black and white men in the U.S. and found equal rates, even though African-Americans have a greater morbidity.[38]

A comparable incidence of latent tumors with varying incidences of clinical disease suggests that initiation of prostate cancer is the same among groups, but there are differences in the rate of promotion or progression to clinically evident prostate cancer.[39] Populations with higher incidences of prostate cancer may be more susceptible to prostate cancer promoting events or may be exposed to different promoting agents. Whittemore and colleagues note that the transformation rate from histologic to clinically evident cancer is similar for black and white men, but that African-American men appear to have a larger volume of latent prostate cancer. Larger volume latent cancers are likely those that progress most rapidly to become clinically evident. While the events that cause the racial differences in incidence of clinically significant prostate cancer are undefined, they are likely to be numerous.[40–42]

When reviewing recent data concerning prostate cancer incidence one must keep in mind that prostate cancer is a significant cause of male death, but newer screening modalities are identifying both indolent and aggressive prostate cancers. The rise in U.S. prostate cancer incidence and changes in diagnostic technology make it difficult to answer the question "Is there a true increase in the number of clinically significant prostate cancers?" A part of the rise in deaths attributed to prostate cancer may be a result of greater prostate cancer awareness and increased medical surveillance among the growing number of persons surviving into the oldest age groups. These groups have a decreasing cardiac mortality and a high prevalence of prostate cancer. It is likely that the higher American incidence cannot be attributed purely to technical improvements in diagnosis, as these improvements have been introduced into practice over the past 15 years. American prostate cancer incidence and mortality have been high for some time when compared to other countries.[43]

RISK FACTORS FOR PROSTATE CANCER

The definitive etiology of prostate cancer is unknown, but much can be surmised from what is known. Autopsy studies demonstrate a similar prevalence of indolent disease among races and cultures, but there are vastly differing incidences of clinically evident disease among races and cultures that cannot be attributed to screening. This fact and the varying prostate cancer death rates (which are less likely to be affected by screening than incidence rates) suggest that environmental stimuli and genetics are important in prostate cancer etiology.

In the previous section, we reviewed the factors of race/ethnicity and age that affect an individual's risk for developing clinically significant prostate cancer. In this section, we review other risk factors that have been suggested for prostate cancer and the evidence supporting them.

Family History

Case control analysis has identified familial patterns of prostate cancer.[44] A Mendelian pattern of inheritance has been identified in several families.[45] Men who have a first-degree relative with prostate cancer are estimated to have a 2.1- to 2.8-fold greater risk of developing prostate cancer when compared to the general population.[46] Those with a first-degree relative and a grandfather or uncle with prostate cancer have a risk that may be sixfold greater than that of the general population. There is suggestion that men from some families with a history of female breast cancer have a higher risk for prostate cancer.[47,48]

A definitive link between prostate cancer and family history has not been made. Some families likely develop prostate cancer due to a yet unidentified inherited genetic susceptibility. Other families may have a high incidence of prostate cancer because members share similar environmental exposures. While family history and genetic factors likely influence one's risk of clinically relevant prostate cancer, the vast majority of victims have no known risk factors other than male gender and age.

Benign Prostatic Hyperplasia

It is difficult to determine whether benign prostatic hyperplasia (BPH) is a risk factor for the development of prostate cancer. The two diseases have a number of similarities and dissimilarities. BPH, like prostate cancer, is common in aging men and both diseases exhibit androgen dependence. BPH is most often found in the central or transitional zone of the prostate, while cancer is most often found in the peripheral zone of the gland. BPH has been linked to the diagnosis of prostate cancer with relative risks of 5.1 to 13.5 in retrospective and prospective studies.[49–52] Other studies looking for associations have failed to find an association between BPH and prostate cancer.[53–55]

Because of the high prevalence of indolent prostate cancer, treatment for BPH likely increases one's risk for being diagnosed with prostate cancer.[5] It is very possible that BPH does not increase one's risk of developing prostate cancer, but increases one's risk of being diagnosed with prostate cancer.

Socioeconomic Factors

Poverty has been correlated with an increased incidence of cancer. In the U.S., race is often a surrogate for poverty. Older studies using a number of methods to correlate prostate cancer risk and socioeconomic status had mixed findings.[49,56–64] Most found that persons of lower socioeconomic status are diagnosed with more advanced disease, but none demonstrate socioeconomic status to be a highly significant factor in cancer etiology. Recently, two groups of investigators, in well-designed studies, attempted to find an association between poverty and risk of prostate cancer in African-Americans and whites. They correlated SEER prostate cancer incidence with population density, education, and income. Both studies found no statistically significant correlation between race or socioeconomic status and prostate cancer incidence.[65,66]

Occupation

Despite a number of studies of prostate cancer incidence among men of various occupations, no occupation has been firmly identified as a risk factor for the disease. Farmers, mechanics, newspaper workers, plumbers, welders, and electroplate and rubber workers have been alleged to have increased incidence. While no occupation can be conclusively linked to prostate cancer, men exposed to cadmium (welders and electroplate workers) are perhaps most interesting. Several reports tend to support the hypothesis that cadmium exposure weakly increases the risk for prostate cancer.[67–73]

There are theoretical reasons why cadmium exposure may be linked to prostate cancer. Cadmium is an antagonist of zinc in a number of reactions. Zinc is necessary in a number of intracellular metabolic pathways.[74,75] Most importantly, it is a crucial cofactor for several DNA repair enzymes. Of all body organs, the prostate has the highest concentration of zinc. Normal and hyperplastic prostate glands have higher concentrations of zinc when compared to glands with prostatitis or cancer.[76–81]

Smoking

The literature on cigarette smoking and prostate cancer risk is conflicting. Several studies have correlated smoking with the diagnosis of prostate cancer.[54,82,83] Indeed, Hsing estimated an increased relative risk of 1.8 for smoking and 2.1 for tobacco chewing. One case control study did not find a link between smoking and prostate cancer.[84] The increased risk of prostate cancer among smokers may be due to health care behavior. When compared to nonsmokers, smokers are more likely to see a physician and be examined for prostate cancer. Those screened for prostate cancer are more likely to be diagnosed.

Infection

There is no clear association between prostate cancer and infection. Increased herpesvirus and cytomegalovirus titers have been reported in prostate cancer patients when compared to control populations. This finding has not been confirmed in a large study, nor do we know of a study of viral pathogenesis using more sensitive techniques such as polymerase chain reaction. A hypothesis involving a viral pathogenesis has not been widely espoused.[85]

Repeated prostatitis has been suggested as a cause for prostate cancer. Some have pointed to the decreased zinc concentration in inflamed prostates and tried to make an association with the same finding in prostates containing cancer. Several studies have failed to show an association between prostatitis and prostate cancer development, and several studies have suggested a possible correlation. Any purported association between prostatitis and prostate cancer remains purely speculative.[86-92]

Sexual Behavior

The relationship between sexual behavior, fertility, and prostate cancer has been repeatedly studied.[49,64,86,87,93] Despite reports dating back to the turn of the century, no clear relationship has been established between sexual activity, sexual behavior, and prostate cancer.

Vasectomy

Vasectomy leads to histologic changes in the prostate and has been associated with higher circulating levels of testosterone. In 1987, Sidney reported on 5,332 men with prostate cancer who were each matched with three nonvasectomized comparison controls.[94] That study found no increase in prostate cancer nor benign prostatic hyperplasia among vasectomized men. Several subsequent studies have demonstrated that vasectomy confers a small increased risk for prostate cancer. Giovannucci and colleagues conducted a prospective study of 10,055 vasectomized men and 37,800 nonvasectomized men. They found that vasectomized men had an increased relative risk of 1.85 when compared to nonvasectomized men.[95] In a separate retrospective cohort study, Giovannucci and colleagues matched 14,607 vasectomized men with 14,607 nonvasectomized men. This study found vasectomy was associated with an age-adjusted increased relative risk of 1.56.[96] Several studies have found that vasectomy increases relative risk by a factor of 1.7 to 2.2. All find a trend in the association between years since vasectomy and risk of prostate cancer.[54,97,98]

An association between vasectomy and prostate cancer is possible, but any in-creased risk, if it exists, is small. The association may be causative or it may be simply related to health care behavior. It is conceivable that the association is actually a screening selection bias, since men who go to physicians (usually urologists) for vasectomies are more likely to be screened by those urologists for prostate cancer. It is well established that men who tend to be screened are more likely to be diagnosed. This issue needs to be studied further, especially in prospective trials. It is important to note that some studies have associated vasectomy and prostate cancer, but no one has suggested that reversing vasectomies decreases risk, and this should not be advocated without further study.

Diet

Numerous migrant studies have associated diet with prostate cancer.[43,99,100-102] Dietary differences have been suggested as the reason why indolent cancers occur at a similar frequency around the world while clinically significant tumors are more common in western Europe, the U.S., and Canada.[100] Armstrong and Doll compared the prostate cancer death rate and average fat consumption in 32 countries.[103] They found that countries with a high average fat consumption also had a higher rate of prostate cancer death. Rose et al. made a similar correlation.[104] These analyses are further supported by studies showing that populations with diets high in fiber and therefore presumably lower in fat are associated with lower incidences of prostate cancer.[105-113]

It has been suggested that dietary fat may lead to the increased production of sexual hormones. An increased production of androgens in men and estrogens in women may lead to an increased risk of hormonally induced tumors.[114-116] Black South African men fed a Western diet had an increased production of both androgens and estrogens, while the opposite trend was demonstrated in African-American men fed a vegetarian diet.[117,118] Dietary fat appears to increase prostate cancer relative risk by a factor of 1.6 to 1.9.[106,119–124]

A relationship between other dietary factors and prostate cancer risk is difficult to identify. It has been reported that intake of vitamin A from plant sources decreases prostate cancer risk[50,51,119,125] and that the intake of vitamin A from animal sources may increase prostate cancer risk.[111,114] The findings in these studies may be due to the lower fat content in the diets of men with high plant vitamin A intake and a higher fat content in the diets of men with high animal vitamin A intake. Investigators have also researched a relationship between prostate cancer and the intake of vitamin C, vitamin B_1, vitamin B_2, niacin, calcium, selenium, zinc, protein, and carbohydrates. There is no clear association between these common dietary factors and prostate cancer.

The results of a number of dietary intake surveys support the concept that a high-fat diet may increase risk of clinically significant prostate cancer. The precise mechanism is not well defined, but increased hormonal bioavailability due to a high-fat diet has been implied. Plasma concentrations of fatty acids are responsive to dietary fat, and these levels, in turn, do correlate with concentrations of bioavailable sex steroids.[126] Fatty acids have been found to inhibit binding of gonadal steroids to serum sex hormone-binding globulin, causing greater bioavailability of gonadal hormones.[127] A low-fat, high-fiber diet may also decrease the enterohepatic circulation of gonadal hormones, resulting in increased fecal excretion of gonadal hormones and possibly lowering serum levels.[128]

Hormones

The precise role of androgens in the etiology of human prostate cancer is unclear, but evidence is accumulating that suggests that androgenic stimulation of the prostate over a prolonged period promotes prostate carcinogenesis. It is well established that androgens promote cell proliferation and inhibit prostate cell death.[129] Exogenous testosterone administration causes prostate cancer in rats[130] and is thought to increase human prostate cancer risk. The hormonal sensitivity of prostate cancer has been exploited clinically since 1941.[131]

It has been suggested that populations with greater androgenic stimulation of the prostate may be more prone to develop clinically significant prostate cancer. Studies testing this hypothesis vary widely in their results, since this is a difficult concept to study.[132] For example, androgens other than testosterone may be responsible for androgenic stimulation of the prostate and serum androgen levels may not correlate with intraprostatic androgen levels.

Several studies have found no difference in baseline circulating testosterone level in prostate cancer patients when compared to controls.[133–135] In a case control study involving 81 men with prostate cancer, Comstock and colleagues assayed archived serum and found no significant association between serum dehydroepiandrosterone or dehydroepiandrosterone sulfate levels prior to diagnosis and prostate cancer risk.[136]

Barrett-Connor and colleagues studied 1,008 men for 14 years.[137] Total serum testosterone, estrone, estradiol, androstenedione, and sex hormone-binding globulin were measured. Only plasma androstenedione showed a positive dose-response correlation for the development of prostate cancer. A linear dose-response gradient persisted even after adjustment for age and body mass index. Men with a serum androstenedione level of 3.2 nanomolar (nM) or greater were nearly twice as likely to be diagnosed with prostate cancer than those with a level less than 2.2 nM ($P < .05$). Meikle et al. observed a higher sex hormone-binding globulin level in men with prostate cancer when compared to controls and noted a higher testosterone conversion rate in patients with prostate cancer.[138] Ross et al. observed a 15% higher circulating testosterone concentration in African-American men when compared to young white men and hypothesized that such differences may affect the incidence of clinically significant prostate cancer later in life.[139]

Ross and colleagues have subsequently observed higher levels of 3-alpha, 17-beta-androstenediol glucuronide, and androsterone glucuronide in black and white American men when compared to Japanese men.[140] These androgens are markers for 5-alpha-reductase activity. Differences in androgenic activity may explain the underlying disparity in the incidence of clinically significant prostate cancer between the two races.[139,141] The populations with higher androgen levels also have higher amounts of fat in their diet.[114,115] Androgenic stimulation is likely a promoter of clinically significant prostate cancer. Prostate cancer is rare in men castrated before puberty.[134,141,142] These facts, combined with the well-known effect of androgen ablation on clinical prostate cancer, form part of the basis for the suggestion that prostate cancer may be prevented if tolerable androgenic reduction, inhibition, or blockade can be applied before prostate cancer becomes clinically evident.

PROSTATE CANCER PREVENTION

An intervention that would prevent prostate cancer or inhibit the progression of indolent, low-volume disease would be quite valuable to society. It would not only save lives by preventing cancer deaths but would save some men the anxiety, morbidity, and mortality of cancer treatment.

Dietary Intervention

Epidemiologic studies indicate that populations with low-fat, high-fiber diets have lower prostate cancer incidence.[143] No study is known to show that a change to a low-fat diet lowers prostate cancer risk after years of a high-fat diet. A change in diet has some appeal and while American dietary habits are improving, the change is slow and future generations may benefit. A low-fat diet is likely to decrease the risk of other cancers and diseases. More scientific studies are needed.

Chemopreventive Agents

There are several agents that have potential as prostate cancer chemopreventives. If effective, a high-risk male could take the agent for a period of time and reduce the risk of developing the disease. In order to be acceptable, such an intervention must be safe and easily tolerated, and additional health benefits such as prevention of prostatism or cardiac disease would be desirable.

Sporn and colleagues have demonstrated that pharmacologic treatment of laboratory animals with the vitamin A analog fenretinide (4-HPR) prevents development of an androgen-responsive adenocarcinoma.[144] The implications of this finding are unknown, as are the mechanisms of 4-HPR. Clinical studies of 4-HPR and other retinoic acids are underway to determine toxicities and usefulness as a chemopreventive agent.

Difluoromethylornithine (DFMO) is a potential prostate cancer chemopreventive agent. DFMO acts as a suicide substrate inactivating the enzyme ornithine decarboxylase (ODC).[145] ODC is responsible for the rate-limiting step in mammalian synthesis of polyamines. The polyamines are normal cell constituents important for cell proliferation. The prostate has very high concentrations of ODC and polyamines.[146] DFMO has been shown to have chemopreventive activity in several animal tumors. Kadmon and associates have demonstrated chemopreventive activity in Dunning R3327 rat prostatic carcinoma models.[147] Several small human trials involving DFMO are currently underway. These trials will primarily assess the drug's adverse effects but will also assess activity in bladder and colon cancer prevention. A large-scale clinical trial, like that necessary to demonstrate effectiveness as a prostate cancer preventative, is premature.

A very attractive approach to prostate cancer prevention is through androgenic inhibition. The current hormonal manipulations used to treat prostate cancer would likely be effective in preventing disease, but the toxicities of these drugs make them undesirable. Inhibition of 5-alpha-reductase may prevent prostate cancer by lowering androgenic stimulation to the prostate, while having limited side effects.[148] The enzyme 5-alpha-reductase is a nuclear membrane-bound NADPH-dependent delta-3-ketosteroid 5-alpha-oxidoreductase that converts testosterone (T) to dihydrotestosterone (DHT). Studies suggest that DHT is the primary androgen in prostate biology.[149] Inhibition of the enzyme decreases androgenic stimulation of the prostate with negligible effects on other androgen-dependent organs. Giving support to this hypothesis is the observation that 5-alpha-reductase activity is low in Asian populations at low risk for prostate cancer compared to American men.[150]

There are two known 5-alpha-reductase isoenzymes. 5-alpha-reductase-1 is present in low levels in a number of tissues and 5-alpha-reductase-2 is found in androgen-sensitive cells of the skin and prostate.[151,152] The testes and adrenal glands secrete T into the bloodstream. A substantial fraction of T diffusing into 5-alpha-reductase containing cells is irreversibly converted to DHT. Although both T and DHT can bind to the cellular prostate androgen receptor and produce androgen-mediated affects, DHT is far more potent than T. When compared to T, DHT exhibits a higher binding affinity for and lower dissociation rate from the androgen receptor. The DHT-receptor complex has greater stability and a higher binding affinity for DNA.[149]

The key role that 5-alpha-reductase-2 and DHT play in prostate development is demonstrated by an observation of nature. Males with inherited homozygous 5-alpha-reductase deficiency are pseudohermaphrodites with a female or ambiguous external genitalia until puberty. The normal increase in T production at puberty induces development of a small phallus and virilization. After puberty, individuals with the enzyme deficiency usually become morphologically and functionally normal males, although they do not develop acne or male pattern baldness. Even though they maintain normal serum testosterone levels after puberty, they have an underdeveloped prostate. Prostate growth has been observed when these individuals are administered very high doses of testosterone or given physiologic doses of DHT.[153,154] Further evidence of DHT's importance to prostate biology is found in studies of normal men administered the 5-alpha-reductase inhibitor finasteride. They have decreased serum and prostatic DHT levels, a reduction in serum PSA, and in many cases regression of benign prostatic hyperplasia.[154–156]

Laboratory testing of the hypothesis that 5-alpha-reductase inhibition will prevent prostate cancer is difficult. Rodent carcinogenesis models are not well suited for this purpose. All major, accepted rodent prostate cancer models involve administration of pulse doses of a chemical carcinogen followed by chronic administration of high doses of androgens.[116,144] The very fact that androgens are necessary to promote prostate cancer development in laboratory animals is, in itself, supportive of the theory that decreasing androgenic stimulation can lower prostate cancer risk.

Blocking 5-alpha-reductase can inhibit the growth of several human prostate cancer cell lines in tissue culture and rodent implant models.[157,158] A decrease in androgenic stimulation, such as DHT inhibition, likely exerts its greatest influence at early stages of tumor development and progression. Nonetheless, the treatment of men with stage D prostate cancer with 5-alpha-reductase inhibitors does cause some decrease in serum PSA. While the clinical significance of this decline is unknown, it demonstrates that DHT inhibition may exert some influence even on metastatic prostate cancer.[159]

While 5-alpha-reductase inhibitors have some antitumor activity, anticancer activity is not necessary in order for a drug to prevent cancer. Carcinogenesis is a process. Decreasing the androgenic stimulation of prostate cells may lower the probability that these cells will enter that process. The fact that androgenic stimulation of the prostate is only partially decreased means that finasteride therapy may not cause a tumor to become resistant to more severe hormonal manipulations.

A number of 5-alpha-reductase inhibitors have been synthesized. Finasteride was the first 5-alpha-reductase inhibitor to enter clinical trials. It is a steroidal analog of testosterone that functions as a reversible competitive inhibitor of 5-alpha-reductase. There is substantial information on the toxicity profile of finasteride. It has been studied extensively for the management of benign prostatic hyperplasia and has been approved by the U.S. Food and Drug Administration for that indication.

Finasteride (5 mg/day, orally) causes a 75% decrease in serum DHT levels, an 80% decrease in intraprostatic DHT, and a 10% increase in serum T. Despite the 10% average increase in serum T, all values were within the clinically normal range in several large trials. While very high concentrations of T can interact with androgen receptors similar to dihydrotestosterone, the increased T levels found in men with 5-alpha-reductase deficiency and men taking finasteride are not high enough to promote prostate growth.[149,160] Finasteride has demonstrated itself to be a very safe drug with minimal side effects. Given its excellent safety profile and the possibility that it may prevent BPH, finasteride may be very suitable for long-term administration as a cancer chemopreventive agent.

The NCI and several of its cooperative oncology groups are sponsoring a randomized, double-blind, placebo-controlled trial to determine if DHT inhibition will reduce the incidence of prostate cancer. The trial will enroll 18,000 men, 55 years of age and older, in good health, with no evidence of prostate cancer. Participants will be randomized to finasteride 5 mg/day orally or placebo and followed for 7 to 10 years. The primary objective is to demonstrate a decreased incidence of prostate cancer in the treatment group, when compared to the placebo group. The trial design allows for a 90% power to detect a 25% difference in prostate cancer incidence between the two groups.

Participants in the trial will be followed with a digital rectal examination and serum PSA annually. Participants and their physicians will be blinded to the PSA values because serum PSA is lowered by finasteride. The values will be reported to the subjects and their physicians as normal or abnormal.

In order to assure an equal opportunity for PSA-driven detection of prostate cancer in both arms, men in the placebo arm with a serum PSA over 4.0 will be evaluated for prostate cancer with a sextant biopsy of the prostate, and the same proportion of compliant men in the finasteride arm (those with the highest PSAs) will also receive a prostate biopsy. In a final effort to reduce biases in prostate cancer detection for or against the finasteride arm, all men in the trial will receive a sextant prostate biopsy at the end of their seventh year on study.

Such a large randomized trial can have a number of other benefits beyond determining if finasteride prevents prostate cancer. Prospectively following a group of men in a well-designed trial can yield valuable data on the epidemiology, etiology, and natural history of prostatic pathologies, the screening and diagnosis of prostate cancer, and quality of life in the aging male. The study also provides a unique opportunity to assess finasteride's ability to prevent benign prostatic hyperplasia.

The value of early detection and the currently available screening technologies are the subject of several ongoing and planned clinical trials. This chemoprevention trial, with a rigorous screening program, will also yield valuable data addressing prostate cancer screening methods in participants on both arms of the trial. The trial will generate data on the effect of prolonged 5-alpha-reductase treatment on serum PSA concentration and help assess serial changes in serum PSA over time as a screening tool. Inhibition of 5-alpha-reductase may increase the sensitivity of serum PSA as a prostate cancer screen or it may decrease it.

SUMMARY

A review of the epidemiology of prostate cancer is really an outline of the questions that have not been answered about prostate cancer. Increasing age is a risk factor for prostate cancer. Incidence and mortality rates are higher in certain countries and among certain races despite rates of indolent cancers being relatively equal and very prevalent. Environmental and especially dietary influences which vary among ethnicities and cultures are likely an important cause of clinically significant prostate cancers.

Rates of prostate cancer diagnosis are increasing, especially among white American men. Much of this is due to advances in technologies that require further study. A number of men with prostate cancer do not benefit from being diagnosed and treated, while some clearly do. Medical science's abilities to distinguish those with prostate cancer needing aggressive treatment from those with cancer requiring no therapy are extremely limited. Further research is needed in this area.

Androgenic stimulation is thought to be of significance in prostate carcinogenesis. Blocking androgenic stimulation of the prostate with 5-alpha-reductase inhibition is being studied in a large clinical trial, the results of which will hopefully address many of the other questions about prostate cancer and its biology.

REFERENCES

1. Gloeckler Ries LA, Hankey BF, Edwards BK (eds): Cancer Statistics Review 1973–1987. Bethesda, MD: NCI (DHHS publication no. NIH 90-2789), 1990.

2. National Cancer Institute, Division of Cancer Prevention and Control. 1987 Annual Cancer Statistic Review: Including Cancer Trends: 1950–1985. Bethesda, MD: National Cancer Institute (NIH publication no. 88-2789), 1988.

3. Seidman H, Mushinski MH, Gelb SK, Silverberg E: Probabilities of eventually developing or dying of cancer—United States. CA 35:36, 1985.

4. Miller BA, Ries LAG, Hankey BF, Kosary CL, Edwards BK (eds): Cancer Statistic Review: 1973–1990. Bethesda, MD: National Cancer Institute. NIH Pub, 1993.

5. Potosky AL, Kessler L, Gridley G, Brown CC, Horm JW: Rise in prostatic cancer incidence associated with increased use of transurethral resection. J Natl Cancer Inst 82:1624–1628, 1990.

6. Mettlin C, Jones GW, Murphy GP: Trends in prostate cancer care in the United States 1974–1990: Observations from the Patient Care Evaluation Studies of the American College of Surgeons Commission on Cancer. CA 43(2):83–91, 1993.

7. Cooner WH, Mosley BR, Rutherford CL Jr, Beard JH, Pond HS, et al.: Prostate cancer detection in a clinical urological practice by ultrasonography, digital rectal examination, and prostate specific antigen. J Urol 143:1146–1152, 1990.

8. Scardino PT: Early detection of prostate cancer. Urol Clin N Am 16:635–655, 1989.

9. Oesterling JE: Prostate specific antigen: a critical assessment of the most useful tumor marker for adenocarcinoma of the prostate. J Urol 145:907–923, 1991.

10. Stamey TA: Cancer of the prostate. Monogr Urol 4(3):1–21, 1983.

11. Franks LM, Durh MB: Latency and progression in tumors: the natural history of prostate cancer. Lancet (ii):1037–1039, 1956.

12. Stemmermann GN: Unsuspected cancer in elderly Hawaiian Japanese: an autopsy study. Hum Pathol 12:1039–1044, 1982.

13. Stemmermann GN, Nomura AMY, Chyou PH, Yatani R: A prospective comparison of prostate cancer at autopsy and as a clinical event: The Hawaii Japanese experience. Cancer, Epidemiology, Biomarkers and Prevention 1:189–193, 1992.

14. Hirst AE, Bergman RT: Carcinoma of the prostate in men 80 or more years old. Cancer 7:136–141, 1954.

15. Dhom G: Epidemiologic aspects of latent and clinically manifest carcinoma of the prostate. J Cancer Res Clin Oncol 106:210–218, 1983.

16. Andrews GS: Latent carcinoma of the prostate. J Clin Pathol 2:197–208, 1954.

17. Franks LM: Latent carcinoma of the prostate. J Clin Pathol 68:603–616, 1954.

18. Lundberg S, Berge T: Prostate carcinoma: an autopsy study. Scand J Urol Nephrol 4:93–97, 1970.

19. Liavag I: Atrophy and regeneration in the pathogenesis of prostatic carcinoma. Acta Pathol Microbiol Scand 73:338–350, 1968.

20. Harbits T, Haugen OA: Histology of the prostate in elderly men. Acta Pathol Microbiol Scand (A) 80:756–768, 1972.

21. Viitanen I, Hellens A: Latent carcinoma of the prostate in Finland. Acta Pathol Microbiol Scand 44:64–67, 1958.

22. Holund B: Latent prostatic cancer in a consecutive autopsy series. Scand J Urol Nephrol 14:29–35, 1980.

23. Oota K: Latent carcinoma of the prostate among the Japanese. Acta Un Int Cancer 17:952–957, 1961.

24. Karube K: Study of latent carcinoma of the prostate in the Japanese based on necropsy material. Tohoku J Exp Med 74:265–285, 1961.

25. Akazaki K, Stemmermann J: Comparative study of latent carcinoma of the prostate among Japanese in Japan and Hawaii. J Natl Cancer Inst 50:1137–1144, 1973.

26. Edwards CN, Steinthosson E, Nicholson D. An autopsy study of latent prostatic cancer. Cancer 6:531–554, 1953.

27. Halpert B, Sheehan E, Schmalhorst W, Scott R: Carcinoma of the prostate: a survey of 5000 autopsies. Cancer 16:737–742, 1963.

28. Baron E, Angrist A: Incidence of occult adenocarcinoma of the prostate after fifty years of age. Arch Pathol 32:787–793, 1941.

29. Guileyardo JM, Johnson WD, Welsh RA, Akazaki K, Correa P: Prevalence of latent prostatic carcinoma in two U.S. populations. J Natl Cancer Inst 65:311–316, 1980.

30. Sakr W, Haas GP, Cassin B, Pontes JE, Crissman J: The frequency of carcinoma and intraepithelial neoplasia of the prostate in young male patients. J Urol 150:379–385, 1993.

31. Yamabe H, ten Kate FJW, Gallee MPW, Schroeder FH, Oisha K, Okada K, et al.: State A prostatic cancer: a comparative study in Japan and the Netherlands. World J Urol 4:136–140, 1986.

32. Breslow N, Chan CW, Dhom G, Drury RAB, Franks LM, Gellei B, et al.: Latent carcinoma of prostate in seven areas. Int J Cancer 20:680–688, 1977.

33. Yatani R, Chigusa I, Akazaki K, Stemmermann GN, Welsh RA: Geographic pathology of latent prostatic carcinoma. Int J Cancer 29:611–616, 1982.

34. Barnetson J: L'epitheliome latent de la prostate. Sem Hosp Paris 30:129–132, 1954.

35. Owen WL: Cancer of the prostate: a literature review. J Chron Dis 29:89–114, 1976.

36. Yatani R, Shiraishi T, Nakakuki K, Kusano I, Takanari H, Hayashi T, et al.: Trends in frequency of latent prostate carcinoma in Japan from 1965–1979 to 1982–1986. J Natl Cancer Inst 80:683–687, 1988.

37. Carter BS, Carter HB, Isaacs JT: Epidemiologic evidence regarding predisposing factors to prostate cancer. Prostate 16:187–197, 1990.

38. Sakr W, Haas GP, Cassin B, Pontes JE, Crissman J: The frequency of carcinoma and intraepithelial neoplasia of the prostate in young male patients. J Urol 150:379–385, 1993.

39. Whittemore AS, Keller JB, Betensky R: Low-grade, latent prostate cancer volume: predictor of clinical cancer incidence? J Natl Cancer Inst 83:1231–1235, 1991.

40. Pienta KJ, Partin AW, Coffey DS: Cancer as a disease of DNA organization and dynamic

cell structure. Cancer Res 49:2525–2530, 1989.

41. Feinberg AP, Coffey DS: The concept of DNA rearrangement in carcinogenesis and development of tumor cell heterogeneity. In Owens AH Jr, Coffey DS, Baylin SB (eds): Tumor Cell Heterogeneity: Origins and Implications. New York: Academic Press, pp 469–488, 1982.

42. Vogelstein B, Fearon ER, Hamilton SR, Kern SE, Preisinger AC, Leppert M, et al.: Genetic alterations during colorectal tumor development. N Engl J Med 319:525–530, 1988.

43. Waterhouse J, Muir C, Shanmugaratnam K: Cancer incidence in five continents. In Cancer Incidence. Lyon, France: International Agency for Research in Cancer. Publ 42, vol 6, 1982.

44. Carter BS, Bova GS, Beaty TH, Steinberg GD, Childs B, Isaacs WB, Walsh PC: Hereditary prostate cancer: epidemiologic and clinical features. J Urol 150:797–802, 1993.

45. Carter BS, Beaty TH, Steinberg GD, Childs B, Walsh PC: Mendelian inheritance of familial prostate cancer. Proc Natl Acad Sci 89:3367–3371, 1992.

46. Steinberg GD, Carter BS, Beaty TH, Childs B, Walsh PC: Family history and the risk of prostate cancer. Prostate 17:337–340, 1990.

47. Arason A, Barkard RB, Egilsson V: Linkage analysis of chromosome 17q markers and breast-ovarian cancer in Icelandic families, and possible relationship to prostatic cancer. Am J Hum Genet 52(4):711–717, 1993.

48. Tulinius H, Egilsson V, Olafsd GH, Sigvaldason H: Risk of prostate, ovarian, and endometrial cancer among relatives of women with breast cancer. Br Med J 305:855–857, 1992.

49. Mishina T, Watanabe H, Araki H, Nakao M: Epidemiological study of prostatic cancer by matched-pair analysis. Prostate 6:423–436, 1985.

50. Graham S, Haughey B, Marshall J, Priore R, Byers T, Rzepka T, et al.: Diet in the epidemiology of carcinoma of the prostate gland. J Natl Cancer Inst 70:687–692, 1983.

51. Kolonel LN, Yoshizawa CN, Hankin JH: Diet and prostatic cancer: a case-control study in Hawaii. Am J Epidemiol 127:999–1012, 1988.

52. Armenian HK, Lilienfeld AM, Diamond EL, Bross ID: Relation between benign prostatic hyperplasia and cancer of the prostate. Lancet (ii):115–117, 1974.

53. West DW, Slattery ML, Robison LM, French TK, Mahoney AW: Adult dietary intake and prostate cancer risk in Utah: a case-control study with special emphasis on aggressive tumors. Cancer Causes Cont 2:84–94, 1991.

54. Honda GD, Bernstein L, Ross RK, Greenland S, Gerkins V, Henderson BE: Vasectomy, cigarette smoking, and age at first sexual intercourse as risk factors for prostate cancer in middle-aged men. Br J Cancer 57:326–331, 1988.

55. Greenwald P, Kirmiss V, Polan AK, et al.: Cancer of the prostate among men with benign prostatic hyperplasia. J Natl Cancer Inst 53:335–340, 1974.

56. Hakky SI, Chisholm GD, Skeet RG: Social class and carcinoma of the prostate. Br J Urol 51:393–396, 1979.

57. Seidman H: Cancer death rates by site and sex for religious and socioeconomic groups in New York City. Environ Res 3:234–250, 1970.

58. Richardson IM: Prostatic cancer and social class. Br J Prev Soc Med 19:140–142, 1965.

59. Great Britain Registrar General: The registrar general's decennial supplement, England and Wales, 1951. Occup Mort, Part II, 1957.

60. Buell P, Dunn JE, Breslow L: The occupational-social class risks of cancer mortality in men. J Chronic Dis 12:600–621, 1960.

61. Ernster VL, Winkelstein W Jr, Selvin S, Brown SM, Sacks ST, Austin DF, et al.: Race, socioeconomic status, and prostatic cancer. Cancer Treat Rep 61:187–191, 1977.

62. Clemmesen J, Nielson A: The social distribution of cancer in Copenhagen, 1943–1947. Br J Cancer 5:159–171, 1951.

63. Graham S, Levin M, Lilienfeld AM: SES distribution of cancer in Buffalo, New York. Cancer 13:180–191, 1960.

64. Greenwald P, Damon A, Kirmis V, Polan AK: Physical and demographic features of men before developing cancer of the prostate. J Natl Cancer Inst 53:341–346, 1974.

65. Baquet CR, Horm JW, Gibbs T, Greenwald P: Socioeconomic factors and cancer incidence among blacks and whites. J Natl Cancer Inst 83:551–557, 1991.

66. McWhorter WP, Schatzkin AG, Horm JW, Brown CC: Contribution of socioeconomic status to black/white differences in cancer incidence. Cancer 63:982–987, 1989.

67. Shaarawy M, Mahmoud KZ: Endocrine profile and semen characteristics in male smokers. Fertility Sterility 38:255–257, 1982.

68. Potts CL: Cadmium proteinuria—the health of battery workers exposed to cadmium oxide dust. Ann NY Acad Sci 271:273–279, 1976.

69. Kipling MD, Waterhouse JAH: Cadmium and prostatic carcinoma. Lancet (i):730–731, 1967.

70. Kolonel L, Winkelstein W: Cadmium and prostatic carcinoma. Lancet 566–567, 1977.

71. Armstrong BG, Kazantzis G: Prostatic cancer and chronic respiratory and renal disease in British cadmium workers: a case control study. Br J Indust Med 42:540–545, 1985.

72. Elghany NA, Schumacher MC, Slattery ML, West DW, Lee JS: Occupation, cadmium exposure, and prostate cancer. Epidemiology 1:107–115, 1990.

73. Lemen RA, Lee JS, Wagoner JK, Blejer HP: Cancer mortality among cadmium production workers. Ann NY Acad Sci 271:273–279, 1976.

74. Wynder EL, Mabuchi K, Whitmore W: Epidemiology of cancer of the prostate. Cancer 28:344–360, 1971.

75. Kerr WK, Keresteci AG, Mayoh H: The distribution of zinc within the human prostate. Cancer 13:550–554, 1960.

76. Whitmore, WF Jr: Comments on zinc in the human and canine prostate. Natl Cancer Inst Monogr 12:337–340, 1963.

77. Schrodt GR, Hall T, Whitmore WR Jr: The concentration of zinc in diseased human prostate glands. Cancer 17:1555–1566, 1964.

78. Gyorkey F, Min K-W, Huff J, Gyorkey P: Zinc and magnesium in human prostate gland: normal, hyperplastic, and neoplastic. Cancer Res 27:1348–1353, 1967.

79. Mawson CA, Fischer MI: The occurrence of zinc in the human prostate gland. Can J Med Sci 30:336–340, 1952.

80. Whelan P, Walker BE, Kelleher J: Zinc, vitamin A, and prostatic cancer. Br J Urol 55:525–528, 1983.

81. Wilden EG, Robinson MRG: Plasma zinc levels in prostatic disease. Br J Urol 47:295–299, 1975.

82. Hsing AW, McLaughlin JK, Schuman LM, Bjelke E, Gridley G, Wacholder S, et al.: Diet, tobacco use, and fatal prostate cancer: results from the Lutheran Brotherhood cohort study. Cancer Res 50:6836–6840, 1990.

83. Shaarawy M, Mahmoud KZ: Endocrine profile and semen characteristics in male smokers. Fertility Sterility 38:255–257, 1982.

84. Fincham SM, Hill GB, Hanson J, Wijayasinghe C: Epidemiology of prostatic cancer: a case control study. Prostate 17:189–206, 1990.

85. Centifaanto YM, Kaufman HF, Zam ZS, Drylie DM, Deardourf SL: Herpesvirus particles in prostatic carcinoma cells. J Virol 12:1608–1611, 1973.

86. Cannon L, Bishop DT, Skolnick M, Hunt S, Lyon JL, Smart CR: Genetic epidemiology of prostate cancer in the Utah Mormon genealogy. Cancer Surv 1:47–69, 1982.

87. Checkoway H, DiFerdinando G, Hulka BS, Mickey DD: Medical, life-style, and occupational risk factors for prostate cancer. Prostate 10:79–88, 1987.

88. Sanford EJ, Geder L, Laychock A, Rohner TJ, Rapp F: Evidence for the association of the cytomegalovirus with carcinoma of the prostate. J Urol 102:789–792, 1977.

89. Ross RK, Deapen DM, Casagrande JT, Paganini-Hill A, Henderson BE: A cohort study of mortality from cancer of the prostate in catholic priests. Br J Cancer 43:233–235, 1981.

90. Ross RK, Shimizu H, Paganini-Hill A, Honda G, Henderson BE: Case-control studies of prostate cancer in blacks and whites in southern California. J Natl Cancer Inst 78:869–874, 1987.

91. Heshmat MY, Herson J, Kovi J, Niles R: An epidemiologic study of gonorrhea and cancer of the prostate gland. Med Ann District of Columbia 42:378–383, 1973.

92. Oishi K, Okada K, Yoshida O, Ohno Y, Hayes RB, Schroeder FH, et al.: A case-control study of prostatic cancer in Kyoto, Japan: sexual risk factors. Prostate 17:269–279, 1990.

93. King H, Diamond E, Lilienfeld AM: Some epidemiological aspects of cancer of the prostate. J Chron Dis 16:117–153, 1963.

94. Sidney S: Vasectomy and the risk of prostatic cancer and benign prostatic hypertrophy. J Urol 138:795–797, 1987.

95. Giovannucci E, Ascherio A, Rimm EB, et al.: A prospective cohort study of vasectomy and prostate cancer in US. JAMA 269(7):873–877, 1993.

96. Giovannucci E, Tosteson TD, Speizer FE, et al.: A retrospective cohort study of vasectomy and prostate cancer in US men. JAMA 269(7):878–882, 1993.

97. Ross RK, Paganini-Hill A, Henderson BE: The etiology of prostate cancer: what does the epidemiology suggest? Prostate 4:333–344, 1983.

98. Mettlin C, Natarajan N, Huben R: Vasectomy and prostate cancer risk. Am J Epidemiol 132:1056–1061, 1990.

99. Dunn JE: Cancer epidemiology in populations of the United States. Cancer Res 35:3240–3245, 1975.

100. Haenszel W, Kurihoro M: Studies of Japanese migrants. J Natl Cancer Inst 40:43–68, 1968.

101. Yu H, Harris RE, Gao Y, Gao R, Wynder EL: Comparative epidemiology of cancers of the colon, rectum, prostate and breast in Shanghai, China versus the United States. Int J Epidemiol 20:76–81, 1991.

102. Muir CS, Nectoux J, Staszewski J: The epidemiology of prostate cancer. Geographical distribution and timetrends. Acta Oncol 30:133–140, 1991.

103. Armstrong B, Doll R: Environmental factors and cancer incidence and mortality in different countries with special reference to dietary practices. Int J Cancer 15:617–631, 1975.

104. Rose DP, Boyar AP, Wynder EL: International comparisons of mortality rates for cancer of the breast, ovary, prostate, and colon, and per capita food consumption. Cancer 58:2363–2371, 1986.

105. Rotkin ID: Studies in the epidemiology of prostatic cancer: expanded sampling. Cancer Treat Rep 61:173–180, 1977.

106. Hutchinson GB: Epidemiology of prostatic cancer. Semin Oncol 3:151–159, 1976.

107. Slattery ML, Schumacher MC, West DW, Robison LM, French TK: Food consumption trends between adolescent and adult years and subsequent risk of prostate cancer. Am J Clin Nutr 52:752–757, 1990.

108. Snowdon DA, Phillips RL, Choi W: Diet, obesity, and risk of fatal prostate cancer. Am J Epidemiol 120:244–250, 1984.

109. Mettlin C, Selenskas S, Natarajan N, Huben R: Beta-carotene and animal fats and their relationship to prostate cancer risk. A case-control study. Cancer 64:605–612, 1989.

110. Mills PK, Beeson WL, Phillips RL, Fraser GE: Cohort study of diet, lifestyle, and prostate cancer in Adventist men. Cancer 64:598–604, 1989.

111. Hirayama T: Epidemiology of prostate cancer with special reference to the role of diet. Natl Cancer Inst Monogr 53:149–155, 1979.

112. Heshmat MY, Kaul L, Kovi J, Jackson MA, Jackson AG, Jones GW, et al.: Nutrition and prostate cancer: a case-control study. Prostate 6:7–17, 1985.

113. Ohno Y, Yoshida O, Oishi K, Okada K, Yamabe H, Schroeder F: Dietary beta-carotene and cancer of the prostate: a case-control study in Kyoto, Japan. Cancer Res 48:1331–1336, 1988.

114. Hamalainen E, Adlercreutz H, Puska P, Pietinen P: Diet and serum hormones in healthy men. J Steroid Biochem 20:459–464, 1984.

115. Coffey DS: Physiological control of prostatic growth. In: Prostate Cancer, an Overview. UICC Workshop on Prostatic Cancer, 1978. Geneva: International Union Against Cancer. Technical Report series, vol 48, pp 4–23, 1979.

116. Noble RL: The development of prostatic adenocarcinoma in Nb rats following prolonged sex hormone administration. Cancer Res 19:1125–1139, 1959.

117. Coffey DS, Pienta KJ: New concepts in studying the control of normal and cancer growth of the prostate. In: Current Concepts and Approaches to the Study of Prostate Cancer. New York: Alan R. Liss, pp 1–73, 1987.

118. Hill P, Wynder EL, Garbaczewski L, Garnes H, Walker ARP: Diet and urinary steroids in black and white North American men and black South African men. Cancer Res 39:5101–5105, 1979.

119. Kolonel LN, Nomura AMY, Hinds MW, Hirohata T, Hankin JH, Lee J: Role of diet in cancer incidence in Hawaii. Cancer Res (Suppl) 43:2397–2402, 1983.

120. Lew EA, Garfinkel L: Variations in mortality by weight among 750,000 men and women. J Chron Dis 32:563–576, 1979.

121. Severson RK, Grove JS, Nomura AM, Stemmermann GN: Body mass and prostatic cancer: a prospective study. Br Med J 297:713–715, 1988.

122. Kaul L, Heshmat MY, Kovi J, Jackson MA, Jackson AG, Jones GW, et al.: The role of diet in prostate cancer. Nutrit Cancer 9:123–128, 1987.

123. Severson RK, Nomura AMY, Grove JS, Stemmermann GN: A prospective study of demographics, diet, and prostate cancer among men of Japanese ancestry in Hawaii. Cancer Res 49:1857–1860, 1989.

124. Berg JW: Can nutrition explain the pattern of international epidemiology of hormone-dependent cancers? Cancer Res 35:3345–3350, 1975.

125. Kolonel LN, Hinds MW, Nomura AMY, Hankin JH, Lee J: Relationship of dietary vitamin A and ascorbic acid intake to the risk for cancers of the lung, bladder, and prostate in Hawaii. Natl Cancer Inst Monogr 69:137–142, 1985.

126. Bruning PF, Bonfrer JMG: Free fatty acid concentrations correlated with the available fraction of estradiol in human plasma. Cancer Res 46:2606–2609, 1989.

127. Street C, Howell RJS, Perry L: Inhibition of binding of gonadal steroids to serum binding proteins by non-esterified fatty acids: the influence of chain length and degree of unsaturation. Acta Endocrinologica 120:175–179, 1989.

128. Pusater DJ, Roth WT, Ross JK, Shultz TD: Dietary and hormonal evaluation of men at different risks for prostate cancer: plasma and fecal hormone-nutrient interrelationships. Am J Clin Nutr 51(3):371–377, 1990.

129. Kyprianou N, Isaacs JT: Activation of programmed cell death in the rat ventral prostate after castration. Endocrinology 122:552, 1988.

130. Noble RL: The development of prostatic adenocarcinoma in NB rats following prolonged sex hormone administration. Cancer Res 37:1929, 1977.

131. Huggins C, Hodges CV: Studies on prostate cancer I: The effect of castration, of estrogen and of androgen injection on serum phosphatases in metastatic carcinoma of the prostate. Cancer Res 1:293–297 1941.

132. Ross RK: The hormonal basis of prostate cancer. Proc Annu Meet Am Assoc Cancer Res 31:457–458, 1990.

133. Meikle W, Stanish WM: Familial prostatic cancer risk and low testosterone. J Clin Endocrin Metab 54:1104–1108, 1982.

134. Ghanadian R, Puah KM, O'Donohue EPM: Serum testosterone and dihydrotestosterone in carcinoma of the prostate. Br J Cancer 39:696–699, 1979.

135. Hammond GL, Kontturi M, Vihko P, Vihko R: Serum steroids in normal males and patients with prostatic diseases. Clin Endocrinol 9:113–121, 1978.

136. Comstock GW, Gordon GB, Hsing AW: The relationship of serum dehydroepiandrosterone and its sulfate to subsequent cancer of the prostate. Cancer Epidemiol Biomarkers Prev 2:219–221, 1993.

137. Barrett-Connor E, Garland C, McPhillips JB, Khaw KT, Wingard DL: A prospective, population-based study of androstenedione, estrogens, and prostatic cancer. Cancer Res 50(1):169–173, 1990.

138. Meikle AW, Smith JA, Stringham JD: Production, clearance, and metabolism of testosterone in men with prostatic cancer. Prostate 10:25–31, 1987.

139. Ross RK, Bernstein L, Judd H, Hanisch R, Pike M, Henderson B: Serum testosterone levels in healthy young black and white men. J Natl Cancer Inst 76:45–48, 1986.

140. Ross RK, Bernstein L, Lobo RA, Shimizu H, Stanczyk FZ, Pike M, et al.: 5-alpha-reductase activity and risk of prostate cancer among Japanese and US white and black males. Lancet 339:887–889, 1992.

141. Hovenian MS, Deming CL: The heterologous growth of cancer of the human prostate. Surg Gynecol Obstet 86:29–35, 1948.

142. Wynder ER, Mabuchi K, Whitmore W: Epidemiology of cancer of the prostate. Cancer 28:344, 1971.

143. Howie BJ, Scultz TD: Dietary and hormonal interrelationships among vegetarian Seventh-Day Adventists and nonvegetarian men. Am J Clin Nutr 42:127–134, 1985.

144. Pollard M, Luckert PH, Sporn MB: Prevention of primary prostate cancer in Lobund-Wistar rats by N-(4-hydroxyphenyl) retinamide. Cancer Res 51(13):3610–3611, 1991.

145. Metcalf BW, Bey P, Danzin, Jung MJ, et al.: Catalytic irreversible inhibition of mammalian ornithine decarboxylase by substrate and product analogues. J Am Chem Soc 100:2551–2553, 1978.

146. Danzin C, Jung MJ, Grove J: Effect of alfa-difluoromethylornithine, an enzyme-activated irreversible inhibitor of ornithine decarboxylase, on polyamine levels in rat tissues. Life Sci 24:519–524, 1979.

147. Kadmon D: Chemoprevention in prostate cancer: the role of Difluoromethylornithine (DFMO). J Cell Biochem (Suppl)` 16H:122–127, 1992.

148. Bruchovsky N, Rennie PS, Batzold FH, Goldenberg SL, Fletcher T, McLoughlin MG: Kinetic parameters of 5-alpha-reductase activity in stroma and epithelium of normal, hyperplastic, and carcinomatous human prostates. J Clin Endocrinol Metab 67:806, 1988.

149. Grino PB, Griffin JE, Wilson JD: Testosterone at high concentration interacts with the human androgen receptor similarly to dihydrotestosterone. Endocrinology 126(2):1165–1171, 1989.

150. Lookingbill DP, Demers LM, Wang C, Leung A, Rittmaster RS, Santen RJ: Clinical and biochemical parameters of androgen action in normal healthy Caucasian versus Chinese

subjects. J Clin Endocrinol Metab 72(6):1242–1248, 1991.

151. Anderson S, Berman DM, Jenkins EP, Russell DW: Deletion of steroid 5-alpha-reductase-2 gene in male pseudohermaproditism. Nature 354(14):159, 1991.

152. Anderson KM, Liao S: Selective retention of dihydrotestosterone by prostatic nuclei. Nature 219:277–279, 1968.

153. Petersen RE, Imperato-McGinley J, Gautier T, Sturla E: Male pseudohermaphroditism due to steroid 5 alpha reductase deficiency. Am J Med 62:170–191, 1977.

154. Imperato-McGinley JL, Cai L, Orlic SD, Markisz JA, Vaughan ED: Long term treatment of benign prostatic hyperplasia with the 5 alpha reductase inhibitor finasteride (MK-906). J Urol 145(4):265A (abstr), 1991.

155. Imperato-McGinley J, Shackleton C, Orlic S, Stoner E: C19 and C21 5 beta/5 alpha metabolite ratios in subjects treated with the 5 alpha metabolite ratios in subjects treated with the 5 alpha-reductase inhibitor finasteride: comparison of male pseudohermaphrodites with inherited 5 alpha-reductase deficiency. J Clin Endocrinol Metab 70(3):777–782, 1990.

156. Fair WR, Presti JC, Sogani P, Andriole G, Seidmon EJ, Ferguson D, Gormley GJ: Multicenter, randomized, double-blind, placebo controlled study to investigate the effect of finasteride (MK-906) on stage D prostate cancer. J Urol 145(4):317A, 1991.

157. Kadoham N, Karr JP, Murphy GP, Sandberg AA: Selective inhibition of prostatic tumor 5 alpha-reductase by a 4-methyl-4-aza-steroid. Cancer Res 44:4947, 1984.

158. Petrow V, Padilla GM, Mukherji S, Marts SA: Endocrine dependence of prostatic cancer upon dihydrotestosterone and not upon testosterone. J Pharm Pharmacol 36:352, 1984.

159. Presti JC, Fair WR, Andriole G, Sogani PC, Seidman, Ferguson D, Ng J, Gormley G: Multicenter, randomized, double-blind, placebo controlled study to investigate the effect of finasteride (MK-906) on Stage D prostate cancer. J Urol 148(4):1201–1204, 1992.

160. Gormley GJ: Role of 5 alpha reductase inhibitors in the treatment of advanced prostatic carcinoma. Urol Clin North America 18(1), 1991.

4

Screening for Cancer of the Prostate

Gregory T. Bales, M.D., and Glenn S. Gerber, M.D.

INTRODUCTION

Carcinoma of the prostate is the most common malignancy and the second leading cause of cancer death in American men.[1] The American Cancer Society has projected that approximately 165,000 new cases will be diagnosed and more than 35,000 deaths due to prostate cancer will occur in 1993.[2] As the life expectancy of Americans increases, it is anticipated that the prevalence and mortality from prostate cancer will increase as well. Therefore, improved detection and treatment methods are necessary to combat the expanding magnitude of this health problem.

Despite recent advances in medical and surgical therapy, there has been little change in the mortality rate from prostate cancer over the past 30 years.[1–3] This is largely due to the significant percentage of men who have either locally or systemically advanced disease at the time of diagnosis. While approximately 60% of patients with prostate cancer have clinically localized disease at the time of diagnosis, the remaining 40% have evidence of metastases (Table 1). However, almost half of these localized patients are found to have locally or systemically advanced disease after surgical staging.[4–6] Consequently, only about a third of patients diagnosed with prostate cancer have organ-confined disease. Therefore, screening efforts have been focused on detecting prostate cancer at an earlier, potentially curable stage.

Effective screening programs must include methods that are safe, accurate, inexpensive, and easy to perform. Traditionally, digital rectal examination (DRE) has been the method used to evaluate the prostate gland. Two new modalities, measurement of prostate-specific antigen (PSA) levels and transrectal ultrasonography (TRUS), have also been proposed as screening tests. Presently, the indications and most appropriate methods for prostate cancer screening remain controversial. While screening using a variety of modalities has been shown to increase the detection of localized tumors,[7,8] the ultimate goal of screening is a decrease in disease-specific mortality. Randomized, prospective studies to address this issue have not been performed. To this end, the National Cancer Institute (NCI) is currently undertaking a large multicenter trial to determine the effect of screening on prostate cancer mortality. This is part of a prostate, lung, colon, and ovarian cancer study that is accruing patients at 10 centers around the country. One hundred forty-eight thousand patients will participate in this trial. However, these results will not be available for many years. As a result, clinicians must counsel patients based on the present state of knowledge. This chapter reviews the risk factors for prostate cancer, and summarizes the advantages and lim-

Prostate Cancer, pages 65–75 © 1994 Wiley-Liss, Inc.

TABLE 1. Clinical Stage at Diagnosis

Stage	Patient (%)
A	20.8–25.9
B	28.9–30.7
C	14.9–17.7
D	21.5–25.9
Unknown	4.3–9.2

From the National Survey of Prostate Cancer in the United States by the American College of Surgeons. J Urol 127:930, 1982.

itations of DRE, PSA, and TRUS in the detection of prostate cancer. In addition, guidelines for the use of these screening modalities are presented.

RISK FACTORS   (see also Chapter 3)

Screening for carcinoma of the prostate is presently recommended by organizations such as the American Cancer Society for all men, regardless of their individual risk for developing the disease. The American Cancer Society's current guidelines are that every man over the age of 50 be screened annually with a DRE and PSA level. However, in an era of limited health care resources, it may be increasingly important to focus screening efforts on high-risk groups. Therefore, clinicians must identify which patients most need to be evaluated.

Prostate cancer is a disease process that is more prevalent in older men. Epidemiologic studies have shown a 40-fold increase in the incidence of prostate cancer from age 50 to 85 years.[9] In the United States, less than 1% of prostate cancers are detected in men younger than 50 years of age, 16% are discovered in men 50 to 64 years old, and the remaining 83% are detected in men older than 64 years of age.[10] A family history of prostate cancer has also been demonstrated to be an important risk factor for the development of prostate cancer. Steinberg et al. demonstrated that ma-lignant prostatic disease was twice as likely to develop in a patient who had one first-degree relative with prostate cancer than in those with no family history of the disease.[11] The risk of developing prostate cancer became 5 to 11 times higher if two or three first-degree relatives were affected.[11] Finally, data from the Surveillance, Epidemiology, and End-Results program of the NCI indicate that the risk of development of prostate cancer is 50% higher in African-Americans than in white males in the United States.[12] American blacks have the highest rate of prostate cancer in the world. A higher testosterone level may account for this difference, although this has not been clearly implicated. Therefore, while prostate cancer screening may ultimately be shown to be appropriate in all men after they reach a certain age (e.g., greater than 50 years), it may be particularly important to focus efforts on African-Americans and those with a family history of the disease.

Another potential high-risk group may be men who have undergone vasectomy. Recent data from the Harvard School of Public Health have suggested that vasectomy is associated with an increased risk of developing prostate cancer.[13] These results were consistent among a variety of epidemiologic studies and suggest an increase in risk over time following vasectomy. Paradoxically, this study also found a lower overall mortality among the men who had undergone vasectomy. However, other large studies have not found an association between vasectomy and prostate cancer.[14,15] Future investigations will be necessary to confirm or refute this association and to determine how vasectomy may increase the risk of developing prostate cancer.

In sum, age, race, and family history all appear to be important factors in determining the risk of development of prostate cancer. In addition, previous vasectomy may also play a role. As further screening trials are performed, it may be particularly important to focus efforts and to study closely the impact of screening in high-risk groups, such as African-Americans and men with a family history of the disease.

SCREENING REQUIREMENTS

Before discussing the individual screening tests, one should consider the limitations and potential sources of error inherent to screening. As noted previously, reducing disease-specific mortality is the primary objective of a cancer screening test. It seems apparent that if routine screening improves survival rates and early detection of disease, then mortality should be reduced. However, this may not necessarily be the case. The results of a lung cancer screening study using sputum cytology provides an example of how screening results can be misleading.[16] The results of this study indicated that by using sputum cytology, lung tumors were detected earlier and patient survival was increased. However, the overall mortality rate from lung cancer was the same in those whose disease was detected by sputum cytology testing as that of an unscreened control population. Consequently, it was concluded that lung cancer screening using sputum cytology is not appropriate.

Why does improved survival and early detection not invariably lead to diminished mortality? This is because there are several potential errors that can occur in uncontrolled screening studies. One of these errors is lead-time bias. Lead time refers to the detection of malignancy from screening methods versus detection due to the development of symptoms. The concept of lead-time bias is best demonstrated using a clinical situation. A 65-year-old man is found to have an elevated PSA during a screening study. He is ultimately diagnosed with carcinoma of the prostate and undergoes treatment. He eventually succumbs to metastatic disease at age 74. Now

assume that the patient in question does not participate in a screening study. He presents to his physician at age 72 with bone pain and work-up reveals metastatic prostate cancer. He undergoes hormonal treatment but dies of his disease at age 74. The screened patient had a nine-year length of survival versus only two years for the unscreened patient. However, the eventual outcome was not changed. Thus, screening suggested benefit when none truly occurred.

Another potential error is length-time bias.[17] Tumors in asymptomatic patients that are detected by screening tend to be less aggressive than those tumors diagnosed by standard methods in men who present with symptoms. Consequently, the difference in survival time between the screened and unscreened populations may be related to inherent tumor biology rather than any benefit from screening.

The final error of screening trials is one of overdetection. Autopsy studies have determined that more than 30% of men over the age of 50 have pathologic evidence of prostate cancer.[18,19] Obviously, most of these tumors are small foci of malignancy that will never result in clinical disease. Yet if screening is able to detect some of these indolent tumors and treatment is initiated, a survival advantage may be demonstrated for screened versus unscreened patients. Again, a randomized, controlled study would prevent this potential error.

ADVERSE CONSEQUENCES OF SCREENING

While the potential benefits of screening are frequently discussed, the potential disadvantages are often overlooked. The most significant adverse consequence of screening involves overdetection. If small foci of malignancy that would never become significant are detected, then patients may potentially be subjected to unnecessary treatment and potential morbidity. Although it has been suggested that available screening methods are incapable of detecting such small tumors,[20] random biopsies performed in some clinical situations will occasionally detect insignificant disease. As a result, patients would suffer the potential morbidity and mortality of treatment without any benefit. For example, the perioperative mortality rate from radical prostatectomy approaches 1%.[21,22] Also, incontinence and impotence rates of at least 2% and 25%, respectively, can be expected.[23,24] Patients receiving radiation therapy also may suffer potential side effects. As a result, the morbidity from screening and detecting insignificant disease may offset the advantage of early diagnosis of some clinically significant tumors. Consequently, until it is shown that disease-specific mortality rates are reduced, patients need to be advised of both the relative benefits and risks of screening.

DIGITAL RECTAL EXAMINATION (DRE)

DRE, the traditional means of evaluating the prostate gland for the presence of malignant disease, is still recommended by the American Cancer Society on an annual basis in men 40 years of age or older.[25] A large-scale study performed by Gilbertson indicated that DRE screening was beneficial. In his study, selected patients found to have prostate cancer by DRE underwent radical prostatectomy. The resulting 5- and 10-year survival rates for this cohort of patients were similar to age-matched controls.[26]

In another study involving 4,367 men, Jenson determined that the survival rate was improved when prostate cancer was diagnosed by DRE in subsequent years rather than in the initial year of screening.[27] It was thought that less advanced tumors were identified in screened men after having had a prior normal examination. Thompson et al. also analyzed the incidence of local versus advanced disease in men with tumors identified before and after the onset of screening by an annual DRE.[28] The findings of this study showed that prostate cancer diagnosed after the initial year of screening was more frequently localized.

In contrast to these studies, the value of routine screening using DRE has been questioned since this examination is very subjective and is dependent on the skill of the examiner in detecting asymmetry and nodularity of the prostate. In addition, although many of the tumors detected by DRE screening are clinically localized, a significant percentage will be upstaged pathologically at the time of surgery. Chodak et al. and Mueller et al. reported that 50% and 42% of screened patients, respectively, have pathologic evidence of tumor spread beyond the prostate when surgically staged.[29,30] In another study of screening using DRE, 56 patients with palpable cancer were identified by examining over 5,000 men during a six-year period.[31] After a median follow-up of 75 months, patients with carcinoma detected in subsequent years of screening after a previously normal examination actually had a greater cancer-specific mortality rate than those diagnosed in the first year of screening. These results indicate that annual DRE may not affect early detection and decrease cancer-specific mortality.

The presence of locally advanced prostate cancer in large numbers of screened patients may arise because DRE lacks sufficient sensitivity. Stamey et al. noted extracapsular disease in 18% of patients with less than 3 cc of cancer volume, as compared with 79% of those with tumor volume greater than 3 cc.[22] DRE may not be sensitive enough to diagnose the presence of these small-volume tumors. Lee et al. performed a study comparing transrectal ultrasound and DRE.[32] In that study, only 41% of cancers less than 1.5 cm in diameter were detected by DRE. Since patients with tumors of this size are believed to have the best prognosis, it was concluded that DRE has limited sensitivity in detecting those tumors with the greatest potential for cure. Thus, routine screening by DRE alone may not confer enough advantage at the present time to be widely offered.

In summary, prostate cancer screening using DRE has been shown to have flaws. While there undoubtedly have been many patients who have benefited from this form of screening, it is unlikely that testing using DRE alone will lead to a decrease in disease-specific mortality. However, the low cost and relative ease of performing the examination ensure the continued use of this test. Further controlled, randomized studies may indicate that DRE has a potentially more useful role in affecting mortality from prostate cancer.

SCREENING USING SERUM MARKERS

The most significant advance in prostate cancer screening has been the identification of prostate-specific antigen, a serine protease demonstrated to be specific for prostatic epithelium. Previously, prostatic acid phophatase (PAP) was the only serum marker with a clinical application in detecting prostate cancer. However, several studies have determined that PAP is normal in 57% to 73% of patients with localized prostate cancer.[33] This limited ability to detect early prostate cancer, coupled with the fact that many patients with abnormal levels of PAP already have advanced disease, limits the usefulness of screening using this tumor marker.

The use of serum PSA levels as a screening test has gained considerable attention. Unlike screening using DRE, PSA testing is not user dependent and does not rely on subjective interpretation. In addition, the overall detection rate of prostate cancer is increased through the use of PSA testing.[34] While large screening studies using DRE alone have led to cancer detection rates of 0.8–1.7%,[26,27,35] recent screening trials using PSA have noted detection rates of 2.2–5%.[36–39] In two large studies of over 1,000 men undergoing routine DRE and PSA testing, it was determined that 30% of the cancers would have been missed if PSA levels had not been performed.[37,38] In addition, screening using PSA may improve the detection of organ-confined tumors. Catalona et al. noted that when PSA was added to DRE for routine screening, 68% more organ-confined prostate cancers were discovered.[37] Furthermore, the incidence of advanced disease at the time of diagnosis was reduced for men whose tumors were detected by serial PSA determinations (79/193—41%) or single PSA determinations (14/46—30%) as compared to men whose cancer was detected by an abnormal DRE (24/36—67%).[40]

Despite these advantages, PSA screening does have limitations. First, since PSA is expressed by normal and malignant cells, patients with benign processes, such as hyperplasia or prostatitis, may have falsely elevated levels. One study determined that the mean serum PSA concentration was 5.61 ng/ml in men with organ-confined prostate cancer and 5.92 ng/ml in men with pathologically documented benign prostatic hyperplasia (BPH).[41] In another study, Brawer et al. found that more than 20% of patients with pathologically proven BPH had elevated PSA levels (normal <4.0 ng/ml by Hybritech assay).[42] If a higher PSA level than 4.0 ng/ml is chosen as the upper limit of normal, then the specificity increases and can more reliably indicate a malignant process. One study determined that with a cut-off of 10.0 ng/ml, the specificity for detecting prostate cancer using PSA is 92%.[36] However, this improved specificity is achieved at the expense of reduced sensitivity and many more cancers would escape detection.

The second major shortcoming of screening using PSA is a low sensitivity. In fact, studies using PSA screening have noted that 14–27% of patients with clinically localized prostate cancer have normal PSA levels.[43,44] As a result, screening with PSA alone will miss many tumors. In an effort to improve sensitivity, Labrie et al. determined that 3.0 ng/ml should be used as the threshold value for PSA testing.[45] However, even with this lower limit, the sensitivity was still only 80.7%, and a greater percentage of false positives resulted. However, despite this limitation, PSA is still the most sensitive individual screening test available.[37]

A new parameter that may be helpful in certain clinical situations is PSA density (PSAD) or index. PSAD is determined by dividing the serum PSA level by the prostatic gland volume, as measured by transrectal ultrasonography. The concept of PSAD is based on the fact that cancerous prostatic epithelium produces higher serum levels of PSA than do benign prostatic conditions on a cell-for-cell basis. It is believed that prostate cancer results in a greater degree of cell architectural destruction, thereby leading to an increased release of PSA into the serum.[46] By using the PSAD, an improved distinction between prostate cancer and BPH may be possible.

Benson et al. compared PSAD in 41 patients with clinically confined prostate cancer and 20 patients with pathologically proven BPH.[47] The cancer group had significantly greater PSAD values compared to the BPH group (0.581 and 0.044, respectively).[47] These authors also reported on 533 patients with PSA levels between 4.1–10 ng/ml who underwent transrectal ultrasound.[48] Two hundred eighty-nine of those men also underwent sonographically guided biopsy.[48] The mean PSA values for the positive biopsy group (7.0 ng/ml) and the negative biopsy group (6.8 ng/ml) were virtually identical, indicating the relative lack of specificity of mild PSA elevations (4.1–10 ng/ml) in assessing the presence of prostate cancer. However, the mean PSAD was significantly higher for the positive biopsy group. Therefore,

PSAD may be helpful in patients with minimal PSA elevations in determining how aggressively to pursue the diagnosis of prostate cancer.

An additional way to use PSA to predict the presence of prostate cancer is to assess the rate of change serially over several years (PSA velocity). Carter et al. retrospectively measured the rate of change of PSA in men later shown to have biopsy-proven BPH, no prostatic disease, or prostate cancer.[49] Using a cut-off value for PSA rate of change as 0.75 ng/ml per year, the specificity for detecting prostate cancer was 90%. In comparison, using a single serum PSA determination of 4.0 ng/ml or more, the specificity for prostate cancer detection was only 60%. Consequently, the rate of change of PSA may be the most sensitive means of differentiating men with prostate cancer from those with benign prostatic enlargement.

In conclusion, PSA screening clearly leads to an increase in the detection of localized prostate cancer. In addition, PSA density and serial measurements of PSA over time may enhance the specificity of prostate cancer detection. Further study is necessary to assess the effectiveness of these approaches and to assess whether PSA screening will lead to a decrease in disease-specific mortality.

SCREENING USING TRANSRECTAL ULTRASOUND

Transrectal ultrasonography has also been suggested as a screening modality for prostate cancer. Both Lee et al. and Cooner et al. have demonstrated that the cancer detection rate using TRUS is approximately twice that of DRE and that some significant, nonpalpable tumors can be detected.[32,50] However, the invasiveness, cost, and nonspecific nature of TRUS severely limits its usefulness as a screening test. Cooner et al. have demonstrated that the positive predictive value of an abnormal TRUS in men with a benign DRE is only 16%.[36] In addition, the cancer detection rate of TRUS when both the PSA and DRE are normal is only 2.5%. An additional study indicating the limitations of screening using TRUS was reported by Carter et al.[51] These authors assessed the contralateral lobe of the prostate by TRUS in men with stage B_1 disease and compared these results with the pathological findings of the subsequently performed radical prostatectomy. The resultant sensitivity and specificity of TRUS were only 52% and 68%, respectively.

The final consideration in determining whether TRUS has a place as a general screening method is the economic impact of such an approach. It is estimated that the cost of obtaining a TRUS in all men older than 50 years of age would be in excess of a billion dollars per year.[46] Since it has been demonstrated that TRUS has very limited sensitivity and specificity, it cannot be considered a cost-effective, efficient screening method. For these reasons, it is generally recommended that TRUS not be used for prostate cancer screening, but rather be reserved for further evaluation of the prostate in men with an elevated PSA and/or an abnormal DRE.

CURRENT GUIDELINES

Since the true benefit of prostate cancer screening remains unknown, how should physicians counsel patients who are concerned about the disease? Clearly, the development of PSA and TRUS has improved the ability to detect localized disease. Therefore, patients should be made aware that the use of these modalities may lead to the diagnosis of organ-confined cancer that is not detectable by DRE. However, patients should also be informed that there are inherent risks to screening and that no studies demonstrating a reduction in disease-specific mortality have been performed.

Because each of the previously mentioned screening modalities has limitations, several authors have studied the combined use of DRE, PSA, and TRUS. It was hoped that by integrating the above methods, increased detection with a superior specificity could be attained. In a large study by Cooner et al., 1,807 men were evaluated using DRE, serum PSA, and TRUS.[36] Two hundred eleven men had prostate cancer diagnosed secondary to an abnormal PSA level. Forty-one (19%) of these patients had a benign DRE and their cancers would have escaped detection if DRE had been performed alone. However, of the 203 men with cancer who had an abnormal DRE, 33 (16%) had a normal PSA level. Therefore, it is clear that PSA and DRE do not always detect the same tumors. Thus, it has been suggested that these tests used in combination may serve as the optimum method for detecting prostate cancer.

Catalona et al. screened a population of 1,653 men 50 years of age or older by measuring serum PSA levels.[37] Those men with an abnormal PSA underwent DRE and TRUS. Ultrasound-directed biopsies were performed in men with an abnormal rectal examination or suspicious ultrasound finding. The results were compared to a control group of 300 men in whom biopsy was performed because of symptoms or abnormal findings on DRE. It was reported that the measurement of PSA levels had the lowest error rate of the tests for predicting prostate cancer. However, 21% of the men with prostate cancer in the control group had a normal PSA level. Therefore, these cancers would have escaped detection if PSA screening alone had been used. Catalona and his associates concluded that serum PSA measurements in combination with DRE are better than either modality alone in optimizing cancer detection.[37]

As a result of these and other studies, investigators now recommend that DRE

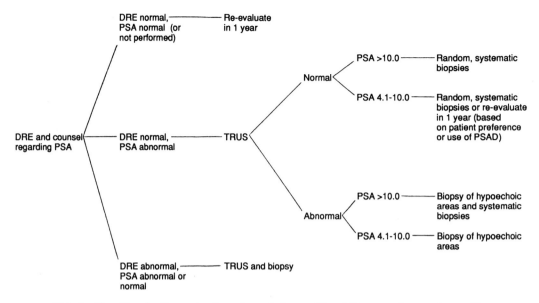

Fig. 1. Algorithm for the evaluation of men between 50 and 70 years of age and men 40–70 years of age with a family history of prostate cancer or who are African-Americans.

and PSA be performed together since their use in combination provides the best overall assessment of the prostate gland.[37,46] For those men who are discovered to have a suspicious prostate examination and/or elevated PSA level, TRUS is recommended and biopsies are performed of all hypoechoic areas. If the PSA alone is elevated and the subsequent TRUS is normal, then a question arises regarding random prostate biopsies. Cooner et al. found that the cancer detection rate in men with a normal rectal examination and a PSA greater than 10 ng/ml was 28%.[36] Conversely, those with a PSA level between 4.1 and 10 ng/ml and a normal DRE had a detection rate of only 7%.[36] Therefore, men with a PSA level greater than 10 ng/ml appear to have a significant risk of harboring malignancy and should undergo routine, systematic biopsies of the prostate as described by Hodge et al.,[52] regardless of the findings of ultrasonography. For patients who have a minimally elevated PSA level between 4.1 and 10 ng/ml, then the PSAD may serve as

a guide. If the PSAD is high (>0.15), then systematic biopsies may be warranted, while a low PSAD may allow a period of observation. However, this approach requires further study and it is clear that if the goal is to optimize prostate cancer detection, then an aggressive approach to prostate biopsy is indicated.

An algorithm that summarizes the guidelines for the screening of men over 50 years of age, and African-Americans or patients with a family history of prostate cancer over 40 years of age, is presented in Figure 1. In general, screening is limited to men less than 70 years of age since recent reports have demonstrated excellent 10-year disease-specific survival of patients with clinically localized, grades 1 and 2 prostate cancer treated with observation or palliative treatment alone.[53] However, general state of health and familial longevity are the most important factors and it is probably best to limit screening to those men with a life expectancy of greater than 10 years.

SUMMARY

Prostate cancer is likely to be a growing health care problem throughout the remainder of this and into the next century. Without the results of randomized, properly controlled studies on large populations of men, it remains unclear whether screening will decrease disease-specific mortality. In addition, because of the prolonged natural history of prostate cancer, the results of studies attempting to address this issue will not be available for many years. While screening may appear to provide an individual patient with benefit, when deployed on a large-scale basis, both the potential morbidity and cost could have a negative overall effect on health care. These are issues that must be taken into consideration if society is to best allocate limited health care resources. Until definitive results of screening trials are available, patients should be counseled regarding the relative risks and benefits of screening so they can decide how aggressively to pursue the diagnosis of prostate cancer. If the decision to screen for prostate cancer has been reached, it appears that this can be achieved in the most cost-effective and efficient manner by combining DRE and PSA, with TRUS reserved for the further evaluation of men with an abnormality noted on initial testing.

REFERENCES

1. Chiarodo, A: National Cancer Institute Round Table on Prostate Cancer: Future research directions. Cancer Res 51:2498, 1991.
2. Boring CC, Squires TS, Tong T: Cancer statistics, 1993. CA Cancer J Clin 43:7, 1993.
3. Silverberg E, Lubera J: Cancer statistics, 1987. CA Cancer J Clin 37:2, 1987.
4. Chodak GW, Keller P, Schoenberg HW: Assessment of screening for prostate cancer using the digital rectal examination. J Urol 141:1136, 1989.
5. Thompson IM, Ernst JJ, Gangai MP, Spence CR: Adenocarcinoma of the prostate: results of routine urological screening. J Urol 132:690, 1984.

6. Thompson IM, Rounder JB, Teague JL, Peek M, Spence CR: Impact of routine screening for adenocarcinoma of the prostate on stage distribution. J Urol 137:424, 1987.
7. Oesterling JE: Prostate specific antigen: a critical assessment of the most useful tumor marker for adenocarcinoma of the prostate. J Urol 145:907, 1991.
8. Shinohara K, Wheeler TM, Scardino PT: The appearance of prostate cancer on transrectal ultrasonography: correlation of imaging and pathological examinations. J Urol 142:76, 1989.
9. Carter HB, Coffey DS: The prostate: an increasing medical problem. Prostate 16:39, 1990.
10. National Cancer Institute. Cancer Statistics Review, 1973–88. Bethesda, MD: National Cancer Institute (Publication No. NIH 91-2789), 1991.
11. Steinberg GD, Carter BS, Beaty TH, Childs B, Walsh PC: Family history and the risk of prostate cancer. Prostate 17:337, 1990.
12. Mebane C, Gibbs T, Horm J: Current status of prostate cancer in North American black males. J Natl Med Assoc 82:782, 1990.
13. Giovannucci E, Ascherio A, Rimm EB, Colditz GA, Stampfer MJ, Willett WC: A prospective cohort study of vasectomy and prostate cancer in US men. JAMA 269:873, 1993.
14. Sidney S: Vasectomy and risk of prostate cancer and benign prostatic hypertrophy. J Urol 138:795, 1987.
15. Nienhuis H, Goldacre M, Seagroatt V, Gill L, Vessey M: Incidence of disease after vasectomy: a record linkage retrospective cohort study. Br Med J 304:743, 1992.
16. Fontana RS, Sanderson DR, Woolner LB, et al.: Lung cancer screening: the Mayo program. J Occup Med 28:746, 1986.
17. Love RR, Camilli AE: The value of screening. Cancer 48:489, 1981.
18. Baron E, Angrist A: Incidence of occult adenocarcinoma of the prostate after fifty years of age. Arch Pathol 32:787, 1941.
19. Edwards CN, Steinthorsson E, Nicholson D: An autopsy study of latent prostatic cancer. Cancer 6:531, 1953.
20. Walsh PC: Why make an early diagnosis of prostate cancer? J Urol 147:853, 1992.
21. Middleton AW Jr: Radical prostatectomy for carcinoma in men more than 69 years old. J Urol 138:1185, 1987.
22. Stamey TA, McNeal JE, Freiha FS, et al.: Morphometric and clinical studies on 68 consecu-

tive radical prostatectomies. J Urol 139:1235, 1988.

23. Boxer RJ, Kaufman JJ, Goodwin WE: Radical prostatectomy for carcinoma of the prostate: 1951–1976. A review of 329 patients. J Urol 117:208, 1977.

24. Pontes JE, Huben R, Wolf R: Sexual function after radical prostatectomy. Prostate 8:123, 1986.

25. Update January 1992: the American Cancer Society guidelines for the cancer related checkup. CA Cancer J Clin 42:44, 1992.

26. Gilbertsen VA: Cancer of the prostate gland: results of early diagnosis and therapy undertaken for cure of the disease. JAMA 215:81, 1971.

27. Jenson CB, Shahon DB, Wangensteen OH: Evaluation of annual examinations in the detection of cancer. Special reference to cancer of the gastrointestinal tract, prostate, breast and female reproductive tract. JAMA 174:1783, 1960.

28. Thompson IM, Rounder JB, Teague JL, et al.: Impact of routine screening for adenocarcinoma of the prostate on stage distribution. J Urol 137:424, 1988.

29. Chodak GW, Keller P, Schoenberg HW: Assessment of screening for prostate cancer using the digital rectal examination. J Urol 141:1136, 1989.

30. Mueller EJ, Crain TW, Thompson IM, et al.: An evaluation of serial digital rectal examinations in screening for prostate cancer. J Urol 140:1445, 1988.

31. Gerber GS, Thompson IM, Thisted R, Chodak GW: Disease-specific survival following routine prostate cancer screening by digital rectal examination. JAMA 269:61, 1993.

32. Lee F, Littrup PJ, Torp-Pedersen ST, et al.: Prostate cancer: comparison of transrectal US and digital rectal examination for screening. Radiology 168:389, 1988.

33. Vihko P, Kontturi M, Lukkarinen O, et al.: Screening for carcinoma of the prostate. Rectal examination, and enzymatic and radioimmunologic measurements of serum acid phosphatase compared. Cancer 56:173, 1985.

34. Catalona WJ: Screening for prostate cancer. Presented to the President's Cancer Panel, Bethesda, MD, October, 1992.

35. Chodak GW, Schoenberg HW: Early detection of prostate cancer by routine screening. JAMA 252:3261, 1984.

36. Cooner WH, Mosley BR, Rutherford CL Jr, Beard JH, Pond HS, Terry WJ, Igel TC, Kidd DD: Prostate cancer detection in a clinical urological practice by ultrasonography, digital rectal examination, and prostate specific antigen. J Urol 143:1146, 1990.

37. Catalona WJ, Smith DS, Ratliff TL, et al.: Measurement of prostate-specific antigen in serum as a screening test for prostate cancer. N Engl J Med 324:1156, 1991.

38. Brawer MK, Chetner MP, Beatie J, Buchner DM, Vessella RL, Lange PH: Screening for prostatic carcinoma with prostate specific antigen. J Urol 147:841, 1992.

39. Brawer MK, Chetner MP, Beatie J, Lange PH: Prostate specific antigen and early detection of prostatic carcinoma. J Urol 145:382A, 1991.

40. Catalona WJ, Smith D, Ratliff TL: Single and serial measurement of serum prostate-specific antigen as a screening test for early prostate cancer. J Urol 147:450A, 1992.

41. Partin AW, Carter HB, Chan DW, Epstein JI, Oesterling JE, Rock RC, et al.: Prostate specific antigen in the staging of localized prostate cancer: influence of tumor differentiation, tumor volume and benign hyperplasia. J Urol 143:747, 1990.

42. Brawer MK, Rennels MA, Schifman RA: Significance of serum PSA in men undergoing prostate surgery for benign disease. Am J Clin Pathol 89:428, 1988.

43. Stamey TA: Prostate specific antigen in the diagnosis and treatment of adenocarcinoma of the prostate. Monogr Urol 10:49, 1989.

44. Lange PH, Ercole CJ, Lightner DJ, et al.: The value of serum prostate-specific antigen determinations before and after radical prostatectomy. J Urol 141:873, 1989.

45. Labrie F, Dupont A, Suburu R, et al.: Serum prostate specific antigen as pre-screening test for prostate cancer. J Urol 147:846, 1992.

46. Cupp MR, Oesterling JE: Prostate-specific antigen, digital rectal examination, and transrectal ultrasonography: their roles in diagnosing early prostate cancer. Mayo Clin Proc 68:297, 1993.

47. Benson MC, Whang IS, Pantuck A, Ring K, Kaplan SA, Olsson CA, et al.: Prostate specific antigen density: a means of distinguishing benign prostatic hypertrophy and prostate cancer. J Urol 147:815, 1992.

48. Benson MC, Whang IS, Olsson CA, McMahon DJ, Cooner WH: The use of prostate specific

antigen density to enhance the predictive value of intermediate levels of serum prostate specific antigen. J Urol 147:817, 1992.

49. Carter HB, Pearson JD, Metter EJ, Brant LJ, Chan DW, Andres R, et al.: Longitudinal evaluation of prostate-specific antigen levels in men with and without prostate disease. JAMA 267:2215, 1992.

50. Cooner WH, Eggers GW, Lichtenstein P: Prostate cancer: new hope for early diagnosis. Ala Med 56:13, 1987.

51. Carter HB, Hamper UM, Sheth S, Sanders RC, Epstein JI, Walsh PC: Evaluation of transrectal ultrasound in the early detection of prostate cancer. J Urol 142:1008, 1989.

52. Hodge KK, McNeal JE, Stamey TA: Ultrasound guided transrectal core biopsies of the palpably abnormal prostate. J Urol 142:66, 1989.

53. Johansson JE, Adami HO, Andersson SW, Bergstrom R, Holmberg L, Krusemo UB: High 10-year survival rate in patients with early, untreated prostatic cancer. JAMA 267:2191, 1992.

5

Clinical Utility of Monoclonal Antibodies in Prostate Cancer

Joseph V. Gulfo, M.D.

BACKGROUND

Antibodies are glycoproteins that selectively bind to molecular targets or antigens. Extensive research has been undertaken in the identification of antibodies directed against antigens expressed by tumor cells. There are a number of potential clinical uses of antibodies in the management of patients with cancer. Depending on the antigen/antibody system, it may be possible to apply this technology to predict the biological behavior of cancers, thereby stratifying patients into prognostically important groups. This may have significant clinical implications. Another clinical application involves the identification of antibodies that when administered to patients (in vivo) will selectively target cancer cells. When coupled to other agents (such as radioisotopes) the antibodies may allow for imaging (immunoscintigraphy) or therapy (radioimmunotherapy) of cancer. Another approach for therapy involves the coupling of antibodies to toxins (immunotoxins) or chemotherapeutic agents (drug conjugates).

Some antibodies have been shown to be of significant benefit in the detection and treatment of several cancers. Recently, OncoScint CR/OV, a radiolabeled immunoconjugate of MAb B72.3 that targets TAG-72, a glycoprotein expressed by a variety of adenocarcinomas, has been approved by the Food and Drug Administration for use in the detection and staging of ovarian and colorectal cancers.[1] Antibody conjugates are being developed (as imaging and therapeutic agents) for use in other malignancies as well, including breast and lung cancer and melanoma and lymphoma.[2-4]

The use of antibody conjugates to detect and treat cancer is a recent technology. Imaging with polyclonal antibodies was first reported in 1948,[5] however, research in the field accelerated with the development of monoclonal antibodies (homogeneous antibodies that recognize a single antigenic epitope) in 1975 with the work of Kohler and Milstein.[6] Since this time, there have been many reports of radiolabeled monoclonal antibodies used in the detection and treatment of malignancies. Hybridoma technology has led to a convenient means by which murine (mouse) antibodies directed against human tumor antigens can be identified and isolated.[7]

What advantages do monoclonal antibodies offer? Have any monoclonal antibodies been used to detect prostate cancer? What is the potential for therapy? Can monoclonal antibodies contribute to the management of individual patients? These

Prostate Cancer, pages 77–94 © 1994 Wiley-Liss, Inc.

questions and others are currently being investigated.

ANTI-PROSTATE CANCER ANTIBODIES

Prostate-specific antigen (PSA) and prostatic acid phosphatase (PAP) are biochemical markers of prostate cancer that have been the subjects of intense investigation. Currently, PSA is being used in a variety of clinical settings, including: (1) in prostate cancer screening, (2) as a means of stratifying patients into high- and low-risk groups for the presence of localized versus distant disease, (3) in quantitating response to various forms of therapy, and (4) in selecting optimal therapy for patients at various stages of disease. Several investigators have evaluated radiolabeled anti-PSA and anti-PAP antibodies for immunoscintigraphy.[8-12] Although some bony and soft tissue sites of metastatic disease and primary lesions were identified, poor sensitivity, the high incidence of human–anti-mouse antibodies (HAMA), and inadequate safety profile have accounted for disappointing results in these early trials.[1]

Recently, other monoclonal antibodies to non-PSA/PAP antigens expressed by prostate cancer cells have been identified and are undergoing investigation.[14-18] (One of these, MAb 7E11-C5.3, under clinical evaluation as an in vivo imaging and therapeutic agent, is discussed later.) MAb PD41 is an $IgG1_k$ generated by hyperimmunization of BALB/c mice with a membrane preparation prepared from a moderately to poorly differentiated prostate cancer surgical specimen.[17] Considering only those cases in which 10% or more of the tumor cells were identified by PD41, immunohistochemical evaluation revealed that it selectively reacts with prostate adenocarcinoma (65% of 130 frozen primary carcinoma tissue specimens tested) with no staining of fetal or benign prostate specimens and minimal reactivity (less than 1% of cells staining positive) with

normal prostate tissues. Undifferentiated primary prostate carcinomas appeared to lose PD41 expression. The antigen was not expressed on any available prostate cancer cell line nor was it expressed in 21 normal tissue types (131 specimens) and 12 non-prostate carcinoma tissue types (80 specimens) tested. PD41 binds to target antigen present in seminal plasma obtained from prostate carcinoma patients but not to seminal plasma from normal donors. Recently, the antigen has been detected in serum and there is evidence to suggest that it may be an independent marker of progression.[19] It appears that PD41 may recognize a prostate carcinoma-associated mucin-like antigen, which is preferentially expressed on prostate carcinomas, and, therefore, may be a useful marker to distinguish benign prostate hyperplasia from prostate cancer.

MAb PR1 is an IgM_k prepared by immunization of BALB/c mice with a primary human prostate carcinoma cell strain cultured from a needle biopsy derived from a cancer of Gleason pattern 4 + 4.[18] Immunohistochemical analysis revealed that it reacts uniformly with the surface of most (25/26) adenocarcinomas of the prostate, normal prostate (10/10), and benign prostatic hyperplasia (BPH) (10/10) specimens. It reacted with two samples of metastatic prostate cancer, one in a lymph node and the other in bladder. Some reactivity was also noted with other normal human tissues, including colon (apical brush border), kidney (collecting ducts), bile and pancreatic ducts, salivary glands (acini and ducts), small bowel (apical brush border), and stomach (parietal cells). There was little or no reactivity with several other types of cancer, including bladder, breast, ovarian, and colon cancers. There was no reactivity with DU145 cell lines; however, PR1 did react strongly with 20% of the cells present in LNCaP cultures and less strongly with about 1% of the cells present in PC-3 cultures. Cloning of the cDNAs encoding the V_H and the V_L regions of MAb PR1 has been accomplished.[20] A recombinant immunotoxin was constructed by connecting the V_H region to the V_L region by a $(Gly_4\text{-}Ser)_3$ linker and fusing this single chain F_V to PE38KDEL, a truncated version of *Pseudomonas* exotoxin. PR1(F_V)-PE38KDEL was shown to bind to cells expressing the PR1 antigen and was very cytotoxic to a subset of LNCaP cells. PR1 and its single chain F_V may be useful for the diagnosis or therapy of prostate cancer.

MAb Prost 30 is one of several IgG1 antibodies that resulted from the immunization of BALB/c mice with mechanically minced tissues from fresh benign hyperplastic and malignant prostate specimens.[16] Immunohistochemical analysis revealed that it reacts with all 35 benign and 30 malignant prostates tested. The reactivity was present in the prostatic epithelial cells and luminal secretions. Of the 22 other normal tissue types tested, weak and heterogeneous reactivity with some tubules in 7 of 19 normal kidney specimens and 1 of 7 lung cancers was noted. There was no reactivity in seven nonprostate human carcinoma tissue types (64 specimens) tested. Circulating antigen has not been detected. MAb Prost 30 may have clinical potential for treatment of localized carcinoma of the prostate, in the treatment of BPH, or even in the prevention of BPH or prostate cancer.

MURINE MABS AND HUMAN ANTI-MOUSE ANTIBODIES

Patients exposed to MAbs of murine origin frequently develop HAMA. The clinical implications of this immunologic response are significant. HAMA may form immune complexes with subsequently administered murine MAbs, altering their biodistribution and neutralizing their effects. Considering radiolabeled murine monoclonal antibody conjugates, typically,

clearance of the antibody from the blood is increased, whole-body clearance of the radiolabel is increased, activity in liver or spleen is enhanced, and uptake by the target tumor is decreased.[21] As a result, the quality of diagnostic images may deteriorate markedly[22,23] and administered therapeutic doses may not reach their target.[24] Very low levels of HAMA may not interfere at all with pharmacokinetics, imaging, or therapy. The upper limit of HAMA that is noninterfering must be determined individually for each assay method, however.

The presence of HAMA might also produce false results (elevated or depressed) of in vitro immunoassays that use murine antibodies.[25,26] Among the tests that could potentially be altered by HAMA are assays for tumor markers (such as PSA and PAP) and for drugs (such as phenobarbital).

Finally, various hypersensitivity-type reactions, including anaphylaxis or serum sickness, could occur as a result of HAMA formation.[22] Some of the symptoms reported with murine antibody administration include chills, fever, urticaria, lymphadenopathy, arthralgias, and renal dysfunction. Reports of these reactions have been extremely rare, however, among patients who have received radiolabeled MAbs.

The frequency of HAMA development among patients with cancer who are given murine MAbs varies greatly. Van Kroonenburgh and Pauwels[24] reviewed studies of patients undergoing diagnostic imaging or immunotherapy with several different radiolabeled MAbs. HAMA responses occurred in 0% to 100% of the patients, with a majority of the studies reporting frequencies of 50% or more. A high rate of HAMA development has also been reported by investigators using anti-PSA or anti-PAP antibodies in patients with prostate cancer. For example, half of the patients in one study who received up to 80 mg of PAY-276, an anti-PAP MAb, developed HAMA.[10]

POTENTIAL IN VIVO USES OF MABS IN PROSTATE CANCER DETECTION

As in all cancers, accurate staging is critical in the selection of the most appropriate form of therapy for each patient. This is true not only in the initial evaluation of a patient who presents with prostate cancer but also throughout the course of his disease. Knowledge of the presence, location, and extent of disease aids in selecting patients who will benefit from radical surgery, radiotherapy (external beam or brachytherapy), and hormonal ablative therapy. In addition, the identification of sites of disease is important in salvage/palliative settings.

Prostate Cancer Screening

Prostate cancer screening is the subject of much debate. Presently, the use of PSA, digital rectal examination (DRE) transrectal ultrasound, and PSAD (PSA density) are being intensely evaluated.[27] To date, no method or combination of methods has been shown to be able to distinguish patients with BPH only from patients with cancer. Once a patient is positively screened, prostate biopsies are performed to evaluate whether cancer is present. Often patients need to undergo repeat biopsies before cancer is documented because visualization of the area of the gland involved with tumor is not always possible. In addition, it has not been possible to distinguish patients in whom aggressive therapy versus watchful waiting would be optimal.

Presumed Localized Disease

When a patient is determined to have biopsy-proven adenocarcinoma of the prostate, complete clinical staging follows. Depending on the institution, this may include radionuclide bone scan, DRE, transrectal ultrasound, computed tomography (CT) or magnetic resonance imaging (MRI) of the pelvis and abdomen, and, recently, transrectal MRI. However, clinical staging falls short in differentiating those patients who have truly organ-confined disease from those with extraprostatic locoregional extension. Only 40% of the patients felt to have clinical stage B disease are found to have truly organ-confined disease at prostatectomy.[28] In addition, the amount of cancer within the prostate gland is very strongly correlated with tumor behavior[28]; however, accurate in vivo assessment of tumor volume is not possible with current noninvasive imaging modalities.

The evaluation of the pelvic lymph nodes is critical in the management of patients with presumed localized disease. The presence or absence of metastases to the pelvic lymph nodes is one of the most important prognostic factors for patients with prostate cancer. Gervasi et al.[29] reported that patients with a single microscopic focus of cancer in a lymph node had patterns of progression and cancer-specific mortality rates similar to those of patients with more extensive nodal disease and much worse than those of patients with no nodal metastases. The risk of metastatic disease at 10 years was 31% ± 7% for those with no lymph node involvement and 83% ± 7% for those with at least one malignant node. Similarly, the risk of dying of prostate cancer within 10 years was nearly three times higher for those with at least one malignant lymph node (57% ± 11%) than for those with no lymph node metastases (17% ± 6%).

Urologists routinely perform staging pelvic lymph node dissections prior to prostatectomy to evaluate the pelvic lymph nodes. In patients at higher risk for nodal involvement (by virtue of clinical stage, grade, PSA level) laparoscopic node dissection is often performed. Lymph node dissection—either open or laparoscopic—is currently the only accurate method for staging pelvic lymph nodes. Hanks et al. recently compared outcomes in 805 patients whose lymph node status was established by lymphangiography or CT (554 patients) or by lymph node dissection (251 patients).[30]

TABLE 1. Clinical vs. Pathologic Staging: Analysis of Clinical Endpoints by Stage of Primary Lesion[30]

	Clin − (%)	Clin + (%)	Path − (%)	Path + (%)
Survival 5 Yr				
B	77	80	84	61
C	65	60	82	66
NED at 5 Yr[a]				
B	63	55	72	32
C	44	38	64	32
Free of mets at 5 Yr[b]				
B	84	85	85	46
C	60	55	75	44

[a]No evidence of disease at 5 years (stage B and C).
[b]Free of metastases at 5 years (stage B and C).

They calculated five-year survival, survival with no evidence of disease, local recurrence, and freedom from metastases for these patients, based on whether their lymph node status was determined clinically or pathologically. The results (Table 1) showed that lymph node status as evaluated by pelvic lymph node dissection divided the patients into prognostically different groups, whereas evaluation by CT or lymphangiography did not. Further, patients with pathologically negative lymph nodes had significantly better outcomes than did patients who were judged clinically to have negative lymph nodes.

CT evaluation of pelvic lymph nodes. CT does not reveal the internal architecture of pelvic lymph nodes and, therefore, the interpretation of CT scans relies on nodal size as the indicator of possible neoplastic involvement.[31–33] There is some variability in the criteria to define enlargement of pelvic lymph nodes, but generally 1.2 or 1.5 cm seems to be the lower limit.[33–35] Small (nonenlarged) nodes with micrometastases and enlarged nodes with benign processes are inaccurately diagnosed by this modality.[31,36] Lymphadenectomy or fine-needle biopsy is required for an accurate diagnosis of suspicious CT findings.[30,31,34] Table 2 summarizes the sensitivity, specificity, and accuracy of CT in the detection of malignant pelvic lymph nodes reported in 10 studies published during the past 12 years. Sensitivity varied widely, from 0% to 100%; the combined results of the 10 studies yielded an overall sensitivity of 45%. The most common cause of false-negative images in these studies was microscopic disease in normal-sized or minimally enlarged lymph nodes. Enlargement of lymph nodes by nonmalignant processes was a source of false-positive images.

MRI evaluation of pelvic lymph nodes. Like CT, MRI evaluation of the pelvic lymph nodes is constrained by nodal size.[43] Thus, only enlarged nodes can be detected, leading to the same inaccuracies in diagnosis as noted for CT.[44,45] Additional negative features of MRI scans are their expense, the fact that they cause some discomfort for the patient, and the need for an extensive protocol to obtaining accurate images. The use of MRI in staging of prostate cancer has not been as thoroughly studied as has the use of CT. Table 3 summarizes the sensitivity, specificity, and accuracy of this procedure in the detection of malignant pelvic lymph nodes in three recent trials. The sensitivity ranged from 4% to 69%, with an overall value of 31%. Because the detection of malignant nodes is based on enlargement, false-negative readings again occurred when the involved nodes were normal size.

TABLE 2. Detection of Pelvic Lymph Node Metastases by Computerized Tomography

Author/Year	Patients			Sensitivity[a]		Specificity[a]		Accuracy[a] (%)
	Total	Node +	Node −	%	No.	%	No.	
Benson, 1981[42]	23	7	16	14	1/7	94	15/16	70
Golimbu, 1981[34]	46	17	29	29	5/17	93	27/29	70
Levine, 1981[41]	15	7	8	100	7/7	88	7/8	93
Morgan, 1981[40]	16	6	10	33	2/6	100	10/10	75
Weinerman, 1982[36]	32	16	16	81	13/16	81	13/16	81
Sawczuk, 1983[39]	8	4	4	25	1/4	100	4/4	63
Weinerman, 1983[33]	19	10	9	70	7/10	78	7/9	74
Salo, 1986[38]	36	7	29	29	2/7	100	29/29	86
Hricak, 1987[37]	55	9	46	22	2/9	100	46/46	87
Platt, 1987[32]	32	5	27	0	0/5	96	26/27	81
Total	282	88	194	45	40/88	95	184/194	79

[a]Sensitivity = number of node+ patients with CT evidence of malignant nodes (true positives)/number with positive nodes; specificity = number of node− patients with no CT evidence of malignant nodes (true negatives)/number with negative nodes; accuracy = true positives + true negatives/total number of patients.

Due to the inadequacies of CT and MRI in the evaluation of pelvic lymph nodes, pelvic lymph node dissection is the only accurate staging modality. The obturator pelvic lymphadenectomy is a *sampling* procedure that includes the medial chain of pelvic nodes only (area bounded by the external iliac vein and obturator nerve). Skip lesions (metastases to nodes outside the medial chain without concomitant metastases to the medial chain) are known to occur. It follows that patients with no histologic evidence of metastases to lymph nodes within the surgical field of the staging obturator lymphadenectomy may, in fact, have metastases. Prostatectomy or radiotherapy would not afford the opportunity for cure in these patients.

Recurrent and Residual Prostate Cancer

The widespread use of PSA in following patients who have undergone or are receiving therapy for prostate cancer has made it possible to identify those who have recurrent disease following potentially curative surgery or radiotherapy.[46–49] Many investigators are attempting to develop treatment algorithms based on PSA level following curative and palliative treatments. Although the pattern of PSA increase, pathological stage, grade of

TABLE 3. Detection of Pelvic Lymph Node Metastases by Magnetic Resonance Imaging

Author/Year	Patients			Sensitivity[a]		Specificity[a]		Accuracy[a] (%)
	Total	Node +	Node −	%	No.	%	No.	
Hricak, 1987[37]	55	9	46	44	4/9	100	46/46	91
Bezzi, 1988[44]	51	13	38	69	9/13	95	36/38	88
Rifkin, 1990[45]	185	23	162	4	1/23	96	155/162	84
Total	291	45	246	31	14/45	96	237/246	86

[a]Sensitivity = number of node+ patients with MRI evidence of malignant nodes (true positives)/number with positive nodes; specificity = number of node− patients with no MRI evidence of malignant nodes (true negatives)/number with negative nodes; accuracy = true positives + true negatives/total number of patients.

tumor, and tumor volume may be useful in identifying those who are more likely to have recurred locally versus at distant sites,[50] there is currently no reliable means of predicting or determining the location and extent of disease in patients in whom biochemical evidence of failure has been established. Noninvasive imaging modalities fall short principally because they are not sensitive in identifying disease in this setting. Also, it is economically impractical to consider use of these (for example, CT or MRI) as a means of assessing the whole body.

Patients with biochemical (PSA) evidence of failure following prostatectomy routinely undergo radionuclide bone scan, DRE, transrectal ultrasound, and CT or MRI in an effort to identify the location and extent of disease. Directed or blind prostatic fossa (peri-urethral-vesical anastomosis area) biopsies are often performed to determine whether local or recurrent/residual disease is present. Many patients are found to have a totally negative clinical work-up despite biochemical evidence of failure. Thus, a significant therapeutic dilemma exists in that the selection of the appropriate course of action is governed by information obtained from inadequate staging modalities.

Distant Disease: D₂ Prostate Cancer

In patients with distant disease (stage D₂), therapeutic options are limited. Hormonal ablation with or without anti-androgens is typically performed (medically or surgically). PSA and bone scan are used to follow patients. Bone scan is not specific for metastatic disease; rather, it indicates areas of osteoblastic activity. Often, bone scans remain unchanged in patients responding to hormonal therapy or in patients who have documented hormone refractory disease as documented by rising PSA. Determination of the active sites of disease would assist in the selection of appropriate therapy. In addition, as systemic therapies that demonstrate significant activity against distant disease are developed, the need to adequately assess disease extent and response will become more acute.

Immunoscintigraphy with Monoclonal Antibodies

Clearly, a need exists for a noninvasive, functional staging modality for accurately assessing the presence, location, and extent of prostatic carcinoma in a variety of settings. Immunoscintigraphy using targeting vehicles specific to prostate cancer may be more useful than the other noninvasive modalities such as ultrasound, CT, or MRI because, theoretically, localization is independent of tumor size. Instead, this method is based on the reactivity of MAbs with tumor-associated antigens. In addition, immunoscintigraphy would not be limited to areas of osteoblastic activity (as radionuclide bone scan); rather, localization would be expected to occur at sites of disease provided that the antigen was expressed.

IMMUNOSCINTIGRAPHY OF PROSTATE CANCER USING MAB 7E11-C5.3

Monoclonal Antibody 7E11-C5.3

7E11-C5.3 is a murine IgG₁ monoclonal antibody (MAb) produced by a hybridoma cell line originating from the fusion of murine myeloma cells with spleen cells of mice immunized with the human prostatic carcinoma cell line, LNCaP. This antibody reacts with cytoplasmic membrane-rich fractions of LNCaP cells, but not with soluble cytosol or secretory glycoproteins such as PSA or PAP. In an original publication, 7E11-C5 was reported to react in frozen sections with epithelial cells from prostatic carcinoma, benign prostatic hypertrophy, and, to a lesser degree, normal prostatic glands.[14] Consistently negative results were obtained on immunospecific staining of numerous fresh frozen sections from a wide range of human nonprostatic normal or malignant tissues. Poorly defined staining of kidney tubules was noted and reactivity (intracellular pattern) was also observed with cardiac and skeletal muscle. The antibody was conjugated with the linker-chelator GYK-DTPA using the site-specific conjugation procedure developed by Rodwell et al.[51] Intravenous studies with the indium-111 labeled immunoconjugate (designated CYT-356) in LNCaP human prostate adenocarcinoma xenografts revealed positive localization of tumor with no unusual accumulation in nontumor tissue or organs.[52]

Ongoing immunohistochemical studies using ex vivo human cancer specimens reveal that there appears to be a gradient of reactivity such that a greater percentage of cells stain positive in poorly differentiated versus well-differentiated disease.[19] Studies have shown that an increased percentage of cells stained positive in the lymph node metastases than in the primary prostate tumor from the same patient.[53]

Phase 1 Study of ^{111}In-CYT-356

A phase 1 clinical study in 80 patients with prostate cancer was conducted using single doses of CYT-356 from 0.1 to 10 mg labeled with approximately 5 mCi of indium-111 (a gamma-emitter used for imaging). Forty-eight of the patients had distant metastases (stage D_2 disease), and 32 patients were presurgical candidates scheduled for a staging pelvic lymphadenectomy.[53]

The results indicate that ^{111}In-CYT-356 localizes to prostatic, soft tissue, and bony tumor lesions in patients with prostatic carcinoma.[54] In the nonsurgical group, 43 of 48 patients had bony metastases, as documented by radionuclide bone scan. Overall, antibody imaging detected bony lesions in 58% of patients with positive bone scans, including 21 of 33 (64%) receiving

concomitant hormonal therapy. In one patient, ^{111}In-CYT-356 immunoscintigraphy detected occult bony lesions in the lumbar spine and the bony pelvis; these lesions were not detected on bone scan and were confirmed by subsequent MRI studies. In another patient (Fig. 1), immunoscintigraphy identified three sites of metastatic disease that were not visualized by radionuclide bone scan. The patient was put on hormonal therapy and underwent serial bone scans that demonstrated disease in these areas 15 months later. Interestingly, these areas were not evident on bone scan until the patient became refractory to the hormonal therapy. Additional occult bony lesions detected in two other patients were not confirmed by other diagnostic imaging modalities. These results suggest that antibody imaging has the potential to detect occult bony lesions.

Eight patients had soft tissue tumor lesions documented by tissue biopsy. ^{111}In-CYT-356 immunoscintigraphy detected soft tissue disease in 5 of these 8 patients; the lesions detected in these five patients included lung metastases (n = 2), retroperitoneal adenopathy (n = 1), mediastinal metastases (n = 1), and supraclavicular lymphadenopathy (n = 1).

Thirty-two patients scheduled to undergo pelvic lymphadenectomy received ^{111}In-CYT-356. Thirty of the 31 patients who underwent surgery were found to have documented prostatic carcinoma; the other patient had benign prostatic hypertrophy. ^{111}In-CYT-356 immunoscintigraphic results indicated radiolocalization in prostatic tissue in 17 of the 30 patients (sensitivity 57%) with documented prostate cancer. The antibody images were correctly negative for the patient with benign prostatic hypertrophy. Pelvic lymph node metastases were histologically confirmed in four patients. Immunoscintigraphic scanning detected pelvic lymph node metastases in two of these patients. Antibody scans were true negative in 25 of 27 patients with histologically negative pelvic lymph nodes. CT or MRI correctly identified 1 of the 4 patients with histologically documented lymph node metastases—the antibody scan was also positive in this patient.

Only one patient experienced an adverse event (mild, transient burning at the injection site) that was associated with the ^{111}In-CYT-356 infusion.

Phase 2 Study: Prepelvic Lymphadenectomy

A phase 2 study of ^{111}In-CYT-356 was completed in 76 patients with a tissue diagnosis of prostate cancer who were at high risk for the presence of lymph node metastases and who were scheduled for pelvic lymphadenectomy. The purpose of the study was to evaluate the utility of immunoscintigraphy in the detection of pelvic lymph node metastases. Patients received 0.5 mg of CYT-356 radiolabeled with 5 mCi of indium-111. Of the patients who underwent both immunoscintigraphy and CT imaging of the pelvis, 21 had histologically confirmed lymph node metastases. The MAb scans were positive for 11 of the 21 patients (sensitivity = 52%); the CT scans were positive for 2 of the 21 patients (sensitivity = 10%). Both patients in whom CT was positive for histologically confirmed metastases were also positive immunoscintigraphically. Of the 44 patients with histologically negative lymph nodes, immunoscintigraphy was negative in 42 patients.

Figure 2 shows the antibody scan in a patient with histologic evidence of nodal disease. In this patient, CT was negative for pelvic/abdominal nodal metastasis; however, immunoscintigraphy revealed a focus of uptake in a left common iliac node. Frozen (and permanent) section analysis of the specimens obtained during the obturator pelvic lymphadenectomy procedure revealed no evidence of disease. The surgeon then explored the left common iliac nodes (the area corresponding to the positive localization seen on the antibody scan). Histologic analysis confirmed the presence of foci of metastatic disease.

Size was recorded for 13 of the 27 lesions in these 21 patients. The MAb scan detected 17% of the lesions that were smaller than 0.5 cm (1/6), 100% of those from 0.5 to 1.0 cm in size (4/4), and 67% of those larger than 1.0 cm (2/3). The size of the lymph node lesions was not recorded for the two patients with positive CT scans because they underwent fine-needle biopsy rather than lymphadenectomy; however, since the cutoff for lymph node positivity on CT is 1.5 cm, it is evident that immunoscintigraphy detected metastatic involvement in 9/10 patients with positive nodes measuring at least 5 mm.

Based on the results of this phase 2 study, a phase 3 study in patients at high risk for developing pelvic lymph node metastases who are scheduled to undergo staging pelvic lymph node dissection has been initiated.

Phase 2 Study in Clinically Occult Patients Postprostatectomy

A phase 2 study in patients who have undergone prostatectomy and present with clinically occult biochemical evidence of recurrent/residual disease (PSA >0.8 ng/mL) is near completion. In order to be eligible, patients had negative bone scans, negative CT or MRI of the pelvis/abdomen, and negative or equivocal DRE and transrectal ultrasound of the prostatic fossa. Immunoscintigraphy using 0.5 mg CYT-356 radiolabeled with 5 mCi indium-111 has demonstrated subsequently documented residual/recurrent and metastatic prostate cancer in the prostatic fossa (biopsy proven), lumbar spine (confirmed by MRI), and mediastinum (confirmed by CT). Other sites positive for disease on immunoscintigraphy for which all other staging modal-

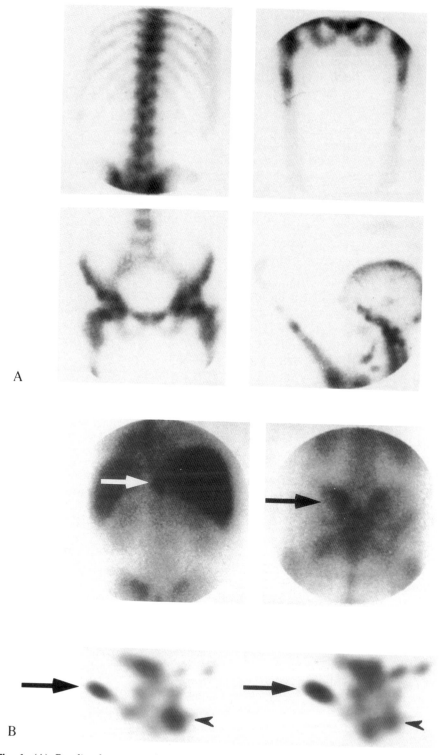

Fig. 1. (A): Baseline bone scan demonstrating diffuse skeletal metastases. (B): Baseline
^{111}In-CYT-356 scan demonstrating uptake in T12 vertebra, right iliac crest, and left sacroiliac joint.

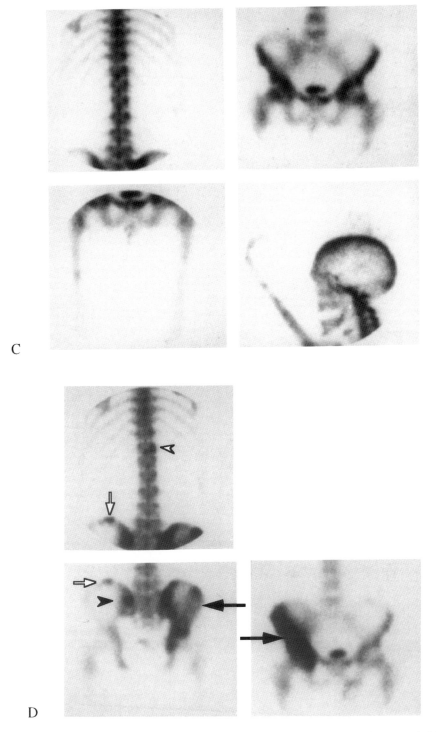

C

D

(C): Bone scan after nine months of maximal androgen ablative therapy (PSA 0.6 ng/mL) demonstrating improvement compared to baseline scan. (D): Bone scan 15 months after initial presentation. Patient with hormone refractory disease (PSA 23 ng/mL). New metastases visible on bone scan—T12 vertebra, right iliac crest, left and right sacroiliac joint. (Courtesy of Drs. Charles Neal and John Texter, Southern Illinois University, Springfield, IL.)

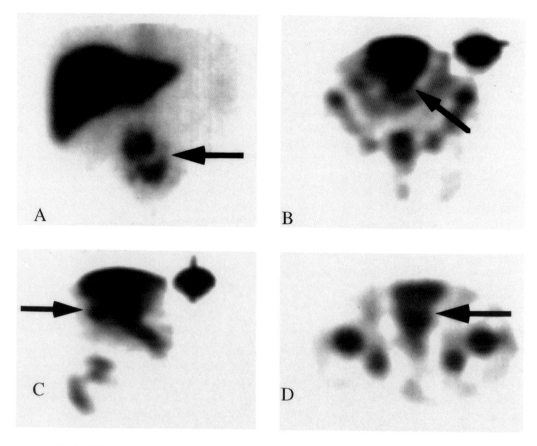

Fig. 2. (A): ^{111}In-CYT-356 planar view of abdomen demonstrating normal liver clearance and retroperitoneal uptake in the lower abdominal/upper pelvic lymph nodes. (B,C): ^{111}In-CYT-356 coronal SPECT (B) and sagittal SPECT (C) demonstrating area of uptake in proximal left common iliac nodes. (D): ^{111}In-CYT-356 transaxial SPECT demonstrating uptake in the prostate. (Courtesy of Drs. Calvin Lutrin and Deepak Chabra, University of California Davis Medical Center, Sacremento, CA.)

ities were negative and biopsy was not performed include pelvic, retroperitoneal, periaortic, axillary, and cervical lymph nodes.

Figure 3 demonstrates the immunoscintigraphy and CT images of a patient with mediastinal adenopathy. He had pathologic stage C_1 cancer and PSA of 4.73 ng/mL (monoclonal assay) at the time of imaging. The clinical work-up was negative; however, findings on the antibody scan in the mediastinum led to a CT scan which demonstrated adenopathy. Figure 4 demonstrates retroperitoneal lymphadenopathy in a patient who presented with a PSA of 7.6 ng/mL (monoclonal assay) eight years postprostatectomy. The clinical work-up was also negative in this patient. CT of the abdomen was originally interpreted as negative. Retrospective review of the CT scan revealed small nodes in the area corresponding to the sites seen on MAb scan. Biopsy of these lesions was not performed; however, follow-up is ongoing. Based on

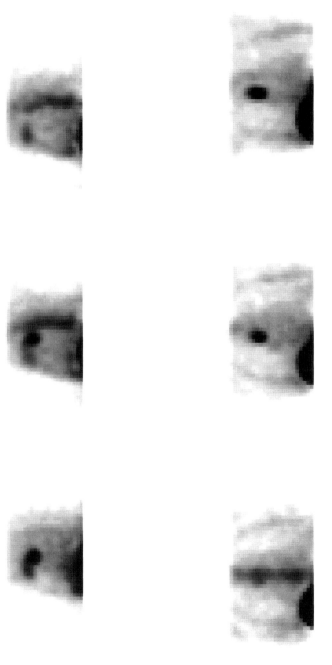

Fig. 3. ^{111}In-CYT-356 scan of the chest demonstrating mediastinal lymphadenopathy. Top, sagittal SPECT view; bottom, coronal SPECT view. (Courtesy of Drs. Richard Williams and Daniel Kahn, University of Iowa Hospitals and Clinics, Iowa City, IA.)

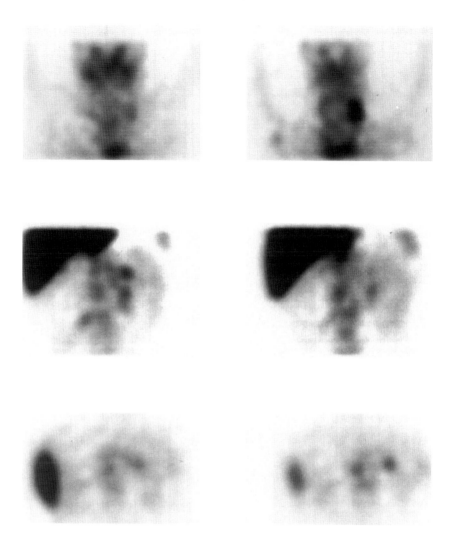

Fig. 4. ^{111}In-CYT-356 scan demonstrating uptake in left cervical and paraaortic lymph nodes and normal liver clearance. Top, coronal neck; middle, coronal abdomen; bottom, transverse abdomen. (Courtesy of Drs. Daniel Petrylak, Alan Yagoda, Carl Olsson, Ronald Van Heertum, and Rashid Fawwaz, Columbia Presbyterian Medical Center, New York, N.Y.)

the data obtained in this study, a phase 3 study in patients with clinically occult recurrent/residual prostate cancer has been initiated.

HAMA Response with ^{111}In-CYT-356

The administration of ^{111}In-CYT-356 has been associated with relatively low levels of HAMA. In clinical studies, the HAMA response was monitored by obtaining serum samples at baseline and at selected intervals for up to 24 weeks after an infusion. The samples were analyzed using the ImmuSTRIP HAMA Test System (Immunomedics; Warren, NJ), a bridging ELISA that measures anticonstant region HAMA.

HAMA results are available from two

completed studies in which patients with prostate cancer received single doses of ^{111}In-CYT-356. Detectable HAMA levels ($\geq 0.4\mu g/mL$) occurred in 2 of 78 patients (3%) in the first study. Refinement of the assay procedure lowered the HAMA-positive level to $\geq 0.2\mu g/mL$ for the next study. Even with the lower cut-off, the frequency of HAMA development was only 7% (5 of 68 patients). The peak titer recorded in these two studies was $1.3\mu g/mL$.

Preliminary results are now available for 16 patients who have received one (n = 11), two (n = 4), or three (n = 1) repeat doses of ^{111}In-CYT-356. Two of the patients who received a single repeat infusion developed HAMA ($\geq 0.2\mu g/mL$) after their second dose, and one patient who received two repeat infusions developed HAMA after both the second and third doses. HAMA was first detected two weeks after an infusion in all three cases, and all patients became HAMA negative by eight weeks. The highest HAMA titer recorded was $0.398\mu g/mL$.

The reason for the low immunogenic potential of ^{111}In-CYT-356 is not yet clear. Currently under development is a HAMA assay that will be specific for the CYT-356 antibody conjugate, to further elucidate the HAMA response to this agent.

POTENTIAL USE OF MABS IN PROSTATE CANCER THERAPY

Except for surgical removal, cancer therapy necessarily involves the use of cytotoxic agents (chemical or radiation). The major hurdle in oncology to date has been the preferential delivery of toxic substances to tumor exclusively, thereby avoiding the consequences of toxic exposure of normal cells. Once disease has spread to distant sites, systemic therapy is required. In this setting, the need for cancer-specific treatment is even more acute.

Monoclonal antibodies that localize to cancer-specific antigens have enormous potential for use as therapeutic agents. The selective delivery of toxic substances to cancer cells would have significant advantages over the currently available therapies. Immunoconjugates labeled with isotopes that have short-range tumoricidal effects have added benefits in that cell kill would not be contingent on delivery of a toxic substance to every cancer cell. Rather, radiation is distributed over an area that may include cancer cells to which no immunoconjugate has localized. This is important when one considers the differential expression of antigens by tumor cells due to tumor heterogeneity.

Radiolabeled monoclonal antibodies will probably be most effective in low-volume disease. The use of monoclonal antibodies may be appropriate in the following settings: (1) in D_2 patients who have had a maximal response to hormone ablative therapy or those who have early refractory D_3 disease, (2) in patients who have clinically occult disease following prostatectomy, (3) in patients with recurrent disease postradiotherapy, or (4) in other settings in which low-volume disease is suspected.

Clinical Studies with ^{90}Y-CYT-356

Based on the results obtained in imaging trials to date, a phase 1 study using CYT-356 radiolabeled with yttrium-90 (beta-emitter used in cancer therapy) has been initiated in hormone refractory prostate cancer patients. The purpose of this study is to determine the maximum tolerated dose of ^{90}Y-CYT-356 and to evaluate in a preliminary fashion the therapeutic potential of this agent in prostate cancer. Upon completion of this study, phase 2 studies designed to evaluate the efficacy of ^{90}Y-CYT-356 in several clinical settings will be initiated.

CONCLUSION

Many investigators are evaluating and developing monoclonal antibodies against prostate cancer antigens for both in vivo and in vitro applications. Monoclonal antibody technology may allow for improvements in our ability to diagnose, differentiate benign from malignant disease, and predict the biologic behavior of cancer. In addition, MAbs may be useful in determining the location and extent of disease, selection of appropriate therapies, and in the treatment of patients. This is a very promising area of investigation and some excellent results have been obtained. Driven by the great potential for developing applications with clinical utility, additional studies evaluating the technology are being pursued with enthusiasm.

ACKNOWLEDGMENTS

The author acknowledges the investigators who have participated in the multicenter studies performed with CYT-356: C. Lutrin and R. White, U.C. Davis Medical Center, Sacramento, CA; D. Podoloff and R. Babaian, M.D. Anderson Cancer Center, Houston, TX; C. Neal and J. Texter, Memorial Medical Center, Springfield, IL; R. Williams and D. Kahn, University of Iowa, Iowa City, IA; C. Olsson, M. Benson, D. Petrylak, R. Fawwaz, Columbia Presbyterian Medical Center, New York; J. Libertino, D. Seldin, Lahey Clinic, Burlington, MA; B. Bodie, S. Bardot, L. Witherspoon, Ochsner Clinic, New Orleans, LA; P. Narayan, D. Gerard, University of California, San Francisco; J. Ryan and G. Chodak, University of Chicago, Chicago, IL; W. Hooser and A. Keller, Cancer Care Associates, Tulsa, OK; J. McAfee and M. Manyak, George Washington University, Washington, DC; E. Cornelius and W. Morgan, Yale University, New Haven, CT; H. Zeissman and J. Lynch, Georgetown University, Washington, DC; D. McLeod, Walter Reed Army Medical Center; Washington, DC; D. Weaver and P. Schellhammer, East Virginia Medical School, Norfolk, VA; H. Abdel-Nabi, E. Rutigliano, and G. Sufrin, Buffalo VAMC, Buffalo, NY; W. Nelp and P. Lange, University of Washington, Seattle, WA; B. McCandless and H. Fisher, Albany Medical Center, Albany, NY; B. Collier and F. Begun, Medical College of Wisconsin, Milwaukee; G. Purnell, University of Arkansas for Medical Sciences, Little Rock; I. Tyson and E. Sanford, University of South Florida College of Medicine, Tampa; G. Winzelberg, Shady Side Hospital, Pittsburgh, PA; E. Mitchell, University of Missouri, Columbia; A. Serafini and R. Vargas, Jackson Memorial Hospital, Miami, FL; S. Harwood, Bay Pines VAMC, Bay Pines, FL; S. Knox and M. Bagshaw, Stanford University Medical Center, Stanford, CA.

REFERENCES

1. Maguire RT, Van Nostrand D (eds): Diagnosis of Colorectal and Ovarian Carcinoma. New York: Marcel Dekker, 1992.

2. Keenan AM: Radiolabeled monoclonal antibodies: current status and future outlook. In: Nuclear Medicine Annual. New York: Raven Press, pp 171–207, 1988.

3. Kaplan EH: The diagnostic and therapeutic use of monoclonal antibodies in colorectal cancer. Hematol Oncol Clin North Am 3:125–134, 1989.

4. Larson SM: Lymphoma, melanoma, colon cancer: diagnosis and treatment with radiolabeled monoclonal antibodies. Radiology 165:297–304, 1987.

5. Pressman D, Keighley G: The zone of activity of antibodies as determined by the use of radioactive tracers: the zone of activity of nephrotoxic antikidney serum. J Immunol 59:141–146, 1948.

6. Kohler G, Milstein C: Continuous cultures of fused cells secreting antibody of predefined specificity. Nature 256:495–497, 1975.

7. Mitchell MS, Oettgen HF (eds): Hybridomas in cancer diagnosis and therapy. In: Progress in Cancer Research and Therapy. New York: Raven Press, pp 1–264, 1982.

8. Goldenberg DM, DeLand FH, Bennett SJ, et al.: Radioimmunodetection of prostatic cancer: in vivo use of radioactive antibodies against prostatic acid phosphatase for diagnosis of prostate cancer by nuclear imaging. JAMA 250:630–635, 1983.

9. Vihko P, Heikkila J, Kontturi M, et al.: Radioimaging of prostate metastases and metastases of prostate carcinoma with ^{99m}Tc-labeled prostatic acid phosphatase-specific antibodies and their Fab fragments. Am Clin Res 16:51–52, 1984.

10. Babaian RJ, Murray JL, Lamki LM, et al.: Radioimmunological imaging of metastatic prostate cancer with 111-indium-labeled monoclonal antibody PAY 276. J Urol 137:439–443, 1987.

11. Halpern SE, Haindl W, Beauregard J, et al.: Scintigraphy with In-111-labeled monoclonal

antitumor antibodies: kinetics, biodistribution, and tumor detection. Radiology 168:529–536, 1988.

12. Abdel-Nabi H, Ortman-Nabi JA, See W, et al.: Clinical experience with intralymphatic administration of ^{111}In-labeled monoclonal antibody PAY 276 for the detection of pelvic nodal metastases in prostatic carcinoma. Eur J Nucl Med 16:149–156, 1990.

13. Babaian RJ, Lamki LM: Radioimmunoscintigraphy of prostate cancer. Semin Nucl Med XIX(4):309–321, 1989.

14. Horoszewicz JS, Kawinski E, Murphy GP: Monoclonal antibodies to a new antigenic marker in epithelial prostatic cells and serum of prostatic cancer patients. Anticancer Res 7:927–936, 1987.

15. Abdel-Nabi H, Vilani J, Cronin V, Evans N: Localization of Prostate Carcinoma with Indium-111 KC4 MoAb: Prelude to Y-90. Diagnostic and Therapeutic Applications of Antibodies, Peptides, and Molecular Recognition Units in Nuclear Medicine, 1993.

16. Bander N: Personal communication.

17. Beckett ML, Lipford GB, Haley CL, Schellhammer PF, Wright GL: Monoclonal antibody PD41 recognizes an antigen restricted to prostate adenocarcinomas. Cancer Res 51:1326–1333, 1991.

18. Pastan I, Lovelace E, Rutherford AV, Kunwar S, Willingham MC, Peehl DM: PR1—a monoclonal antibody that reacts with an antigen on the surface of normal and malignant prostate cells. J Natl Cancer Inst 85(14):1149–1154, 1993.

19. Wright GL: Personal communication.

20. Brinkmann U, Gallo M, Brinkmann E, Kunwar S, Pastan I: A recombinant immunotoxin that is composed of the F_v region of monoclonal antibody PR1 and a truncated form of *Pseudomonas* exotoxin. Proc Natl Acad Sci USA (90):547–551, 1993.

21. Larson SM, Brown JP, Wright PW, et al.: Imaging of melanoma with I-131-labeled monoclonal antibodies. Clin Sci 24(2):123–129, 1983.

22. Pimm MV, Perkins AC, Armitage NC, et al.: The characteristics of blood-borne radiolabels and the effect of anti-mouse IgG antibodies on localization of radiolabeled monoclonal antibody in cancer patients. J Nucl Med 26(9):1011–1023, 1985.

23. Perkins AC, Pimm MV: Immunological responses to monoclonal antibodies. In: Immunoscintigraphy—Practical Aspects and Clinical Applications. New York: Wiley-Liss, pp 111–128, 1991.

24. van Kroonenburgh MJPG, Pauwels EKJ: Human immunological response to mouse monoclonal antibodies in the treatment or diagnosis of malignant diseases. Nucl Med Commun 9:919–930, 1988.

25. Morton BA, O'Connor-Tressel M, Beatty BG, et al.: Artifactual CEA elevation due to human anti-mouse antibodies. Arch Surg 123:1242–1246, 1988.

26. Muto MG, Lepisto EM, Van den Abbeele AD, et al.: Influence of human antimurine antibody on CA 125 levels in patients with ovarian cancer undergoing radioimmunotherapy or immunoscintigraphy with murine monoclonal antibody OC 125. Am J Obstet Gynecol 161:1206–1212, 1989.

27. Cooner WH: Prostate cancer detection: a practical approach. Primary Care and Cancer 13(2):25–31, 1993.

28. Stamey TA, McNeal JE: Adenocarcinoma of the prostate. In Walsh PC, Retik AB, Stamey TA, Darracott Vaughn E (eds): Campbell's Urology. Philadelphia: WB Saunders, pp 1159–1221, 1992.

29. Gervasi LA, Mata J, Easley JD, Wilbanks JH, Seale-Hawkins C, Carlton CE Jr., et al.: Prognostic significance of lymph nodal metastases in prostate cancer. J Urol 142:332–336, 1989.

30. Hanks GE, Krall JM, Pilepich MV, Asbell SO, Perez CA, Rubin P, et al.: Comparison of pathologic and clinical evaluation of lymph nodes in prostate cancer: implications of RTOG data for patient management and trial design and stratification. Int J Radiat Oncol Biol Phys 23:293–298, 1992.

31. Hricak H: Noninvasive imaging for staging of prostate cancer: magnetic resonance imaging, computed tomography, and ultrasound. NCI Monogr 7:31–35, 1988.

32. Platt JF, Bree RL, Schwab RE: The accuracy of CT in the staging of carcinoma of the prostate. Am J Rad 149:315–318, 1987.

33. Weinerman PM, Arger PH, Coleman BG, Pollack HM, Banner MP, Wein AJ: Pelvic adenopathy from bladder and prostate carcinoma. Detection by rapid-sequence computed tomography. Am J Rad 140:95–99, 1983.

34. Golimbu M, Morales P, Al-Askari S, Shulman Y: CAT scanning in staging of prostatic cancer. Urol XVIII(3):305–308, 1981.

35. Einstein DM, Singer AA, Chilcote WA, Desai RK: Abdominal lymphadenopathy: spectrum

of CT findings. RadioGraphics 11:457–472, 1991.

36. Weinerman PM, Arger PH, Pollack HM: CT evaluation of bladder and prostate neoplasms. Urol Radiol 4:105–114, 1982.

37. Hricak H, Dooms GC, Jeffrey RB, Avallone A, Jacobs D, Benton WK, et al.: Prostatic carcinoma: staging by clinical assessment, CT, and MR imaging. Radiology 162:331–336, 1987.

38. Salo JO, Kivisaari L, Rannikko S, Lehtonen T: The value of CT in detecting pelvic lymph node metastases in cases of bladder and prostate carcinoma. Scand J Urol Nephrol 20:261–265, 1986.

39. Sawczuk IS, White RD, Gold RP, Olsson CA: Sensitivity of computed tomography in evaluation of pelvic lymph node metastases from carcinoma of bladder and prostate. Urol XXI(1):81–84, 1983.

40. Morgan CL, Calkins RF, Cavalcanti EJ: Computed tomography in the evaluation, staging, and therapy of carcinoma of the bladder and prostate. Radiology 140:751–761, 1981.

41. Levine MS, Arger PH, Coleman BG, Mulhern CB, Pollack HM, Wein AJ: Detecting lymphatic metastases from prostatic carcinoma: superiority of CT. AJR 137:207–211, 1981.

42. Benson KH, Watson RA, Spring DB, Agee RE: The value of computerized tomography in evaluation of pelvic lymph nodes. J Urol 126:63–64, 1981.

43. Schnall MD, Bezzi M, Pollack HM, Kressel HY: Magnetic resonance imaging of the prostate. Magn Reson Q 6(1):1–16, 1990.

44. Bezzi M, Kressel HY, Allen KS, Schiebler ML, Altman HG, Wein AJ, et al.: Prostatic carcinoma: staging with MR imaging at 1.5 T. Radiology 169:339–346, 1988.

45. Rifkin MD, Zerhouni EA, Gatsonis CA, Quint LE, Paushter DM, Epstein JI, et al.: Comparison of magnetic resonance imaging and ultrasonography in staging early prostate cancer. N Engl J Med 323(10):621–626, 1990.

46. Ritter MA, Messing EM, Shanahan TG, et al.: Prostate-specific antigen as a predictor of radiotherapy response and patterns of failure in localized prostate cancer. J Clin Oncol 10:1208–1217, 1992.

47. Lightner DJ, Lange PH, Reddy PK, Moore L: Prostate specific antigen and local recurrence after radical prostatectomy. J Urol 144:921–926, 1990.

48. Kaplan ID, Cox RS, Bagshaw MA: Prostate specific antigen after external beam radiotherapy for prostate cancer: followup. J Urol 149:519–522, 1993.

49. Killian CS, Yang N, Emrich LJ, et al.: Prognostic importance of prostate-specific antigen for monitoring patients with stages B2 to D1 prostate cancer. Cancer Res 45:886–891, 1985.

50. Partin A: Rate of change of serum prostate specific antigen (PSA) after radical prostatectomy distinguishes local recurrence from distant metastases. American Urologic Association Annual Meeting, May 1993.

51. Rodwell JD, Alvarez, VL, Lee C, et al.: Site-specific covalent modification of monoclonal antibodies: in vitro and in vivo evaluations. Proc Natl Acad Sci USA 83:2632–2636, 1986.

52. Lopes AD, Davis WL, Rosenstrauss MJ, Uveges AJ, Gilman SC: Immunohistochemical and pharmacokinetic characterization of the site-specific immunoconjugate CYT-356 derived from antiprostate monoclonal antibody 7E11-C5. Cancer Res 50:6423–6429, 1990.

53. Abdel-Nabi H, Wright GL, Gulfo JV, Petrylak DP, Neal CE, Texter JE, et al.: Monoclonal antibodies and radioimmunoconjugates in the diagnosis and treatment of prostate cancer. Semin Urol X(1):45–54, 1992.

54. Neal CE, Baker MR, Texter JH: Prostate imaging with antibodies. Appl Radiol 21:39–46, 1992.

6

The Use of Tumor Markers
in Prostate Cancer

David W. Keetch, M.D., and Gerald L. Andriole, M.D.

INTRODUCTION

Because metastatic prostate cancer is without cure, the best hope for decreasing the mortality rate from the disease is to detect tumors that are still confined to the prostate gland. The conventional digital rectal examination is notoriously insensitive at detecting cancer at early stages, with up to 70% of cases advanced beyond the prostate at the time of diagnosis. Development of serum tumor markers that allow the early detection, improved staging, and monitoring of response to therapy have done much to aid clinicians caring for patients with this disease. Serum prostatic acid phosphatase (PAP) was the first serum marker for prostate cancer; more recently, serum prostate-specific antigen (PSA) has been identified. These tumor markers are extremely useful in the early diagnosis, staging, and monitoring of therapy for patients with prostate cancer. In this chapter, we review the clinical roles that these markers play in the diagnosis and management of this common disease.

PROSTATIC ACID PHOSPHATASE

The acid phosphatases are a group of nonspecific enzymes that hydrolyze phosphate esters to inorganic phosphates in an acidic environment. Acid phosphatases are found in the majority of human tissues, including platelets, granulocytes, osteoclasts, liver, spleen, kidney, brain, lung, skeletal muscle, and prostate.[2-5] There are five different isoenzymes, each of which has a different substrate specificity and distinct immunochemical properties. The acid phosphatases produced by the prostate are collectively referred to as "prostatic acid phosphatase." Prostatic acid phosphatase is composed principally of isoenzyme 2 and, to a lesser degree, isoenzyme 4. These isoenzymes are found in greatest concentration in the prostate but are also produced by granulocytes, spleen, and pancreas. For this reason, other disease processes (Table 1) may also lead to elevation of serum PAP.[6-9] PAP is composed of two identical subunits and has a molecular weight of 100,000 kdal.[10] It is rapidly cleared from the serum, with a calculated half-life ranging from 0.5 to 2.5 hours.[11,12] PAP is produced by the epithelial cells lining the prostatic acini and is secreted directly into the prostatic ductal system. Under normal conditions, very little is found in the serum. The PAP level is 500 to 1,000 times higher in prostatic fluid than in the serum of other tissues of patients with normal prostates.[2,13] In patients with abnormal prostates, however

Prostate Cancer, pages 95–112 © 1994 Wiley-Liss, Inc.

TABLE 1. Possible Causes of Prostatic Acid Phosphatase Elevation

Polycythemia vera
Granulocytic leukemia
Neutrophilia
Thromboembolism
Thrombocytopenia
Gaucher's disease
Osteosarcoma
Pancreatic cancer

(benign prostatic hyperplasia, prostatitis, prostatic infarction, or prostate cancer), serum PAP may be significantly elevated.[7,14–18] This is most likely due to disruption of the basal cell layer and basement membrane of the prostatic acini with back leakage of PAP into lymphatics and capillaries.

Kutscher and Wolbergs[19] were the first investigators to define the relationship between acid phosphatase and the prostate by demonstrating high concentrations of this substance in human ejaculate. Gutman and associates[20] subsequently reported a high concentration of acid phosphatase in both prostatic tissue and bony metastasis from prostate cancer. In 1938, Gutman and Gutman[18] found that 11 of 15 (73%) patients with metastatic prostate cancer but only 1 of 85 (1.2%) men with nonprostatic disease had an elevated serum acid phosphatase level. For nearly 50 years, serum PAP has been used extensively in the clinical management of patients with adenocarcinoma of prostate.

Assays for Prostatic Acid Phosphatase

The initial assays for acid phosphatase measured the enzymatic activity necessary to hydrolyse an added substrate. The patient's serum is incubated with an organic substrate and the timed release of phosphate is measured to assess the acid phosphatase activity. L-tartrate has been used to increase the specificity of the enzymatic assay, as it inhibits the prostatic iso-

enzymes of acid phosphatase with minimal inhibition of other tissue isoenzymes.[21,22] Specificity has also been increased by the discovery of substrates that were preferentially hydrolyzed by PAP and not by other acid phosphatases. Of these substrates, thymolphthalein monophosphate appears to have the greatest specificity for PAP and is the one most commonly used.[13]

In 1975, Foti and associates[23] introduced an immunologically specific radioimmunoassay for human PAP. Antiserum is produced by immunizing rabbits with purified PAP from prostatic fluid. This antibody to PAP is then absorbed to a fixed surface, allowing rapid and accurate separation of the antibody–antigen complex.[24] This radioimmunoassay is considered to be more sensitive than the traditional enzymatic assay in the detection of PAP.

Monoclonal immunoradiometric assays (IRMA) for PAP employ two monoclonal antibodies directed at different epitopes on the PAP molecule. It was hoped that the monoclonal antibodies would significantly enhance the measurement of serum PAP, but when compared to other methods, IRMA is as good but not significantly better than the other available assays.[25] Counterimmunoelectrophoresis has also been used to measure serum PAP.[26]

Specimen Collection for Acid Phosphatase Determination

It is exceedingly important that samples collected for PAP determination be handled properly. Prompt separation of clot from serum is essential, as both platelets and leukocytes contain acid phosphatase. Failure to expeditiously separate these two components may cause a falsely elevated PAP by both the enzymatic and immunologic assays.[27] Once collected, samples should be stored on ice, as enzyme activity rapidly decreases at room temperature.[28]

Acid phosphatase concentrations have been shown to exhibit diurnal variation.[29,30] Deviations from the baseline value of up to 70% have been reported.[31] For this reason it is felt that serial PAP determination may provide a more accurate assessment of the clinical situation when compared to a single value.

Various forms of prostatic manipulation have been shown to alter serum PAP concentration. The effect of digital rectal examination was reviewed by Brawer and associates,[32] showing 16% of patients having a transient increase in serum PAP after rectal examination. Prostatic massage, urethral catheterization, cystoscopy, and prostate biopsy have also been shown to increase serum PAP.[33,34] For this reason, samples for PAP determination should be obtained before or 48 to 72 hours after any examination or procedure involving the prostate.

Detection by Prostatic Acid Phosphatase

Initially there was considerable enthusiasm that PAP would be useful for the early detection of prostatic carcinoma. It rapidly became apparent, however, that enzymatic acid phosphatase lacked the sensitivity necessary to detect early prostate cancer. Sullivan and associates[35] and Nesbit and Baum[36] reported that only 10% to 20% of patients with clinically localized prostate cancer had abnormal acid phosphatase levels. Measuring the L-tartrate inhibitable fraction of serum acid phosphatase is not more sensitive for the early detection of prostate cancer when compared to total serum acid phosphatase.[37]

Initial studies comparing the traditional enzymatic assays to radioimmunoassays (RIA) showed that the RIAs were more sensitive for the early detection of prostate cancer. Foti and associates[24] reported that of 113 patients with prostate cancer, 33% with stage A, 79% with stage B, 71% with stage C, and 92% with stage D cancer had an elevated serum PAP level by RIA compared to only 12% with stage A, 15% with stage B, 29% with stage C, and 60% with stage D as determined by the Roy enzymatic assay. Other studies also suggested that RIA assays were superior to enzymatic assays in detecting early prostate cancer.[38,39] Subsequent investigations, however, have failed to confirm the superiority of the RIA assay. Williams and colleagues[40] compared three different RIAs with the Roy enzymatic assay in 180 patients, of whom 70 had varying stages of prostate cancer. No difference in specificity was found between the two different types of assays. Currently there is no data to support the use of serum PAP as a primary screening test for prostate cancer.

PAP in Staging Prostate Cancer

The original work by Foti and associates[24] demonstrates a direct correlation between serum PAP elevation and extent of disease. Clinically the enzymatic assays have been useful in predicting stage, while the RIA–PAP levels have not been helpful in this regard. Bahnson and Catalona[41] reported on 96 patients, 19 (20%) of whom had a PAP value in the upper one-half of the reference range. Sixteen of these 19 patients (84%) had extracapsular extension or positive pelvic lymph nodes. Of the 77 men with an enzymatic serum PAP value in the lower one-half of normal range, only 41 (53%) had either pathologic stage C or D1 disease. Five of six (83%) patients with an elevated serum PAP value by the Roy enzymatic assay had pathologic stage C or D1 disease. Work by Oesterling et al.[42] showed that among 275 patients undergoing pelvic lymph node dissection and radical prostatectomy, all patients with an elevated serum enzymatic PAP had either extracapsular disease or lymph node metastasis. Whitesel and associates[43] established the so-called "stage D_o" of prostate cancer. Of 343 patients who underwent pelvic lymph node dissection during treatment of prostate cancer, 25 were found to have a persistently elevated serum enzymatic PAP preoperatively. Fifteen of these 25 patients (60%) had metastases to the pelvic lymph nodes. In the patients with positive lymph nodes followed for a minimum of two years, 10 of 12 (83%) developed bone metastases. In the patients with an elevated enzymatic PAP and negative lymph nodes followed for a minimum of two years, 5 of 7 patients (71%) developed bone metastases. They concluded that a persistently elevated serum enzymatic PAP in patients with prostate cancer indicates subclinical metastases.

With the advent of serum PSA testing, many authors believe serum PAP testing is not routinely necessary. Stamey and Kabalin[44] compared serum PSA to PAP in 230 untreated prostate cancer patients and found serum PSA to be more sensitive for all stages of disease. Burnett and associates[45] reported on 460 men, 21 (4.6%) of whom had elevations of serum enzymatic PAP. All 19 men with elevations who were fully evaluated proved to have either positive bone scans, extraprostatic disease, PSA greater than 100 ng/ml, positive lymph nodes, or positive seminal vesicles. In 17 of the 21 (81%) men, however, advanced disease was detected by either abnormal digital rectal examination or PSA alone. Serum enzymatic PAP provided unique information in only four cases (0.9%) of the entire study population.

Based on these findings, many institutions no longer recommend serum enzymatic PAP in the staging of prostate cancer, especially if the serum PSA is less than 10 ng/ml.

PAP in Monitoring Disease Treatment and Progression

Huggins and Hodges were first to report that serum acid phosphatase levels decrease after antiandrogen therapy for prostate cancer.[46] A decrease in serum PAP of 50% or more indicates a partial response to treatment. If the serum PAP level falls to the normal range after treatment, it is considered a favorable prognosis for a prolonged response.[47] A normal serum PAP level after treatment does not signify an absence of cancer. An increasing level of serum PAP after treatment indicates disease progression. Serial testing to document the increase is necessary. Most authors feel that even though serum PAP is useful in predicting response and monitoring disease progression, serum PSA is a more appropriate means of following patients. Thus, most patients with prostate cancer are serologically monitored only with PSA testing.

Serum PAP: Summary

Serum enzymatic prostatic acid phosphatase currently plays a limited role in the diagnosis and management of prostate cancer. The sensitivity and specificity of this tumor marker are far too low for it to be used as a screening test for prostate cancer. The only current role for PAP testing (using the enzymatic assay) may be in staging patients with clinically localized disease, although some authors question the legitimacy of PAP in this setting, especially if the serum PSA is less than 10 ng/ml. Serum PSA testing has nearly completely supplanted serum PAP testing in most aspects of prostate cancer diagnosis, staging, and management.

PROSTATE-SPECIFIC ANTIGEN

Prostate-specific antigen is rapidly becoming the most widely used tumor marker in oncology (Table 2). PSA was first described by Hara and associates in 1971[48] in the seminal plasma. It was purified by Wang and associates[49] in 1979 from prostatic tissue. Wang and coworkers[50] subsequently demonstrated that the PSA found in seminal plasma is immunologically and biochemically identical to that isolated

TABLE 2. Possible Clinical Uses of Serum PSA Testing

1. Early detection of prostate cancer
2. Calculation of PSA density
3. Calculation of PSA slope
4. Staging of prostate cancer
5. Monitoring prostate cancer after therapy

from the prostate gland. PSA was then detected in the serum and found to be the same as that isolated from the prostate.[51] It was once thought that PSA is produced only by the prostate, but evidence is accumulating that it may be produced by other body tissues[52] and in females with renal cell carcinoma.[53]

PSA is a kallikrein-like serine protease that is produced by the epithelial lining cells of the prostatic acini and ducts. Functionally, it is thought to liquify the seminal coagulum by proteolysis of the predominant protein component. It has been demonstrated to be present in the serum of men with both benign and malignant prostatic conditions. Numerous factors interact to determine serum PSA concentration (Table 3). PSA is a single-chain glycoprotein that is 93% amino acids and 7% carbohydrates.[54] Structurally, it is a monomer with 240 amino acid residues and four side chains. The molecular weight of PSA is approximately 34,000 daltons with isoelectric points ranging from 6.8 to 7.2.[55] The complete gene that encodes for PSA is found on chromosome 19 and has been found to comprise about 6 kilobases. Two major

TABLE 3. Factors that Determine Serum PSA Concentration

Number of viable normal prostatic epithelial cells
Number and differentiation of neoplastic prostatic epithelial cells
Hormonal milieu
Architectural integrity of the prostate
Location of malignant prostatic epithelium—intraprostatic or metastatic
Rate of clearance

transcription initiation sites have been identified.[56] The half-life of PSA in the serum is between 2.2 and 3.3 days.[57,58]

PSA Assays

PSA is measured by RIA methods. Three commercially produced kits are currently available in the United States. The Pros-Check RIA kit (Yang Laboratories, Bellevue, WA) is a polyclonal double antibody RIA test based on the principle of competitive binding between radiolabeled antigen and free antigen in solution. In studies by Stamey[58] and Yang,[59] the upper limit of normal using this assay was calculated to be 2.5 ng/ml. The Tandem-R PSA assay (Hybritech, Inc., San Diego, CA) is a solid-phase, two-site IRMA that uses two noncompeting murine monoclonal antibodies to separate epitopes of the PSA molecule. PSA in the sample binds to a unique monoclonal antibody fixed on a plastic bead. Simultaneously, a separate distinct epitope of the PSA molecule is detected with a second radiolabeled mouse monoclonal antibody in solution. Myrtle and associates[60] have determined the normal range for PSA using this assay to be 0.0 to 4.0 ng/ml. The Tandem-R PSA assay is currently the most widely used serum PSA assay. Its lowest limit of detection is 0.1 ng/ml.

The Tandem-E PSA assay is similar to the Tandem-R assay in that it also uses two mouse monoclonal antibodies in a solid-phase two-site immunometric assay. The difference is that instead of using a radiolabeled antibody, the Tandem-E assay employs the enzyme alkaline phosphatase which is attached to the unbound antibody. No radioactive products are used.

The performances of the monoclonal (M-PSA) Tandem-R assay and the polyclonal (P-PSA) Pros-check assay were evaluated by Chan and associates[61] in patients with benign and malignant conditions of the prostate. Both assays performed comparably well both analytically and clinically. The P-PSA values were consistently 1.5 times higher than the M-PSA values. In patients with benign prostatic hyperplasia, 67% of P-PSA values and 63% of M-PSA values were elevated. In patients with cancer, 78% of the P-PSA values and 75% of the M-PSA values were elevated. The M-PSA assay was thought to be more specific at low serum levels. Graves and colleagues[62] also compared the Pros-Check polyclonal assay to the monoclonal Tandem-R assay but used independently purified antigen as the calibrator. They found the P-PSA assay yielded values 1.4 to 1.9 times higher than the M-PSA assay when using the kit calibrators. When the independent PSA calibrator was substituted for the respective kit calibrators, both assays yielded essentially identical results. They concluded that the differences in assay values arise from differences in the assigned values of the kit calibrators. Otherwise both assays had similar responses in the high and low range.

Ultrasensitive PSA Assay

Ultrasensitive assays allow for detection of extremely low serum concentrations of PSA when compared to the conventional PSA assays. The IMx PSA assay (Abbott Laboratories) has Food and Drug Administration approval and is commercially available. It is a microparticle enzyme immunoassay that correlates well with the radioimmunometric Tandem-R assay (Hybritech) with an overall correlation coefficient of 0.988.[63] The minimal detectable level of the IMx-PSA assay, however is 0.03 ng/ml. A third Hybritech assay employing chemoluminescent may have a lowest limit of detection of 0.004 ng/ml.[64] In each of eight postradical prostatectomy patients who later suffered clinical recurrence, the authors estimated that, using 0.1 ng/ml as an indication of recurrence, this assay provided between several

months' and three years' lead time. The ability to detect tumor recurrence or persistence sooner after radical prostatectomy using an ultrasensitive assay may allow for earlier institution of adjuvant therapy. It should be emphasized, however, that no study has demonstrated that earlier institution of adjuvant therapy results in improved cause-specific survival. Further clinical trials are needed to evaluate this issue.

PSA Specimen Collection

Blood samples for PSA determination are collected into a nonheparinized tube. The serum component is then separated. If samples are not tested within 24 hours, they should be stored at $-20°C$, as serum PSA values have been shown to decline if samples are stored at room temperature.[65] It is recommended that blood samples for serum PSA determination be obtained prior to any prostatic manipulation (Table 4).

The effect of digital rectal examination (DRE) on serum PSA levels was reported by Chybowski and associates.[66] The median change in serum PSA after DRE was 0.4 ng/ml compared to negative 0.1 ng/ml in a control group having a repeat PSA determination after no DRE. In 76% of the patients having a DRE, the repeat PSA value was greater than the initial PSA value. In the control group that had no intervening DRE, the repeat PSA value was greater than the initial PSA value in only 32% of cases. Only four patients, however, with an initial PSA value in the normal reference range (0.0 to 4.0 ng/ml) had a post-DRE value of greater than 4.0 ng/ml. The

---

TABLE 4. Possible Causes of Serum PSA Elevation

1. Prostatitis
2. Benign prostatic hyperplasia
3. Prostate cancer
4. Prostatic massage
5. Prostate biopsy
6. Urethral manipulation

---

change in serum PSA after DRE was independent of diagnosis (benign prostatic hyperplasia [BPH] cancer, prostatitis). Yuan and associates[67] examined the effect of DRE, prostate massage, transrectal ultrasonography, and transrectal needle biopsy on serum PSA levels in 199 men. DRE had no clinically significant effect on serum PSA levels either immediately or 90 minutes after the examination. Falsely increased PSA levels (to greater than 4.0 ng/ml) were found in 1 of 17 men (6%) following prostatic massage and in 3 of 27 men (11%) following ultrasonography. Transrectal needle biopsy caused an immediate increase in serum PSA in 92 of 100 men. The immediate increase varied from 1- to 52-fold with a mean of 5.91 times the baseline level. The degree of PSA increase was related to the number of biopsies: three or fewer cores caused a smaller initial increase in the serum PSA level than four cores or more. In 29 of 92 men (32%) followed weekly, the serum PSA levels did not return to baseline as expected from calculations using the published serum PSA half-life of 2–3 days. This occurs because there may be ongoing "leakage" of PSA from the prostate to the serum ("PSA fistula") for a few weeks after biopsy. The likelihood of a persistently elevated serum PSA level four weeks after transrectal biopsy was 7%. The authors recommend postponing PSA measurements for one week following DRE, prostatic massage, or prostatic ultrasound and at least four weeks after a prostate biopsy.

When collecting serum PSA samples, it is essential to know the patient's current and recent medications, as drugs that interfere with androgen production or action lower the serum PSA level. Specifically, luteinizing hormone-releasing agonists such as Lupron and Zoladex, antiandrogens such as Flutamide (Eulexin), and the 5-alpha reductase inhibitor, finasteride (Proscar), may profoundly lower serum PSA levels. For example, Proscar causes a 50%

decrease in serum PSA levels after six months of therapy.[68] There is some concern that these agents may delay the diagnosis of prostate cancer by artifactually lowering the serum PSA.

PSA in the Early Detection of Prostate Cancer

The ideal tumor marker for screening of malignant diseases should meet several essential criteria: the disease being searched for is common, an effective treatment is available, and the test is inexpensive and well accepted by the screening population. If all of these criteria are fulfilled, screening should result in decreased morbidity and mortality from the disease process. There is a great deal of controversy as to whether serum PSA and prostate cancer fulfill these criteria, although early experience has suggested that PSA testing detects pathologic organ-confined cancer in a high proportion of cases and that radical prostatectomy nearly always completely eradicates pathologically confined prostate cancer. There is an urgent need to evaluate PSA as a screening tool, as prostate cancer is the most common cancer among American males and is responsible for the death of about 35,000 men annually.[1] Using conventional diagnostic techniques (i.e., prostate biopsy if suspicious DRE or prostatic symptoms) only about 30% of prostate cancers are organ confined and curable by radical prostatectomy. To increase the proportion of new prostate cancers that are curable, either new, effective treatments for advanced disease are needed (unhappily, none are on the horizon) or intensive screening programs that detect disease before it leaves the prostate must be implemented.

Several large-scale studies have been conducted to evaluate the role of PSA as a screening tool for prostate cancer. Brawer and coworkers[69] measured serum PSA levels in 1,249 men over 50 years and performed digital rectal examination and ultrasound-guided prostate biopsy of those who had a PSA level of greater than 4.0 ng/ml. Serum PSA was elevated in 187 (15%) patients. Cancer was detected in 32 patients for an overall cancer detection rate of 2.6%. In a series of 1,002 men between 45 and 80 years, Labrie and associates[70] performed digital rectal examination, transrectal ultrasonography of the prostate, and serum PSA testing independent of each other. They found 57 cancers for an overall detection rate of 5.7%. Of these 57 patients with cancer, 46 (81%) had a serum PSA value of greater than 3.0 ng/ml. At a threshold of 3.0 ng/ml, the sensitivity and specificity of PSA were 80.7% and 89.6%, respectively. Catalona et al. screened 1,653 men aged 50 or older using serum PSA.[71] Patients with an elevated serum PSA value (≥4.0 ng/ml) underwent DRE and transrectal ultrasonography with biopsy if either or both of these tests were abnormal. The serum PSA was elevated, ranging from 4.0 to 9.9 in 107 (6.5%) patients. Of these patients, 19 of 85 (22%) were found to have cancer. Serum PSA levels were 10.0 ng/ml or higher in 30 (1.8%) patients. Twenty-seven of these patents underwent prostate biopsy, 18 (67%) of whom were found to have cancer. The overall detection rate in the study was 2.2%. The combination of serum PSA and DRE with transrectal ultrasonography if either is abnormal seems to provide a better method of detecting prostate cancer than DRE alone. These findings are supported by Cooner and associates,[72] who reported 1,807 patients who had been *referred* for prostate evaluation. Prostate biopsy was performed in 835 of these patients (46.2%) for an abnormal transrectal ultrasound. Cancer was found in 263 (14.6%) patients. Of the patients with an elevated serum PSA value by the Tandem-R assay, 35% were found to have cancer. Of those patients with a serum PSA value of above 10.0 ng/ml, 58% were found to have cancer. The combination of serum PSA plus DRE was found to be superior in predicting prostate cancer when compared to either modality alone.

Although serum PSA determination appears to be helpful in the early diagnosis of prostate cancer, it is by no means perfect. Of the cancers detected in the Cooner study,[72] 20% had a normal PSA value. Likewise, 21% of the cancers in the Catalona study[71] control population and 28% of the cancers reported by Labrie[70] had normal PSA values.

Other studies have called into question the utility of serum PSA as a screening tool for the early detection of prostate cancer. Wang and associates,[73] using the polyclonal PSA assay and a normal range of 0.0 to 5.0, found 70 of 99 patients (70%) with values ≥5.0 ng/ml to have prostate cancer. Only 1 of 46 patients (2%) with a serum PSA value of <5 ng/ml was found to have prostate cancer. However, 25 of these 99 patients (25%) were found to have BPH or prostatitis. They concluded that PSA is not a good test to detect early prostate cancer. Bhatti and colleagues[74] used the monoclonal assay to measure serum PSA levels in 118 patients with prostate cancer, 69 patients with BPH, and 69 control patients. Using 24 ng/ml as an arbitrary upper limit of normal, they calculated the sensitivity and specificity of PSA to be 68% and 32%, respectively. Only 6 of 69 patients (9%) with BPH had a serum PSA greater than 24 ng/ml; however, 66 of 72 (92%) of prostate cancer patients with a serum PSA value of greater than 24 ng/ml had stage D disease. In this study, levels of PSA in early prostate cancer were not statistically different from values of PSA in men with BPH. Stamey and associates[58] compared the levels of polyclonal PSA (normal <2.5 ng/ml) in 127 patients with untreated prostate cancer to 73 patients undergoing TURP for pathologically documented BPH. Serum PSA was elevated in 63 of 73 (86%) men with BPH compared to 122 of 127 (96%) men with prostate cancer.

Even though the exact role of serum PSA in early detection of prostate cancer is yet to be defined, several generalizations may be made. Overall, serum PSA can be useful in the earlier diagnosis of prostate cancer. Serum PSA in combination with digital rectal examination is superior to serum PSA alone in the diagnosis of prostate cancer. Men with prostate cancer may have a normal serum PSA. Screening for prostate cancer appears to be appropriate, as early stage disease is curable by currently available treatments, whereas advanced disease is not curable.

PSA Density

Although PSA is a specific marker for the prostatic epithelium, it is not a specific marker for prostate cancer. Attempts to increase the accuracy of PSA as a diagnostic tool for prostate cancer have led to the concept of PSA density (PSAD).[75] PSAD is calculated by dividing the serum PSA by the prostatic volume. The rationale for this concept is based on the premise that prostate cancer cells leak more PSA into the serum (3.5 ng/ml/gram tissue) than BPH cells (0.3 ng/ml/gram tissue).[58,76,77] Therefore, men with small prostates and an elevated serum PSA level are more likely to have prostate cancer, compared to men with a large prostate with an elevated PSA level. Benson and associates[75] reported the PSAD on 61 patients, 41 (67%) of whom had prostate cancer and 20 (33%) of whom had BPH. The mean PSAD for the cancer group was 0.581 compared to a mean of 0.044 for the BPH patients. In those patients with a PSAD of 0.1 or greater, 33 of 34 (97%) had cancer. All patients with a PSAD of greater than 0.12 had prostate cancer. All patients with BPH had a PSAD of less than 0.1 except for one (PSAD = 0.117). Benson and associates further evaluated the value of PSAD in patients with an intermediate elevation in serum PSA levels (4.1 to 10.0 ng/ml).[78] Of 533 patients with a PSA level between 4.1 and 10.0 ng/ml, 289 (54%) underwent prostate biopsy. Cancer was found in 98 (34%). PSAD was 0.297 ± 0.153 in the cancer group compared to 0.188 ± 0.104 in the no cancer group. This difference was statistically significant ($P < 0.0000$). They conclude that PSAD offers some advantages over PSA alone in the evaluation of patients with intermediate elevations of serum PSA values. Ramon and coworkers[79] also concluded that PSAD was superior to serum PSA values in the evaluation of men with intermediate levels of PSA elevation.

Not all investigators agree that PSAD is superior to PSA alone in screening for prostate cancer. Over the last four years, approximately 20,000 men over the age of 50 have been evaluated in PSA-based screening programs at Washington University. All patients have been evaluated with an initial PSA. The ROC curves for both PSA and PSA density for men undergoing screening program overlap, suggesting that PSAD does not help predict which patients have cancer any more than PSA alone. Analysis of various subgroups of men undergoing screening also fails to show any significant benefit of PSA density rather than PSA alone to guide the decision for biopsy. The failure of PSA density to be useful in the screening setting probably occurs because relatively few of the men in screening programs have significant BPH; therefore, these serum PSA levels are more reflective of the presence of cancer.

The role of PSAD has also been evaluated in the setting of patients who have a persistently elevated serum PSA value and an initial negative prostate biopsy.[80] In this setting, patients with a PSAD >0.15 had a 50% probability of having cancer detected on subsequent biopsy compared to a 9% probability if the PSAD was <0.15.

Overall, PSAD appears to offer a slight advantage compared to serum PSA values alone in distinguishing benign from malignant disease. This advantage may be most useful in those patients who have an intermediate elevation (4.0–10.0 ng/ml) in their PSA level. Further investigations are needed to delineate precisely the role of PSAD in the detection of prostate cancer.

PSA Slope

Using serum samples from the Baltimore Longitudinal Study of Aging, Carter and associates[81] evaluated the concept of PSA slope, that is, the rate of change of PSA. They retrospectively analyzed 54 men who had been followed for at least seven years prior to the diagnosis of BPH or prostate cancer. Three groups of men were studied: 18 who had biopsy-proven prostate cancer, 20 who underwent simple prostatectomy for BPH, and 16 who had no prostatic disease. Men in the study had undergone serum PSA testing every 2 to 2.5 years. The median PSA value [ng/ml(range)] at the time of histologic diagnosis differed significantly among the groups: 0.9 (0.2–6.7), 2.8 (1.1–6.5), and 7.7 (0.6–47.7), for control, BPH, and cancer patients, respectively. There was also a significant difference in the rate of PSA change between men with prostate cancer and BPH but not between men with BPH and normal prostates. The specificity of PSA slope above 0.75 ng/ml/year for distinguishing prostate cancer and BPH was 90% and for distinguishing between prostate cancer and controls was 100%. Work by Beatie and Brawer[82] suggests that an increase in serum PSA exceeding 20% per year may indicate cancer. These studies suggest that PSA slope may play an important role in the early detection of prostate cancer, as health-conscious individuals return for annual PSA determinations.

PSA Doubling Time

PSA is produced only by the prostatic epithelium and is related to the volume of prostatic epithelium that is present. Eval-

uation of the rate of change of PSA (slope) may provide a means of determining prostatic growth and improve the management of men with prostatic diseases. Stamey and Kabalin[83] estimated the PSA doubling time in men with stage A and B prostate cancer to be approximately two years based on PSA changes that occurred after diagnosis. From the Baltimore Longitudinal Study of Aging, Carter and associates[84] estimated PSA doubling time for men without prostate disease to be 74 ± 13 years at age 60 and 99 ± 13 years at age 85. Patients with BPH had PSA doubling times of 12 ± 5 and 17 ± 5 years at ages 60 and 85, respectively. In patients with prostate cancer, PSA change was found to have both a linear and an exponential phase. During the exponential phase, the doubling time for patients with local/regional and advanced/metastatic disease ranged from 1.5 to 6.6 (median, 3 years) and 0.9 to 8.5 (median, 2 years), respectively.

The estimation of prostatic growth rates by PSA slope may be helpful in distinguishing different prostatic diseases. Further studies are needed to define the potential use of prostatic growth rates in guiding the diagnosis and treatment of prostatic disease processes.

Serum PSA as a Staging Tool in Prostate Cancer

Serum PSA values increase with advancing stages of prostate cancer. Stamey et al.[76] have shown a direct correlation between serum PSA concentration and the volume of prostate cancer. Myrtle and associates[85] reviewed 553 patients with varying clinical stages of prostate cancer. The serum PSA value was elevated above 4.0 ng/ml in 63% of stage A, 71% of stage B, 81% of stage C, and 88% of stage D prostate cancers. Hudson and colleagues[86] have also demonstrated that serum PSA concentration is directly proportional to clinical stage of prostate cancer. However, these studies show considerable overlap among serum PSA values and the various clinical stages. Serum PSA is therefore insufficient to determine the clinical stage on an individual basis.

A critically important question is if serum PSA concentration is able to distinguish intracapsular, organ-confined prostate cancer from extracapsular and advanced disease. Partin and associates[87] have evaluated the role of serum PSA concentration in the pathologic staging of prostate cancer. They found that there was no difference in the serum PSA levels in 72 men with BPH and 185 men with organ-confined prostate cancer. Serum PSA levels were greater than or equal to normal (2.8 ng/ml) in 44 of 72 men (61%) with BPH compared to 101 of 185 (58.4%) with organ-confined disease, 71 of 87 (81.6%) with capsular penetration, 23 of 24 (96%) with seminal vesical involvement, and 53 of 54 (98%) with pelvic lymph node involvement. The mean serum PSA level for patients with prostate cancer increased as pathologic stage increased. The mean PSA values (ng/ml) for organ-confined disease, capsular penetration, seminal vesical involvement, and lymph node involvement were 5.6, 7.7, 23.2, and 26.2, respectively. Although serum PSA correlated well with pathologic stage, it was less useful to predict pathologic stage in individual patients. They concluded that this was because of the unpredictable contribution from the BPH component of the gland and and possibly the decreasing production of PSA by higher grade lesions. Stamey et al.[58] report that 27 of 37 (73%) patients having a serum PSA value of above 15 ng/ml (normal <2.8 ng/ml) had microscopic capsular penetration, while 16 of 37 (43%) of patients with a serum PSA in this same range had seminal vesical invasion. At the same time, nearly 50% of patients with a serum PSA concentration of <15 ng/ml also had microscopic capsular penetration. Ercole and associates[88] also report that

lower PSA values are less predictive of localized cancer. Of 46 patients with PSA levels of less than 10 ng/ml, 18 (39%) had extracapsular disease. Oesterling and colleagues[89] report that only 9 of 21 patients (43%) with a PSA >10.0 ng/ml and 3 of 8 patients (38%) with a PSA of >16 ng/ml had pathologically confined tumors. Based on these data, we can conclude that although serum PSA levels correlate well with tumor volume, PSA values are of limited value in accurately predicting preoperative pathologic stage in individual patients.

More recently, prebiopsy serum PSA levels have been used to guide the selection of patients for laparoscopic pelvic lymph node dissection. While the overall incidence of positive pelvic lymph node has fallen substantially among men participating in early detection programs (to less than 5%), patients with occult microscopic metastases would benefit appreciably if they could be identified by laparoscopy rather than by open lymphadenectomy. No specific level of PSA reliably predicts lymphatic metastases. In general, however, serum PSA levels above 40 ng/ml in patients with high Gleason score tumors (≥7) may be associated with positive nodes 30–50% of the time. This combination of PSA and tumor grade appears to offer an acceptable cut-off for laparoscopic node dissection.[103]

Chybowski and colleagues[90] evaluated the ability of serum PSA to predict bone scan findings in 521 cases of newly diagnosed prostate cancer. In 306 men with a serum PSA level of 20 ng/ml or less, only one had a positive bone scan (negative predictive value of 99.7%). No patient with a serum PSA value of <10.0 ng/ml had a positive bone scan. Further work by Oesterling and associates[91] has shown that of 852 cases of newly diagnosed cancer, only seven (0.8%) had a positive bone scan. One of the seven patients with a positive bone scan had a serum PSA value of

<10.0 ng/ml. Based on this, the authors calculated the false-negative rate to be approximately 1.5%. These studies would suggest that a staging radionuclide bone scan may be unnecessary in cases of previously untreated prostate cancer with a low serum PSA value.

PSA in Monitoring Therapy

After radical prostatectomy. PSA is essentially prostate specific. If all prostate tissue is removed at radical prostatectomy, the serum PSA concentration should approach female levels. The definition of an undetectable PSA level will vary depending on the laboratory and ranges from 0.0 to 0.6 ng/ml. Lange and associates[92] evaluated the relationship between early postoperative PSA concentration and clinical course. Of 36 patients with undetectable PSA levels, 92% remained without evidence of recurrence on follow-up ranging from 6 to 70 months. All 16 patients with a PSA concentration of >0.4 ng/ml had recurrence of disease. Paulson and Frazier[93] reported on 189 radical prostatectomies, dividing them into three groups: organ confined (94), specimen confined (54), and positive margins (41). By conventional criteria of recurrence, 2 of 94, 3 of 54, and 5 of 41, respectively, failed within a short follow-up period. Using a PSA value of 0.5 ng/ml (Hybritech assay) as a criterion for failure, however, 16 of 94, 24 of 54, and 29 of 41, respectively, failed. Performing random needle biopsies of the vesicourethral anastomosis in postradical prostatectomy patients, Lightner and associates[94] found cancer in 42% of patients with an elevated serum PSA value compared to no positive biopsies in 30 patients with undetectable PSA values. An undetectable serum PSA value has been reported, however, in a patient with recurrent cancer after radical prostatectomy.[99] Serum PSA, therefore, may not be 100% sensitive of predicting early cancer recurrence after definitive

therapy. Following mean PSA values after radical prostatectomy allows for earlier detection of failure or recurrence with the possibility of adjuvant therapy when tumor burden is small. Whether this early institution of adjuvant therapy translates into increased disease-free survival remains to be determined.

After radiation therapy. PSA has proven useful in determining local failure after radiation therapy. Stamey and associates[95] studied PSA levels in 183 patients following radiation therapy for prostate cancer. PSA levels decreased in 82% of patients during the first year. During the second year, however, PSA values continued to decrease in only 8% of patients. PSA values reached undetectable levels in only 11% of patients. Among 80 patients followed for more than one year, 51% had increasing and 41% stable PSA values. Kabalin et al.[96] performed prostatic biopsies on patients with rising PSA more than 18 months following radiation therapy. Ninety-two percent were found to have persistent cancer. Using 10.0 ng/ml as a cut-off value, 82% of patients with a value below 10 were found to have persistent cancer compared to all patients with a value above 10. Russell and associates[97] demonstrated that an increasing pretreatment PSA was associated with a decreasing chance of remaining a complete responder after definitive radiation therapy. If the serum PSA value was greater than 4 times normal, only 30% of patients were complete responders, compared to 82% if the pretreatment PSA was elevated to less than 4 times normal. If the serum PSA remained elevated beyond 12 months after therapy, 39% and 61% were clinical and chemical failures, respectively. These studies demonstrate that serum PSA levels correlate well with disease status in patients undergoing radiation therapy for prostate cancer.

After hormonal therapy. Numerous studies have documented the usefulness of PSA in monitoring patients with advanced prostate cancer. In 49 patients with stage D2 prostate cancer who underwent hormonal therapy, Ercole and associates[88] found a decrease in the median serum PSA value from 85 to 2.1 ng/ml in the 31 patients achieving a favorable long-term response. Those with an unfavorable response had a decrease from 160 to only 155 ng/ml. Miller and colleagues[98] reviewed 48 patients with stage D2 prostate cancer who underwent hormonal therapy. Patients whose posttreatment nadir PSA level decreased below 4 ng/ml had a significantly longer remission duration than those whose nadir PSA remained elevated. No cases were observed to progress while their serial posttreatment PSA levels continued to decrease or remained at a plateau after reaching the nadir. The time at which the PSA began to increase once the nadir had been reached predated clinical evidence of progression in all patients except two in whom PSA elevation and clinical progression occurred simultaneously. The mean lead time of the serum PSA predicting progression was 7.3 months. Table 5 lists the relative utility of various PSA parameters in predicting response to hormonal therapy in men with previously untreated prostate cancer.

The role of PSA in monitoring patients undergoing chemotherapy for hormone refractory prostate cancer has been nicely addressed by Kelly and associates.[104] They evaluated 110 patients with histologically confirmed metastatic hormone refractory prostate cancer treated on seven consecutive treatment programs. There were 108 patients who had four or more serial PSA determinations one week or more apart. A significantly larger median survival rate was observed for patients with a ≥50% decline in serum PSA (median not reached) when compared to patients with a less than 50% decline in serum PSA (median 8.6 months; $P = 0.0001$). A multivariate analysis demonstrated that serum PSA and the natural log of serum LDH were the variables most predictive of survival. This study further demonstrates the usefulness of serum PSA in monitoring the treatment of prostate cancer.

Urinary PSA

Only limited data exist on the subject of urinary PSA levels and their clinical relevance. Tremblay and associates[100] have demonstrated that low levels of urinary PSA can be reliably detected. De Vere White and colleagues[101] reported the urinary PSA values of patients after radical prostatectomy. Of the 18 patients having stage B or C disease who had positive margins, 15 (83%) had elevated urinary PSA levels compared to only 6 of 14 (43%) having elevated serum levels. Of the margin-negative patients, 72% had elevated urinary PSA levels while only 28% had elevated serum levels. Breul et al.[52] report that there is no difference in urinary PSA

TABLE 5. The Relative Utility of PSA in Predicting Response to Hormonal Therapy in Men with Previously Untreated Prostate Cancer

Parameter	Value Indicating Better Prognosis	Reliability Prognostication
Absolute pretreatment PSA	<300 ng/ml	Poor
3 month posttreatment PSA	<4.0 ng/ml	Excellent
6 month posttreatment PSA	<4.0 ng/ml	Very good
Nadir posttreatment PSA	<4.0 ng/ml	Very good
Rate of posttreatment PSA decline ("half-life")	Half-life <2 weeks	Good

values in patients with localized prostate cancer and BPH. Patients with metastatic prostate cancer had decreased levels compared to those with organ-confined cancer. Iwakiri et al.[102] have shown that the first voided urine sample better reflects local PSA production by the prostate than the midstream sample. The first voided urine PSA decreases significantly in response to radical prostatectomy but is still present even in surgically cured prostate cancer patients. They feel that urethral secretion of low levels of PSA persists after radical prostatectomy and that, overall, urinary PSA is highly unlikely to be clinically useful. Presently, the clinical implications of urinary PSA are uncertain and further extensive investigation is necessary to delineate what role, if any, it will play in the diagnosis and management of prostate cancer.

SUMMARY

Tumor markers play an important role in the diagnosis and management of prostate cancer. Prostatic acid phosphatase, once the mainstay of prostate cancer management, is now infrequently useful. The only remaining role for PAP is in defining stage D_0 prostate cancer. Serum prostate-specific antigen is currently the tumor marker of choice for evaluating men with known or suspected prostate cancer. Although not perfect, it is useful in the early diagnosis of prostate cancer. The combination of serum PSA testing and digital rectal examination as screening tools results in the detection of pathologically organ-confined disease in a high proportion of cases. The fact that PSA lacks high specificity for prostate cancer may be overcome by calculating the PSA density or PSA velocity. PSA values increase with advancing stages of prostate cancer although no particular level will precisely stage individual patients. One of the most useful roles of serum PSA is in monitoring treatment re-

sults and disease progression. Further studies will continue to define the exact role of PSA testing in patients with prostate cancer.

REFERENCES

1. Boring CC, Squires TS, Tong T: Cancer statistics: 1993, CA Cancer J Clin, 4:7–26, 1993.
2. Woodard HQ: Quantitative studies of beta-glycerophosphatase activity in normal and neoplastic tissues. Cancer 9:352–366, 1956.
3. Beckman L, Beckman G: Individual and organ-specific variations of human acid phosphatase. Biochem Genet 1:145–153, 1967.
4. Hanker JS, Hammarstrom LE, Toverud SU: Functional distribution of acid phosphatases in developing bones and teeth. J Dent Res 50:1502–1503, 1971 (abstr).
5. Lam KW, Li O, Li CY, et al.: Biochemical properties of human prostatic acid phosphatase. Clin Chem 19:483–487, 1973.
6. Henneberry MO, Engel G, Grayhack JT: Acid phosphatase. Urol Clin North Am 6:629–641, 1977.
7. Huber PR, Scholer A, Linder E, et al.: Measurement of prostatic acid phosphatase in serum and bone marrow: radioimmunoassay and enzymic measurement compared. Clin Chem 28:2044–2050, 1982.
8. Yam LT, Janckila AJ, Li CY, et al.: Presence of "prostatic" acid phosphatase in human neutrophils. Invest Urol 19:34–38, 1981.
9. Choe BK, Pontes EJ, Rose NR, et al.: Expression of human prostatic acid phosphatase in a pancreatic islet cell carcinoma. Invest Urol 15:312–318, 1978.
10. Heller JE: Prostatic acid phosphatase: its current clinical status. J Urol 137:1091, 1987.
11. Wadstrom J, Wenk M, Huber P: Serum half life of prostatic acid phosphatase. Urol Res 13:131–132, 1985.
12. Vihko P, Schroeder FH, Lukkarinen O, et al.: Secretion into and elimination from blood circulation of prostate specific acid phosphatase, measured by radioimmunoassay. J Urol 128:202–204, 1982.
13. Catalona WJ: Prostate Cancer. Orlando, FL: Grune & Stratton, pp 57–83, 1984.
14. Fair WR, Heston WDW, Kadmon D, et al.: Prostatic cancer, acid phosphatase, creatine kinase-BB, and race: a prospective study. J Urol 128:735–738, 1982.

15. Fleischman J, Catalona WJ, Fair WR, et al.: Lack of value of radioimmunoassay for prostatic acid phosphatase as a screening test for prostatic cancer in patients with obstructive prostatic hyperplasia. J Urol 129:312–314, 1983.

16. Vihko P, Kontturi M: Transient high serum prostate-specific acid phosphatase measured by radioimmunoassay in prostatic infarction. Scand J Urol Nephrol 15:213–214, 1981.

17. Van Cangh PJ, Opsomer R, De Nayer P: Serum prostatic acid phosphatase determination in prostatic disease. A critical comparison of an enzymatic and a radioimmunologic assay. J Urol 128:1212–1215, 1982.

18. Gutman AB, Gutman EB: "Acid" phosphatase occurring in serum of patients with metastasizing carcinoma of prostate gland. J Clin Invest 17:473–478, 1938.

19. Kutscher W, Wolbergs H: Prostata phosphatase. Hoppe-Seylers Z Physiol Chem, 236:237, 1935.

20. Gutman EB, Sproul EE, Gutman AB: Significance of increased phosphatase activity of bone at the site of osteoblastic metastases secondary to carcinoma of the prostate gland. Am J Cancer 28:485–495, 1936.

21. Yam LT: Clinical significance of the human acid phosphatases: a review. Am J Med 56:604–616, 1974.

22. Brendler CB: Isoenzymes in prostate cancer. In Ratliff TL, Catalona WJ (eds): Genitourinary Cancer: Basic and Clinical Aspects. Boston: Martinus Nijhoff, pp 1–18, 1987.

23. Foti AG, Herschman H, Cooper JF: A solid-phase radioimmunoassay for human prostatic acid phosphatase. Cancer Res 35:2446, 1975.

24. Foti AG, Cooper JF, Herschman H, et al.: Detection of prostatic cancer by solid-phase radioimmunoassay of serum prostatic acid phosphatase. N Engl J Med 297:1357–1361, 1977.

25. Davies SN, Gochman N: Evaluation of a monoclonal antibody-based immunoradiometric assay for prostatic acid phosphatase. Am J Clin Pathol 79:114–119, 1983.

26. Chu TM, Wang MC, Scott WW, et al.: Immunochemical detection of serum prostatic acid phosphatase: methodology and clinical evaluation. Invest Urol 15:319–323, 1978.

27. King EJ, Jegatheesan KA: A method of the determination of tartrate-labile prostatic acid phosphatase in serum. J Clin Pathol 12:85, 1959.

28. Ladenson JH: Nonanalytical sources of variation in clinical chemistry results. In Sonnenwirth AC, Jarett L (eds): Gradwohl's Clinical Laboratory Methods and Diagnosis, 8:1. St. Louis: CV Mosby, pp 149–192, 1980.

29. Doe RP, Mellinger GT: Circadian variation of serum acid phosphatase in prostatic cancer. Metabolism 13:445–452, 1964.

30. Brechman WD, Lastinger LB, Sedor F: Unpredictable fluctuations in serum acid phosphatase activity in prostatic cancer. JAMA 245:2501, 1981.

31. Schifman RB, Ahmann FR, Elvick A, et al.: Analytical and physiological characteristics of prostate-specific antigen and prostatic acid phosphatase in serum compared. Clin Chem 33:2086, 1987.

32. Brawer MK, Schifman RB, Ahmann FR, et al.: The effect of digital rectal examination and of serum levels of prostatic-specific antigen. Arch Pathol Lab Med 112:1110, 1988.

33. Hock E, Tessier RN: Elevation of serum acid phosphatase following prostatic massage. J Urol 62:488–491, 1949.

34. Marberger H, Segal SJ, Flocks RH: Changes in serum acid phosphatase levels consequent to prostatic manipulation or surgery. J Urol 78:287–293, 1957.

35. Sullivan TJ, Gutman EB, Gutman AB: Theory and application of the serum "acid" phosphatase determination in metastasizing prostatic carcinoma: early effects of castration. J Urol 48:426, 1942.

36. Nesbit RM, Baum WB: Serum phosphatase determination in diagnosis of prostatic cancer. A review of 1,150 cases. JAMA 145:1321, 1951.

37. Heller JE: Prostatic acid phosphatase: its current clinical status. J Urol 137:1091, 1987.

38. Cooper JF, Foti A, Herschman HH, et al.: A solid-phase radioimmunoassay for prostatic acid phosphatase. J Urol 119:388–391, 1978.

39. Murphy GP, Chu TM, Karr JP: Prostatic acid phosphatase—the developing experience. Clin Biochem 12:226–227, 1979.

40. Williams RD, Dombrovskis S, Dreyer J, et al.: Prostatic acid phosphatase by radioimmunoassay: sensitivity compared with enzymatic assay. JAMA 244:2071–2073, 1980.

41. Bahnson RR, Catalona WJ: Adverse implications of acid phosphatase levels in the upper range of normal. J Urol 137:427–430, 1987.

42. Oesterling JE, Brendler BC, Epstein JI, et al.: Correlation of clinical stage, serum prostatic

acid phosphatase and preoperative Gleason grade with final pathologic stage in 275 patients with clinically localized adenocarcinoma of the prostate. J Urol 138:92–97, 1987.

43. Whitesel JA, Donohue RE, Mani JH, et al.: Acid phosphatase: its influence on the management of carcinoma of the prostate. J Urol 131:70–72, 1984.

44. Stamey TA, Kabalin JN: Prostate specific antigen in the diagnosis and treatment of adenocarcinoma of the prostate: I. Untreated patients. J Urol 141:1070, 1989.

45. Burnett AL, Chan DW, Brendler CB, et al.: The value of serum enzymatic acid phosphatase in the staging of localized prostate cancer. J Urol 148:1832–1834, 1992.

46. Huggins C, Hodges CV: Studies on prostatic cancer. I. The effect of castration, of estrogen and of androgen injection of serum phosphatases in metastatic carcinoma of the prostate. Cancer Res 1:293–297, 1941.

47. Schacht MJ, Garnett JE, Grayhack JT: Biochemical markers in prostatic cancer. Urol Clin North Am 11:253–267, 1984.

48. Hara M, Koyanagi Y, Inoue T, et al.: Physiochemical characteristics of "y-seminoprotein", an antigenic component specific for human seminal plasma. J Legal Med 25:322–324, 1971.

49. Wang MC, Valenzuela LA, Murphy GP, et al.: Purification of a human prostate specific antigen. Invest Urol 17:159, 1979.

50. Wang MC, Valenzuela LA, Murphy GP, et al.: A simplified purification procedure for human prostate antigen. Oncology 39:1–5, 1982.

51. Papsidero LD, Wang MC, Valenzuela LA, et al.: A prostate antigen in sera of prostatic cancer patients. Cancer Res 40:2428–2432, 1980.

52. Breul J, Pickl U, Hartung: Prostate-specific antigen in urine and saliva. J Urol 149:302A, 1993.

53. Pummer K, Wirnsberger G, Purstner P, Stettner H, et al.: False positive prostate specific antigen values in the sera of women with renal cell carcinoma. J Urol 148:21–23, 1992.

54. Chu TM, Kawinski E, Hibi N, et al.: Prostate-specific antigenic domain of human prostate specific antigen identified with monoclonal antibodies. J Urol 141:152–156, 1989.

55. Wang MC, Kuriyama M, Papsidero LD, et al.: Prostate antigen of human cancer patients. In Busch H, Yeoman LC (eds): Methods in Cancer Research: Tumor Markers, 19:179–197, 1982.

56. Riegman PH, Vietstra RJ, van der Korput JA, et al.: Characterization of the prostate-specific antigen gene: a novel human kallikrein-like gene. Biochem Biophys Res Commun 159:95–102, 1989.

57. Stamey TA: Prostate specific antigen in the diagnosis and treatment of adenocarcinoma of the prostate. Monogr Urol 10:50, 1989.

58. Stamey TA, Yang N, Hay AR, et al.: Prostate-specific antigen as a serum marker for adenocarcinoma of the prostate. N Engl J Med 317:909, 1987.

59. Yang N: Pros-Check PSA: a double antibody radioimmunoassay for prostate-specific antigen. In Catalona WJ, Coffey DS, Karr JP (eds): Clinical Aspects of Prostate Cancer. New York: Elsevier, pp 172–178, 1989.

60. Myrtle JF, Klimley PG, Ovor LP, et al.: Clinical utility of prostate-specific antigen (PSA) in the management of prostate cancer. Advances in Cancer Diagnostics, Hybritech, Inc., 1986.

61. Chan DW, Bruzek DJ, Oesterling JE, et al.: Prostate-specific antigen as a marker for prostate cancer. Clin Chem 331:1916–1920, 1987.

62. Graves HCB, Wehner N, Stamey TA: Comparison of a polyclonal and monoclonal immunoassay for PSA: need for an international antigen standard. J Urol 144:1516–1522, 1990.

63. Vessella R, Noteboom J, Lange P: Clinical trial of an ultrasensitive prostate specific antigen (PSA) immunoassay. Clin Chem 37:1024, 1991.

64. Vessella RL, Noteboom J, Lange PH: Ultrasensitive PSA immunoassays: how low do we need to go? J Urol 149:355A, 1993.

65. Brawer MK: Laboratory studies for the detection of carcinoma of the prostate. Urol Clin N Am 17:4, 1990.

66. Chybowski FM, Bergstralh EJ, Oesterling JE: The effect of digital rectal examination on the serum prostate specific antigen concentration: results of a randomized study. J Urol 148:83–86, 1992.

67. Yuan JJJ, Coplen DE, Petros JA, Figenshau RS, et al.: Effects of rectal examination, prostatic massage, ultrasonography and needle biopsy on serum prostate specific antigen levels. J Urol 147:810–814, 1992.

68. Gormley GJ, Stoner E, Bruskewitz RC, et al.: The effect of finasteride in men with benign prostatic hyperplasia. N Engl J Med 327:17, 1992.

69. Brawer MK, Chetner MP, Beatie J, Buchner DM, et al.: Screening for prostatic carcinoma with prostate specific antigen. J Urol 147:841–845, 1992.

70. Labrie F, Dupont A, Suburu R, et al.: Serum prostate specific antigen as pre-screening test for prostate cancer. J Urol 147:846–852, 1992.

71. Catalona WJ, Smith DS, Ratliff TL, et al.: Measurement of prostate-specific antigen in serum as a screening test for prostate cancer. N Engl J Med 324:1156–1161, 1991.

72. Cooner WH, Mosley BR, Rutherford CL, et al.: Prostate cancer detection in a clinical urological practice by ultrasonography, digital rectal examination and prostate specific antigen. J Urol 143:1146–1154, 1990.

73. Wang TY, Kawaguchi TP: Preliminary evaluation of measurement of serum prostate-specific antigen level in detection of prostate cancer. Ann Clin Lab Sci 16:461–466, 1986.

74. Bhatti PG, Ray P, Guinan P: An evaluation of prostate specific antigen in prostatic cancer. J Urol 137:686–689, 1987.

75. Benson MC, Whang IS, Pantuck A, et al.: Prostate specific antigen density: a means of distinguishing benign prostatic hypertrophy and prostate cancer. J Urol 147:815–816, 1992.

76. Stamey TA, Kabalin JN, McNeal JE, et al.: Prostate specific antigen in the diagnosis and treatment of adenocarcinoma of the prostate. II. Radical prostatectomy treated patients. J Urol 141:1076, 1989.

77. Perrin P, Francois O, Maquet Bringeon JH, et al.: Circulating prostate-specific antigen in benign hypertrophy and localized cancer of the prostate: can PSA be considered as a screening examination for localized cancer? Progres en Urologie 2 (April), 1991.

78. Benson MC, Whang IS, Olsson CA, et al.: The use of prostate specific antigen density to enhance the predictive value of intermediate levels of serum prostate specific antigen. J Urol 147:817–821, 1992.

79. Ramon J, Billebaud T, Boccon-Gibod L, et al.: Prostate specific antigen density: a means to enhance detection of prostate cancer in men with elevated PSA levels. J Urol 149:300A, 1993.

80. Andriole GL, Telle WB, Coplen DE, Catalona WJ: PSA index (PSAI) as a predictor of prostate cancer (CaP) in men with persistent serum PSA elevation. J Urol 147:387A, 1992.

81. Carter HB, Pearson JD, Metter EJ, et al.: Longitudinal evaluation of prostate specific antigen levels in men with and without prostate disease. JAMA 267:2215–2220, 1992.

82. Beatie J, Brawer MK: Prostate specific antigen as the initial test in the early detection of carcinoma, results of the second year screening. J Urol 147:386A, 1992.

83. Stamey TA, Kabalin JN: Prostate specific antigen in the diagnosis and treatment of adenocarcinoma of the prostate. I. Untreated patients. J Urol 141:1070–1075, 1989.

84. Carter HB, Morrell CH, Pearson JD, et al.: Estimation of prostatic growth using serial prostate-specific antigen measurements in men with and without prostate disease, Cancer Res 52:3323–3328, 1992.

85. Myrtle JF, Kimley PG, Ivor LP, et al.: Clinical utility of prostate-specific antigen (PSA) in the management of prostate cancer. Adv Cancer Diag Hybritech, Inc., 1986.

86. Hudson MA, Bahnson RR, Catalona WJ: Clinical use of prostate specific antigen in patients with prostate cancer. J Urol 142:1011–1017, 1989.

87. Partin AW, Carter HB, Chan DW, et al.: Prostate specific antigen in the staging of localized prostate cancer: influence of tumor differentiation, tumor volume and benign hyperplasia. J Urol 143:747–752, 1990.

88. Ercole CJ, Lange PH, Mathisen M, et al.: Prostatic specific antigen and prostatic acid phosphatase in the monitoring and staging of patients with prostate cancer. J Urol 138:1181–1184, 1987.

89. Oesterling JE, Chan DW, Epstein JL, et al.: Prostate specific antigen in the pre- and postoperative evaluation of localized prostate cancer treated with radical prostatectomy. J Urol 139:766–772, 1988.

90. Chybowski FM, Keller JJL, Bergstralh EJ, et al.: Predicting radionuclide bone scan findings in patients with newly diagnosed untreated prostate cancer: prostate specific antigen is superior to all other clinical parameters. J Urol 145:313–318, 1991.

91. Oesterling JE: PSA leads the way for detecting and following prostate cancer. Contemp Urol, pp 60–81, February, 1993.

92. Lange PH, Ercole CJ, Lightner DJ, et al.: The value of serum prostate specific antigen determination before and after radical prostatectomy. J Urol 141:313–318, 1991.

93. Paulson DF, Frazier HA: Is PSA of clinical importance in evaluating outcome after radical surgery? J Urol 149:516–517, 1991.

94. Lightner DJ, Lange PH, Reddy PK, Moore L: Prostate specific antigen and local recurrence after radical prostatectomy. J Urol 144:921, 1990.

95. Stamey TS, Kabalin JN, Ferrari M: Prostate specific antigen in the diagnosis and treatment of adenocarcinoma of the prostate: III. Radiation treated patients. J Urol 141:1084, 1989.

96. Kabalin JN, Hodge KK, McNeal JE, et al.: Identification of residual cancer in the prostate following radiation therapy: role of transrectal ultrasound guided biopsy and prostate specific antigen. J Urol 142:326, 1989.

97. Russell KJ, Dunatov C, Hafermann MD, et al.: Prostate specific antigen in the management of patients with localized adenocarcinoma of the prostate treated with primary radiation therapy. J Urol 146:1046–1052, 1991.

98. Miller JI, Ahmann FR, Drach GW, et al.: The clinical usefulness of serum prostate specific antigen after hormonal therapy of metastatic prostate cancer. J Urol 147:956–961, 1992.

99. Takayama TK, Krieger JN, True LD, Lange PH: Recurrent prostate cancer despite undetectable prostate specific antigen. J Urol 148:1541–1542, 1992.

100. Tremblay J, Frenett G, Tremblay RR, et al.: Excretion of three major prostatic secretory proteins in the urine of normal men and patients with benign prostatic hypertrophy or prostate cancer. Prostate 10:235, 1987.

101. De Vere White R, Meyers FJ, Soares SE, et al.: Urinary prostate specific antigen levels: role in monitoring the response of prostate cancer to therapy. J Urol 147:947–951, 1992.

102. Iwakiri J, Grandbois K, Wehner N, et al.: An analysis of urinary prostate specific antigen before and after radical prostatectomy: evidence for secretion of prostate specific antigen by the periurethral glands. J Urol 149:783–786, 1993.

103. Danella JF, deKernion JB, Smith RB, Steckel J: The contemporary incidence of lymph node metastases in prostate cancer: implications for laparoscopic lymph node dissection. J Urol 149:1488–1491, 1993.

104. Kelly WK, Scher HI, Mazumdar M, Vlamis V, et al.: Prostate-specific antigen as a measure of disease outcome in metastatic hormone-refractory prostate cancer, J Clin Oncol 11:4, 1993.

7

Pathological Predictors of Prognosis in Prostate Cancer

Ruth D. Goldberg, M.B.B.Ch., and Francis H. Straus II, M.D.

INTRODUCTION

Prostate cancer is enigmatic in its natural history and highly unpredictable in its clinical course in the individual patient. Treatment of the tumor, while it remains confined to the prostate, offers the best chance of cure of the disease. However, the problem remains of differentiating those small prostate tumors requiring immediate therapy from those morphologically similar lesions that behave in a more indolent manner. This chapter highlights observable features that may be of value in predicting the possible outcome of the disease and thus influencing the therapeutic options offered to the patient.

PROSTATIC INTRAEPITHELIAL NEOPLASIA

The recognition of a "premalignant" lesion in the prostate is important in understanding the pathobiology of the disease. Prostatic intraepithelial neoplasia (PIN) is characterized by foci of epithelial cell proliferation and anaplasia of cells lining the prostatic ducts and acini.[1] A continuous layer of basal cells surrounds the intraacinar neoplastic cells, although frequently the basal layer is discontinuous or even absent in the higher grades. There is no new gland formation (Figs. 1 and 2). When reporting PIN, the terms low and high grade are now used. Low-grade PIN includes PIN I and most PIN II or mild to moderate dysplasia, while high-grade PIN encompasses PIN III or severe dysplasia and carcinoma in situ.

PIN is associated with invasive carcinoma in 87% of patients 60 years of age or younger. In patients older than 60 years, the association between PIN and BPH and between PIN and carcinoma is about equal.[2]

PIN was found mostly in the periphery of the gland in 68.8% of cases, while in 3.2% of cases it was identified in the inner region of the gland, which corresponds to the distribution of invasive cancer.[2] In each location where PIN was identified, carcinoma was closely associated, but remember most of these studies are retrospective, looking at tissue adjacent to known adenocarcinoma. In one study it has been suggested that patients with PIN may have an elevated PSA[3]; however, a more recent study by Ronnett et al.[4] found that high-grade prostatic intraepithelial neoplasia in and of itself does not account for elevated serum PSA levels. BPH may account for the raised serum levels of PSA in patients with high-grade PIN. More likely, because of the association between high-grade PIN

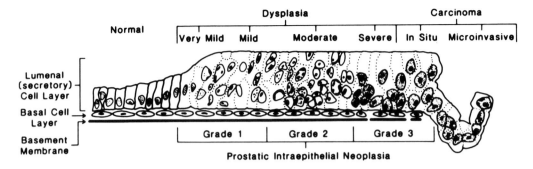

Fig. 1. Diagram of carcinogenesis in the human prostate. PIN grades I, II, and III correspond to mild dysplasia, moderate dysplasia, and severe dysplasia to carcinoma in situ, respectively. Invasion occurs when the basement membrane is disrupted. The dysplastic changes occur in the lumenal secretory cell layer. Reprinted with permission.[1]

and carcinoma, the likely source of the raised PSA is the undiagnosed malignancy.[4]

Although considered a preinvasive stage of cancer, its natural history and the interval between the discovery of PIN and the development of clinical carcinoma is unknown. In patients younger than 60 years of age, it is more frequently associated with invasive prostate cancer and if identified in biopsy or TUR material, the

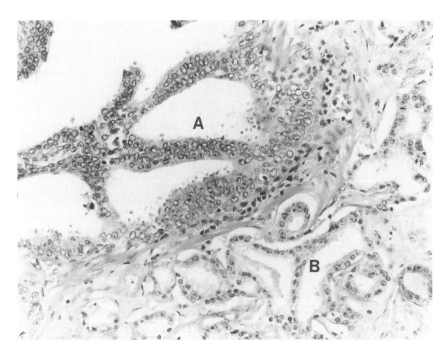

Fig. 2. Prostatic intraepithelial neoplasia and infiltrative adenocarcinoma. **A:** High-grade PIN with trabecular bars. **B:** Infiltrating Gleason grade 3 adenocarcinoma (×180).

patient may have invasive disease else-where or may develop carcinoma in the future.[5]

HISTOLOGICAL DIAGNOSIS OF PROSTATE CANCER

The histological diagnosis of prostate cancer is based on three major criteria, which are nuclear anaplasia, stromal inva-sion, and architectural disturbances.[5,6]

Nuclear anaplasia may be defined as nuclear enlargement, when compared to benign nuclei. There is some variation within a given tumor in the shape, size, and staining characteristics of the nuclei, but they are usually rather uniform. There is peripheral chromatin condensation and nuclear vacuolization. Within the nuclei, there is a large, centrally placed, promi-nent nucleolus, which is recognized as the most important criterion for the diagnosis of prostate cancer. Occasionally multiple nucleoli are visible.

If the nuclei are small and there is little anaplasia, the diagnosis of malignancy will be made on the basis of stromal invasion. Invasion may be into the stroma, peri-neural spaces, vascular or lymphatic chan-nels, periprostatic tissues, bladder neck, or the seminal vesicles. There can be no vas-cular or lymphatic invasion without stro-mal invasion, as the vascular spaces are only identified within the stroma. Another finding suggestive of stromal invasion is the absence of basal cells, which at the light microscopic level is recognized by the loss of acinar–stromal interaction, or by the ab-sence of high molecular weight keratin an-tibody staining cells at the gland periph-ery.

Architectural disturbances also charac-terize prostatic adenocarcinoma. The acini are lined by a single layer of cells. The acini are small, may be closely packed together, with a back-to-back arrangement, or may be large without convolutions, or there

may even be a mixture of large and small glands side by side. Fused glands, a cri-briform pattern, or sheets of cells without definite gland formation may also be en-countered.

Of the three criteria, the nuclear an-aplasia, especially with the prominent nu-cleolus, is the most important diagnostic criterion. Generally, several of these fea-tures are seen in malignancy, but at least one of the three criteria is necessary for the diagnosis of malignancy.

LOCATION AND SITE OF ORIGIN OF THE TUMOR

The prostate has been divided into three major regions: the peripheral zone (PZ), the central zone (CZ), and the transition zone (TZ).[7,80] McNeal maintains that the CZ is relatively resistant to the develop-ment of carcinoma, while most tumors oc-cur in the PZ (Fig. 3). Transurethral resec-tion specimens usually contain tumor

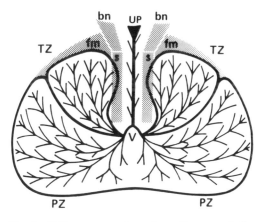

Fig. 3. Oblique coronal section diagram of the prostate, as viewed from the rectal surface, show-ing location of peripheral zone (PZ) and transition-al zone (TZ) in relation to proximal urethral seg-ment (UP), verumontanum (V), preprostatic sphincter (s), bladder neck (bn), and periurethral region with periurethral glands. The anterior fi-bromuscular stroma (fm) is shown as a shaded area. Reprinted with permission.[80]

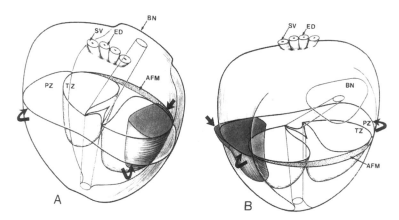

Fig. 4. Transparent three-dimensional images of prostate showing the two zones of cancer origin. A representative cancer in each zone is related to a transverse section through the mid-prostate (curved arrows). Transition zone cancer is on left (**A**) is viewed from the rectal surface and base. Cancer conforms to TZ boundary but invades anteriorly into anterior fibromuscular stroma (arrow). Nontransition zone cancer on right (**B**) is viewed from anterior surface. Cancer conforms to TZ boundary but invades posterolaterally through the capsule (arrow) in the region where nerve penetration of capsule is common. TZ = transition zone, PZ = peripheral zone, AFM = anterior fibromuscular stroma, B = bladder neck, ED = ejaculatory duct, SV = seminal vesicle. Reprinted with permission.[11]

derived from the TZ in association with BPH nodules. These TZ tumors have a slightly different morphologic appearance, in that the acini are wide, variable in size and contour, and are lined by tall columnar clear cells.[7]

The TZ appears to act as a barrier to the spread of non-TZ cancer. TZ tumors arise in the region more commonly associated with BPH and most stage A (TUR) cancers are TZ tumors (Fig. 4).

Histologic grade shows no clear relationship to invasion of the boundary between the transition and peripheral zones. There is no correlation either between the ability of a malignancy to penetrate this boundary and show capsular penetration. Most TZ tumors are less than 1 cc in volume and usually are composed of an admixture of Gleason grades 1 and 2, although some larger tumors may be classified as grade 3 and still retain the clear cell pattern.[8]

Other studies have confirmed the predominantly central or anterior location

(TZ) of stage A2 tumors, which are of low histological grade, as compared with clinical stage B lesions, which are mostly posterior and peripheral and of intermediate grade.[9] Clinical stage B tumors rarely infiltrate the central zone and if they do, the tumors are usually of large size. It is extremely uncommon to find a stage B lesion mostly centrally located.

TUMOR VOLUME

The assessment of tumor volume has been found to be of prognostic importance when assessing the likelihood of prostatic cancer dissemination.[8,10,11] There are several methods of assessing tumor volume. Clinical examination, transrectal ultrasonography, computerized tomography (CT) scanning, magnetic resonance imaging (MRI), and from the proportion of positive to negative chips in TUR specimens, or numbers of positive cores and greatest tumor length in cores from needle core biopsies. All of these methods are limited in their accuracy and the most reliable way is to examine the entire prostate by the method adopted by the Stanford group using computer-assisted morphometric analysis.[12] This method involves determining the cancer volume from an ink tracing on each glass slide of the exact tumor outline as seen at low magnification (40×); doubtful areas are confirmed at higher magnification. Sequential outline maps of the prostate and carcinoma are traced for each level of section through the gland at a magnification of 3×. A computer with a digitizing pad is used to determine the area of tumor at each level of sectioning. The volume is calculated as the sum of the tumor areas at different levels multiplied by the section thickness (0.3 cm). This figure is multiplied by a factor of 1.5 to correct for tissue shrinkage during processing.

If PIN is seen in a biopsy or TUR specimen, its extent is not predictive of tumor volume in the individual patient. Fourteen percent of patients with stage A1 tumors and minimal tumor volume had extensive high-grade PIN.[13] If radical prostatectomy follows a diagnosis of stage A1 disease by TUR, residual tumor was identified in 86% of the specimens, 24% of these being substantial in amount. Therefore it is recommended that tumor volume should not be assessed solely on the TUR specimen, nor can the amount of residual tumor in the radical prostatectomy specimen be predicted.[14]

When discussing the value of tumor volume as a prognostic factor, the site of the tumor plays an important role. In over 200 radical prostatectomy specimens studied by McNeal,[8] he observed that approximately 66% of TZ carcinomas, less than 4 cc in volume, were confined to the zone of origin. Non-TZ tumors of similar volume did not breach the boundary between the peripheral and transition zones. However, the frequency of boundary penetration was strongly related to tumor volume,

with 50% of non-TZ tumors larger than 4 cc penetrating the boundary.

In needle biopsies it is extremely difficult to estimate tumor volume. Dhom[15] suggested that an estimate of the percentage of the core involved may be of clinical use, albeit somewhat crude, and others are measuring greatest length of tumor involvement in a core biopsy as another indication of tumor volume.

McNeal et al.[11] established three important volume ranges in terms of the relationship of multiple morphologic features. Tumors less than 4 cc in volume were unlikely to have positive surgical margins, capsular penetration, seminal vesicle involvement, and lymph node metastases. Tumors with volumes greater than 12 cc were likely to have all of the above features. Those in the 4–12 cc range may or may not have any of these parameters. These relationships are expanded upon in the following paragraphs.

TUMOR VOLUME, CAPSULAR PENETRATION, AND SURGICAL MARGINS

These three entities are closely interrelated and correlate with prognosis of prostate cancer. The term capsular penetration refers to spread of the tumor beyond the prostatic capsule into the extraprostatic adipose tissue. The extent of penetration is defined in terms of the maximum length of tumor that has penetrated the capsule. The surgical margins are regarded as positive if tumor is seen touching the inked edge of the specimen. The presence of seminal vesicle involvement and lymph node metastases, which may be viewed as evidence of extraprostatic spread, are often linked with more distant dissemination.

In tumors greater than 12 cc in volume, capsular penetration is extensive, the surgical margins are positive, and lymph node and seminal vesicle involvement are usual.[11] However, in tumors less than 12 cc in volume, with positive margins, the correlation between tumor volume and extraprostatic spread is not as strong. In this situation, the positive margins represented areas where the capsule had been surgically resected or penetrated at the apex of the gland on the anterior surface, where the sphincter anatomy makes surgery with wide margins almost impossible.[16] It is not surprising that the commonest site for positive margins is the apex (48% of cases), followed by rectal and lateral surfaces, bladder neck, and superior pedicles (24%, 16%, and 10%, respectively).[16] Christensen et al.[9] had a 60% incidence of positive margins in clinical A2 lesions with capsular penetration as compared with 17% incidence of positive margins with clinical stage B tumors with capsular penetration. Most of the A2 tumors were located in the central/anterior portion of the gland, where the previous remarks regarding surgical difficulties pertain. Positive margins are related to tumor volume, but the relative risk is different in different anatomical locations and positive margins at some sites may prove to be less biologically significant.[16] If the tumor is seen entering the prostatic capsule, but there is no complete capsular penetration, then prognosis is unaltered.

In non-TZ tumors, 51% of tumors showed areas of complete capsular penetration, with 30% of these tumors showing greater than 1 cm length of penetration. The extent of capsular penetration and whether it was present or not was strongly correlated with tumor volume. Only 7% of cases with tumor volumes less than 4 cc had capsular penetration of greater than 1 cm, whereas capsular penetration was seen in 56% of cases with tumor volumes measuring 4–12 cc, and 86% of cases had capsular penetration when the tumor was greater than 12 cc in volume.[11]

With regard to positive margins in non-TZ tumors, the apex of the gland is the site most frequently involved, regardless of tumor volume or extent of capsular penetration. When examining radical prostatectomy specimens, the presence of a positive margin should be related to an adjacent area of capsular penetration, but remember the apex of the prostate strays into the urogenital diaphragm causing a diffuse, poorly identifiable capsule. McNeal et al.[11] noted that 47% of prostates with capsular penetration had positive margins, but only 24% had margin positivity within a demonstrated area of capsule penetration. In our experience the surgeon's resected margin is sometimes within the prostate gland parenchyma, thus showing a positive resected margin without capsular penetration.

Capsular penetration was seen in 25% of TZ tumors as compared with 51% of non-TZ lesions. The extent of capsular penetration in TZ tumors rarely exceeded 3 cm, while greater degrees of capsular penetration were more frequently seen in non-TZ tumors. TZ tumors, because of their anterior location and inferior growth (Figs. 3 and 4), are however associated with positive margins more frequently than non-TZ tumors. In TZ tumors with positive margins, the tumor volume in all cases was greater than 4 cc.[8,11]

The differences between TZ and non-TZ tumors are clear with respect to sites of capsular penetration, positive margins, and their potential for dissemination. Capsular penetration as an independent prognostic factor could not be confirmed; however, when its presence in conjunction with tumor volume and seminal vesicle involvement were assessed, capsular penetration was found to have a strong correlation with these other factors. Only when capsular penetration coincided with a positive margin was there some correlation with the clinical course of the disease.[17]

In many instances an accurate assessment of tumor volume is not routinely performed on surgical specimens. Mapping the extent of disease in the prostatectomy specimen may suffice as a semiquantitative evaluation and terms such as small volume, moderate volume, or large volume of tumor may roughly correspond to the three volume subdivisions used by McNeal et al.,[11] but without the difficulties of careful measurement and the use of computer programs to determine quantitative volume figures.

It may be that capsular penetration is simply a reflection of cancer volume, which in turn correlates highly with histologic grade. Histologic grade, tumor volume, and positive margins in areas of capsular penetration are closely correlated with the likelihood of tumor dissemination. In a recent multivariate analysis on radical prostatectomy specimens performed by Epstein et al.,[18] Gleason score was found to be the best predictor of progression, while the surgical margin was the only other variable that added to the prediction. Although an accurate preoperative assessment of tumor volume remains desirable for management of patients, the study shows that measurement of tumor volume in prostatectomy specimens need not be performed as part of the routine pathological analysis, as it does not add information beyond that of Gleason score and the status of capsular margins.

SEMINAL VESICLE AND LYMPH NODE INVOLVEMENT

Seminal vesicle involvement is thought to be a reflection of tumor progression and when taken into account with histologic grade and tumor volume, it is an important prognostic factor. Villers et al.[19] studied 243 radical prostatectomy specimens and found 22% of stage B (non-TZ) tumors were associated with seminal vesicle involvement, while no stage A (TZ) tumors had evidence of seminal vesicle involvement. It was observed that the frequency of seminal vesicle invasion increased progressively with volume, being found in 33% of cases with volumes between 4 and 12 cc, and in 82% of tumors larger than 12 cc in volume. The higher the tumor volume, the higher the chance of bilateral seminal vesicle involvement.

The seminal vesicles are located posterior and superior to the prostate (Fig. 4). The ejaculatory ducts run between the seminal vesicles and join the seminal vesicle ducts just inside the prostatic parenchyma, in the central zone. In a study by Villers et al.,[19] 43 of 47 tumors had seminal vesicle involvement. The tumor invaded through the midbase region to reach the sheath of the ejaculatory ducts within the prostate. In 42 cases, the ejaculatory duct sheath was breached and tumor penetrated its muscular wall. The tumor extension was found in continuity along the ejaculatory duct and into the muscular wall of the seminal vesicle. The portion of the seminal vesicle most commonly involved was the proximal segment, in the region closest to the junction of the seminal vesicle and vas deferens.

The same study[19] demonstrated that tumors 4 cc or less in volume were associated with nodal metastases in 1% of cases. In the group 4 to 12 cc, metastases were identified in 13% of cases, while tumors 12 cc or larger had evidence of nodal metastases in 46% of cases.

Seminal vesicle invasion and the percentage involvement by cancer of each seminal vesicle were related to cancer volume, histological grade, and the presence or absence of lymph node metastases. The frequency and extent of seminal vesicle invasion was strongly correlated with cancer volume, with minimal invasion noted in only 6% of the cases less than 4 cc. The relationship of seminal vesicle involvement to lymph node metastases was statistically significant, but cancer volume and histological grade were much stronger predictors of lymph node metastasis.[19]

In a recent multivariate analysis, Epstein et al.[20] evaluated the relationship between seminal vesicle invasion, tumor volume, grade, and margins with respect to prognosis. The results indicated that patients with seminal vesicle invasion had a significantly worse prognosis than those with capsular penetration. Gleason grade, surgical margins, and seminal vesicle invasion were all independent predictors of progression, whereas tumor volume was not. This finding is in contrast to that of Villers et al.[19] In addition, in those patients with seminal vesicle involvement, there was a trend for surgical margins and Gleason grade to predict progression, while with tumor volume, no such trend was observed.[20]

The general relationship of tumor volume to the extent of disease based on morphologic parameters is represented in Table 1.

HISTOLOGICAL GRADING AND ITS PROGNOSTIC IMPLICATIONS

The importance of histopathologic grading in malignant disease was recognized by Broders in 1926,[21] and since then numerous grading systems for prostate cancer have been devised. The problems of reproducibilty and reliability of each system have been obstacles to the general acceptance of any one system over another. In addition, the limitations inherent in the small sample of needle biopsies further compounds the difficulty of accurately grading prostatic adenocarcinoma.

In Broders's protocol,[22] the extent of tumor differentiation was of prognostic value in terms of patient survival. Mostofi uses both nuclear anaplasia and glandular differentiation in his classification.[23] His system provides good prognostic information on its own or in combination with clinical stage.[24,25]

In 1979 the National Prostate Cancer project recommended that the Gleason grading system[26,77] be used as the standard grading system, but in conjunction with one other system. Over the years the Gleason system has received increasing acceptance. The system utilizes a primary and secondary pattern and, in each, five different patterns. The sum of the two constitutes the grade or score (Fig. 5). With any system the problem of reproducibility exists. Gleason maintains that he can reproduce his diagnoses 80% of the time,[27] while others have reported only 70% reproducibility, even after tutoring from Gleason in using the grading system.[24] The Gleason grading system is also difficult to apply in needle biopsies and biopsy specimens[28] and there is sometimes a discrepancy between the initial biopsy grade and that given to the final specimen (TUR or radical prostatectomy)[37]; however, the practice of grading needle biopsies is still

TABLE 1. Pathology Predictors of Prognosis in Prostate Cancer[a]

	Tumor Volume ≤4 cc (%)	Tumor Volume 4–12 cc (%)	Tumor Volume ≥12 (%)
Capsular penetration (non-TZ/TZ)	7/0	56/25	86/≥86
Seminal vesicle involvement	6	33	82
Pelvic node involvement	1	13	46
Gleason >7	4–25	25–64	>64

[a]Reprinted from refs. 11, 19 with permission of W.B. Saunders Co.

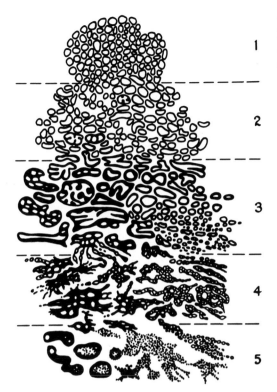

Fig. 5. Prostatic adenocarcinoma (histologic patterns). Standardized drawing for grading system. Reprinted with permission.[79]

performed because of its perceived prognostic value. A variation of one in the 2–10 range frequently occurs between different observers but seldom is the variation greater than this. Such small differences are often meaningless when deciding on the most optimal therapy.

Several papers have studied the relationship between the histological grade and clinical stage of the disease,[29,30] and these combined parameters with respect to long-term survival[31] and lymph node metastases.[32] In a study by Kramer et al.,[33] no patient with a tumor of Gleason score 2 to 4, irrespective of clinical stage, had lymph node metastases, whereas those tumors with scores of 8 to 10 showed 93% of patients had lymph node metastases. In contrast, Zincke et al.[32] found that 38% of pa-

tients with tumors of Gleason score 8 to 10 had lymph node metastases, but some patients with tumors of 2 to 4 Gleason score were found to have nodal metastases. Tumors with a score of 8 to 10 were associated with capsular penetration in 78% of cases and seminal vesicle involvement in 57% of cases.[32] When combining grade and clinical stage, the correlation with positive lymph nodes is strong, rather than using one or other parameter alone.[30,34]

The relationship between tumor volume, lymph node metastases, and histologic grade was studied in 209 patients with clinical stage A and B disease who had undergone radical prostatectomy.[10] A correlation was found between the amount (percent) of poorly differentiated tumor, which corresponded to a Gleason pattern 4 or 5, and nodal status. Positive nodes were found in 22 of 38 patients with more than 3.2 cc of Gleason pattern 4 to 5 (58%), while in tumors less than 3.2 cc of Gleason pattern 4 to 5, only 1 out of 171 patients had lymph node involvement. Gleason pattern 3, excluding the cribriform pattern, averaged 76% of the total tumor volume, in the smallest tumors, and it remained the dominant pattern at all larger cancer volumes (Fig. 6). Generally if the tumor volume is less than 2 cc, no Gleason pattern 4 or 5 will be found, whereas with tumors greater than 2 cc there is a steep increase in the amount of tumors with pattern 4 or 5. Lymph node metastases were identified with tumor volumes greater than 4 cc or when the amount of tumor pattern 4 or 5 was approximately 50% or greater. McNeal[8] noted that 44% of patients had positive lymph nodes when two-thirds of the tumor had Gleason patterns 4 or 5 and the tumor volume was greater than 4 cc.

As noted previously, Gleason grading is performed on biopsy and needle core specimens with some limitations. Foster and Mostofi advocate that grading biopsy specimens should be discontinued.[35] In

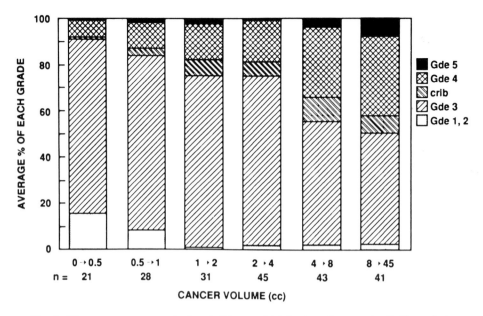

Fig. 6. Mean average percent of each Gleason histologic pattern and cribriform (intra-ductal) cancer compared between cancers in six consecutive volume ranges. The number of cases in each volume range is indicated at the bottom of each column. The volume scale is logarithmic. Reprinted with permission.[10]

Epstein's study[36] of 21 cases with a diagnosis of low-grade carcinoma, 15 of these were followed by radical prostatectomy. In 7 of 15 patients (47%), low-grade cancer was confirmed, but in addition multifocal higher grade tumor was found elsewhere in the specimen, or high- and low-grade tumor were identified in the initial area biopsied. Similar observations regarding the differences between initial and final grading have been recorded.[37] Possible explanations may include undergrading of the initial biopsy or sampling error. Patients with low-grade tumors, on biopsy, may have lymph node metastases. This may be due to tumor grade heterogeneity within a tumor nodule sampled or due to the presence of multifocal higher grade tumor. Therefore basing therapeutic recommendations on the grade of the biopsy specimen alone should be done cautiously.

Histologic grading in conjunction with other parameters such as clinical staging is useful in terms of predicting disseminated disease or survival. There is a good correlation between tumor grade and stage with regard to "survival" of populations of patients irrespective of therapy employed and which grading system is used.[31] However, these prognostic factors cannot be easily applied to therapeutic decisions for the individual patient.

Whatever grading system is used, good and bad tumors may be identified. In terms of reliability and reproducibility, the major disagreements will occur in the intermediate group of tumors, which usually accounts for the majority. Tumor grading does not reliably predict the lethal potential of a tumor in an individual patient, nor the responsiveness of an individual tumor to various forms of therapy.[35,38] Therefore, basing therapy on the grade alone should be cautioned and other parameters should be evaluated in addition to histologic grade when therapeutic options are being considered.

HISTOLOGIC SUBTYPES OF PROSTATIC CARCINOMA

There are several different histologic varieties of prostate cancer. They include small acinar prostatic adenocarcinoma, mucinous adenocarcinoma, prostatic duct adenocarcinoma (endometrioid), transitional and squamous cell carcinoma, basal cell carcinoma, adenoid cystic carcinoma, and neuroendocrine tumors.[6,39]

Kovi[40] and Srigley[41] described the entity of small acinar prostatic adenocarcinoma, but they do not comment if this tumor behaves differently from the usual prostatic adenocarcinoma. One would judge not, as they describe a typical midgrade adenocarcinoma of the prostate.

A diagnosis of mucinous adenocarcinoma of the prostate, as a distinct entity, should only be considered when at least 25% of the tumor resected contains lakes of extracellular mucin. These tumors behave slightly differently from the usual prostatic adenocarcinoma, in that they do not respond well to hormonal therapy and they have an aggressive clinical course.[42] In terms of histologic grading, they are mostly intermediate grade, with the cribriform pattern predominating in the mucinous areas. Other patterns seen in this tumor include tubular, papillary, or solid areas, and a signet ring pattern.[43]

Prostatic duct adenocarcinoma (endometrioid adenocarcinoma)[44,45] arises in the prostatic ducts in and around the verumontanum, which is of Mullerian origin, and has a predominantly papillary growth pattern, thus accounting for the name "endometrial." Epstein also recognizes solid, comedo, or ductal patterns of prostatic duct adenocarcinoma.[42] The tumor cells typically have a tall columnar appearance

with vacuolated cytoplasm.[39] The tumor is positive for PSA and PAP. This may be the sole tumor present, but more often they are admixed with regular acinar adenocarcinoma. This tumor is associated with a more aggressive clinical course, with the average survival being about 36 months, with most patients dying of disseminated disease. A small proportion of these tumors respond to estrogen therapy.[42]

Primary transitional cell carcinomas of the prostate account for 1% to 4% of all prostatic carcinomas.[46] The tumor behaves more like a transitional cell carcinoma of the bladder rather than a prostatic adenocarcinoma, with a 34% five-year survival for stage C disease.[47]

Neuroendocrine cells have been identified in normal, hyperplastic, and neoplastic prostate glands. These cells have been described in prostate cancer in three settings[48,49]: Firstly as a small cell carcinoma, secondly as a carcinoid or carcinoid-like tumor, and finally in ordinary prostate acinar adenocarcinoma, with the latter pattern being the most common. Approximately 10% of prostatic adenocarcinomas show marked neuroendocrine differentiation and up to 47% of adenocarcinomas show some neuroendocrine differentiation.[48]

Small cell carcinoma of the prostate is similar to small cell carcinoma of the lung in terms of their morphological appearances. These tumors are positive for neuron-specific enolase and chromogranin A, but negative for PSA and PSAP. They may produce ACTH, ADH, or other polypeptide hormones. Like small cell carcinomas elsewhere, these tumors pursue an aggressive clinical course, with average survival of less than one year. This histologic variant is in itself a poor prognostic factor. These tumors are also usually insensitive to hormone therapy.[50]

A pure carcinoid tumor of the prostate is yet to be reported; however, prostate adenocarcinomas evolving into carcinomas[51] or adenocarcinomas showing admixed carcinoid features have been observed.[52] No report of a carcinoid syndrome, associated with a prostatic tumor, is documented. Tumors with carcinoid features have been reported to be somewhat resistant to hormonal therapy.[51]

In regular adenocarcinoma with neuroendocrine differentiation, di Sant'Agnese did not find any correlation between grade and histologic pattern with respect to amount of neuroendocrine differentiation. Glezerson and Cohen,[53] in an extension of an initial study, found 41 of 82 cases with neuroendocrine differentiation. Adenocarcinomas that showed prominent neuroendocrine cells had a 35% two-year survival, and none were alive at six years. Those cases which were neuroendocrine negative had a 97% two-year survival, and 94% of patients were alive at six years. These results were highly significant ($P < 0.0001$), and would suggest that the presence of neuroendocrine cells is a poor prognostic indicator, but whether it is an independent factor better than histological grade, as claimed by Cohen et al.,[54] is yet to be confirmed by other investigators. Di Sant'Agnese makes the point that the greater the amount of neuroendocrine differentiation identified, the higher the histological grade.[55] The presence of neuroendocrine differentiation is important to document within any given tumor, as it, with other parameters like grade and stage, can be important prognostic factors when applied in combination.

NUCLEOLAR ORGANIZER REGIONS, NUCLEAR SURFACE AREA, AND ROUNDNESS

Nucleolar organizer regions (NORs) are loops of ribosomal DNA occurring in nucleoli of cells that ultimately process RNA genes. These are special areas in chromosomes 13, 14, 15, 21, and 22. These regions, which can be stained by silver techniques in paraffin-embedded tissue (AgNORs), have been found to correlate with S-phase activity, as determined by flow cytometry, and Ki-67 activity, which is an immunohistochemical marker of nuclear proliferation. There is a distinct difference in AgNOR staining as seen in benign prostatic hyperplasia and prostatic carcinoma, but only slight differences between PIN and prostatic carcinoma.[56] This technique cannot predict biologic aggressiveness once a prostatic cancer has developed, nor is it a useful prognostic indicator in established prostatic carcinoma.[54]

Nucleolar surface area, measured morphometrically, was studied by Tannenbaum et al. in 52 patients with localized and metastatic prostate cancer and compared with Gleason grade.[57] In patients without evidence of disease three or more years after radical prostatectomy, the initial biopsy demonstrated nucleolar surface areas that averaged 1.28 μm^2 (range 0.60–2.27 μm^2), in comparison with patients with metastatic disease or dying of cancer, whose average nucleolar surface area was 5.17 μm^2 (range 2.49–10.01 μm^2). With a single exception in 52 patients, progressive disease was associated with nucleolar surface area measurements larger than 2.40 μm^2. The initial measurement done on the needle biopsy compared closely with measurements done from the prostatectomy specimen. Only 56% of patients with aggressive disease ever had Gleason scores above 6. The investigators claim that this computer measurement is more objective and specific, when compared to light microscopic grading, in terms of predicting tumor progression. Using a nucleolar surface area of greater than 2.40 μm^2 was a good level to distinguish patients likely to have a poor prognosis. In addition, this level may be found in tumors of low Gleason score, which may indicate a more aggressive malignancy than the Gleason score would suggest. These observations, however, have not been confirmed by other studies.

The reported nuclear roundness factor for all malignant prostate cells was 1.059, compared with mean nuclear roundness factor of all normal epithelial nuclei, which was 1.034.[58] The nuclear roundness factor for tumors that had metastasized was 1.069, whereas the factor was 1.047 for tumors that had not metastasized 14 years after the initial diagnosis. No overlap was seen between the two groups; however, there was significant overlap of the Gleason grade between the groups. Determination of nuclear roundness factor requires computer-assisted image analysis, reading 300 randomized nuclei from each case.[59]

Although measuring nuclear roundness is objective, reproducible, and is applicable to individual patients, its usefulness is limited to low-grade tumors, and it is not reliably applicable to needle biopsies.[60]

DNA FLOW/IMAGE CYTOMETRY

DNA flow cytometry studies have provided clinical information shown to be important for the management of solid tumors, including prostate adenocarcinoma. Most low-grade prostate cancers are diploid tumors; however, these tumors may deviate from normal by the DNA content of one or two average chromosomes, without a distinct aneuploid peak being detectable by DNA flow cytometry.[61]

With increasing tumor grade, tetraploid tumors are recognized. Tribukait[62] postulated that prostate cancers progress from diploid to tetraploid to aneuploid to nontetraploid aneuploid. He found most stage A tumors were diploid, while stage C tumors were nontetraploid aneuploid. He observed that tumors may change ploidy with time and this was related to tumor grade and stage. Only 5% of those with diploid tumors at diagnosis died within four years, while approximately 30% of those with tetraploid tumors, 60% of those with single nontetraploid aneuploid cell line, and 75% of those with multiple aneuploid cell lines died within the same time period (Fig. 7).

While the frequency of local progression was not significantly different for those with diploid or nondiploid tumors, the

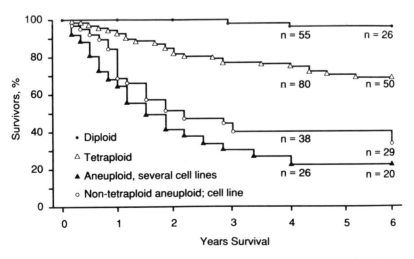

Fig. 7. Survival of patients with newly detected prostatic carcinoma of various DNA categories (n: number of cases). Deaths from intercurrent disease have been excluded. Reprinted with permission.[61]

time to local progression was significantly shorter for those with nondiploid tumors.[62] Only 3% of patients with diploid tumors developed metastases, as compared with 12% of those with tetraploid aneuploid or nontetraploid aneuploid tumors, during the four-year study period.

In patients who presented with lymph node metastases initially, diploid tumors were identified in 7% of patients, 17% had tetraploid tumors, 25% had nontetraploid aneuploid tumors, and 52% had multiple aneuploid stem cell lines.[63] From retrospective studies 70% or 80% of diploid tumors were identified in localized prostate cancer, but increasing numbers of nondiploid tumors were identified in later disease stages.[64]

Approximately 15% of diploid tumors can be expected to progress within five years, a finding that appears to be independent of stage.[65–67] In general the prognosis for nontetraploid aneuploid tumors is worse than for tetraploid aneuploid lesions. Aneuploid tumors of all stages have a higher risk of disease progression, at least until the disease becomes widely disseminated. However, once the tumor has metastasized, DNA ploidy is of no significance.

Most investigators agree that in carcinoma of the prostate there is a correlation between DNA ploidy pattern and conventional histologic grading. Abnormal DNA ploidy patterns were more frequently found in tumors of higher grade.[68] When comparing DNA ploidy with Gleason grading and clinical stage, as an independent variable, it does not add significantly to the grading system, although ploidy and Gleason score combined improves the predictive values of histological grade in higher stage lesions.[69] The addition of the DNA index to the Gleason score separated most of the patients with localized disease from those with advanced disease.[17] In this respect DNA analysis may be of particular value in distinguishing tumors with a higher malignant potential, which would on morphological grounds be graded as Gleason score 5, 6, or 7, which usually form the bulk of prostatic adenocarcinomas, and is the group in which it is most difficult to prognosticate.

DNA ploidy is correlated with tumor volume and stage of the disease. If a tumor has an abnormal DNA content, then the tumor volume is likely to be greater than 4 cc.[70]

DNA flow/image cytometry can provide useful prognostic information; however, the interpretation of the results should be standardized and the criteria, especially those used for DNA histograms of tetraploid and aneuploid tumors, needs to be defined. When assessing the results, they should be evaluated in conjunction with the clinical stage and histologic grade. DNA analysis, at the present time, cannot be regarded as an independent prognostic variable, nor should therapeutic decisions, in an individual patient, be based only on the presence of an aneuploid tumor.[71] The biological significance of ploidy status and prostate tumor progression remains uncertain, particularly with respect to individual prostate cancer, and therefore further study is required.

The S-phase fraction of a tumor, which indicates its proliferative activity, may be measured by several methods. Flow cytometry, AgNORs, and immunohistochemical staining with Ki67 and bromodeoxyuridine (BUDR) are some examples. These are all quantitative techniques and therefore are believed to be objective methods in assessing a tumor's biologic proliferative potential. The immunohistochemical tests are applied to tissue sections. Tumor sampling is important, particularly in prostate cancer, which is known for its tumor heterogeneity. Generally, the higher the S-phase fraction, the higher the tumor proliferation rate. There is also a correlation between high proliferation rates and Gleason score. In one study[72] utilizing

BUDR labeling, the average S-phase fraction of those tumors confined to the prostate was significantly different from those with metastases, perhaps giving some indication of the likely clinical course of the disease. However, 20% of patients with extensive local and metastatic disease had a lower value of proliferation activity, implying that BUDR labeling as a measure of S-phase fraction is not entirely reliable as an independent prognostic factor. Other studies will have to be done to determine the prognostic significance of S-phase fraction quantification in prostate cancer, relating specifically the S-phase fraction value to the clinical course of the disease.

CHROMOSOMES IN PROSTATE CANCER

Adenocarcinoma of the prostate, like adenocarcinoma arising in other solid tissues, contains chromosome rearrangements consisting mainly of deletions rather than translocations. Loss of chromosomes 1, 2, 5, and Y and gain of chromosomes 7, 14, 20, and 22 are recorded. Also rearrangements of chromosome arms 2p, 7q, and 10q are frequent.[73]

In one study of primary prostatic tumors, all had one chromosomal abnormality in common. There was a terminal deletion of the long arm of chromosome 10.[74,75] Others have also reported deletions of chromosome 10.[76]

Tumors that have clonal karyotypic abnormalities were associated with a shorter patient survival time (1.3 years) than those with normal or a mixture of normal and abnormal karyotypes (>3 years). This study suggested that the presence of clonal karyotypic changes in tumor cells may be an independent prognostic factor in prostate cancer patients.[77]

Loss of heterozygosity as reflected in allelic loss is a common event in prostate cancer, with the highest frequency being at 10q and 16q, as seen in 30% of tumors studied. It suggests that chromosomes 16q and 10q may contain sites of tumor suppressor genes important in the pathogenesis of some prostate cancers.[78]

Nevertheless, assignment of a single chromosomal aberration as the primary (specific) one responsible for prostate cancer development is difficult to assess at the present time and requires further investigation. In summary, the chromosomes that appear to be particularly involved in the genesis or promotion of primary prostate cancer include 2, 7, 10, and 16.[73]

CONCLUSION

The ability to identify malignant tumors that will behave in a particular manner is one of the most difficult issues to resolve and is the goal of current investigation. The need for detailed study is obvious; however, for the data to be meaningful, standardization of approach, definitions, and criteria need to be set.

There is no prognostic variable that may be independently applied. The clinical dilemma of which definitive therapy to recommend to an individual patient still remains. There are ever-increasing efforts to diagnose prostate cancer early. The nonpalpable lesions are difficult to assess in terms of tumor volume and representative histological grading, thus making prognostic predictions even more unreliable and problematic.

If in each case of diagnosed prostatic malignancy a histologic variant diagnosis, a tumor grade (if glandular adenocarcinoma), a rough estimate of tumor stage and volume (low, moderate, high), a determination of extraprostatic spread, and evaluation of regional node involvement are all recorded, a fairly accurate assessment of biologic virulence can be made. Unfortunately pathologic verification of extraprostatic spread and regional node involvement require added surgical procedures, and until MRI or other noninvasive techniques are perfected, that will remain the case. Certainly higher grade lesions, larger volume lesions, or carcinoma in younger men carry greater risk for clinically significant disease.

The question remains: Are there biologically virulent malignancies still lurking in the low grade and low volume of disease cases? It is in this group that use of more sophisticated evaluation such as DNA content, chromosomal abnormalities, proliferation potential, and nuclear roundness studies might be of use.

A routine approach is suggested for dealing with tissue from patients with prostatic adenocarcinoma.[35] If these proposals are adopted, valuable information may be obtained and, in time, allow for optimal selection of patients for definitive therapy.

No matter what therapeutic decision is arrived at and followed, continued surveillance with PSA determinations, bone scans, CT scans, and skeletal X-rays is necessary to monitor the patient's well-being and assess the use of further therapeutic modalities.

REFERENCES

1. Bostwick DG, Brawer MK: Prostatic intra-epithelial neoplasia and early invasion in prostate cancer. Cancer 59:788–794, 1987.

2. Kovi J, Mostofi FK, Heshmat MY, Enterline JP: Large acinar atypical hyperplasia and carcinoma of the prostate. Cancer 61:555–561, 1988.

3. Brawer MK, Lange PH: Prostate-specific antigen and pre-malignant change: implication for early detection. Ca Cancer J Clin 39:361–375, 1989.

4. Ronnett BM, Carmichael MJ, Ballentine Carter H, Epstein JI: Does high grade prostatic intraepithelial neoplasia result in elevated serum prostate specific antigen levels? J Urol 150:386–389, 1993.

5. Mostofi FK, Davis CJ, Sesterhenn IA: Pathology of carcinoma of the prostate. Cancer 70:235–253, 1992.

6. Mostofi FK, Sesterhenn IA, Davis CJ: Prostatic carcinoma: problems in the interpretation of prostatic biopsies. Hum Pathol 23:223–241, 1992.

7. McNeal JE, Redwine EA, Freiha FS, Stamey TA: Zonal distribution of prostatic adenocarcinoma. Correlation with histologic pattern and direction of spread. Am J Surg Pathol 12:897–906, 1988.

8. McNeal JE: Cancer volume and site of origin of adenocarcinoma of the prostate. Relationship to local and distant spread. Hum Pathol 23:258–266, 1992.

9. Christensen WN, Partin AW, Walsh PC, Epstein JI: Pathologic findings in clinical stage A2 prostate cancer. Relation of tumor volume, grade and location to pathologic stage. Cancer 65:1021–1027, 1990.

10. McNeal JE, Villers AA, Redwine EA, Freiha FS, Stamey TA: Histologic differentiation, cancer volume, and pelvic lymph node metastases in adenocarcinoma of the prostate. Cancer 66:1225–1233, 1990.

11. McNeal JE, Villers AA, Redwine EA, Freiha FS, Stamey TA: Capsular penetration in prostate cancer. Significance for natural history and treatment. Am J Surg Pathol 14:240–247, 1990.

12. Stamey TA, McNeal JE, Freiha FS, Redwine EA: Morphometric and clinical studies on 68 consecutive radical prostatectomies. J Urol 139:1235–1241, 1988.

13. Epstein JI, Cho KR, Quinn BD: Relationship of severe dysplasia to stage A (incidental) adenocarcinoma of the prostate. Cancer 65:2321–2327, 1990.

14. Epstein JI, Oesterling JE, Walsh PC: The volume and anatomical location of residual tumor in radical prostatectomy specimens removed for stage A1 cancer. J Urol 139:975–979, 1988.

15. Dhom G: Classification and grading of prostate carcinoma—recent results. Cancer Res 60:14–26, 1977.

16. Stamey TA, Villers AA, McNeal JE, Link PC, Freiha FS: Positive surgical margins at radical prostatectomy: importance of apical dissection. J Urol 143:1166–1173, 1990.

17. Pontes JE, Wajsman Z, Huben RF, Wolf RM, Englender LS: Prognostic factors in localized prostate carcinoma. J Urol 134:1137–1139, 1985.

18. Epstein JI, Carmichael M, Partin AW, Walsh PC: Is tumor volume an independent predictor of progression following radical prostatectomy? A multivariate analysis of 185 clinical stage B adenocarcinomas of the prostate with 5 years of followup. J Urol 149:1478–1481, 1993.

19. Villers AA, McNeal JE, Redwine EA, Freiha FS, Stamey TA: Pathogenesis and biological

significance of seminal vesicle invasion in prostatic adenocarcinoma. J Urol 143:1183–1187, 1990.

20. Epstein JI, Carmichael M, Walsh PC: Adenocarcinoma of the prostate invading the seminal vesicle: definition and relation of tumor volume, grade and margins of resection to prognosis. J Urol 149:1040–1045, 1993.

21. Broders AC: Carcinoma grading and practical application. Arch Pathol 2:376–381, 1926.

22. Broders AC: Epithelioma of the genito-urinary organs. Ann Surg 75:574–604, 1922.

23. Mostofi FK: Grading of prostate carcinoma. Cancer Chemother Rep, 59:111–117, 1975.

24. Harada M, Mostofi FK, Corle DK, Byar DP, Trump BF: Preliminary studies of histological prognosis in cancer of the prostate. Cancer Treat Rep 61:223–225, 1977.

25. Schroeder FH, Hop WCJ, Blom JHM, Mostofi FK: Grading of prostate cancer III. Multivariate analysis of prognostic parameters. Prostate 7:13–20, 1985.

26. Gleason DF: Histologic grading and clinical staging of prostatic carcinoma. In Tannenbaum M (ed): Urologic Pathology: The Prostate. Philadelphia: Lea & Febiger, pp 171–198, 1977.

27. Murphy GP, Whitmore WF: A report of the workshops on the current status of histologic grading of prostate cancer. Cancer 44:1490–1494, 1979.

28. Lange PH, Narayan P: Understaging and undergrading of prostate cancer. Argument for postoperative radiation as adjuvant therapy. Urology 21:113–118, 1983.

29. Gleason DF, Mellinger GT, and the Veterans Administration Cooperative Urological Research Group: Prediction of prognosis for prostatic adenocarcinoma by combined histological grading and clinical staging. J Urol 111:58–64, 1974.

30. Sharkey FE, Dusenberry DM, Moyer JE, Barry JD: Correlation between stage and grade in prostatic adenocarcinoma: a morphometric study. J Urol 132:602–605, 1984.

31. Sogani PC, Israel A, Lieberman PH, Lesser ML, Whitmore WF: Gleason grading of prostate cancer: a predictor of survival. Urology 25:223–227, 1985.

32. Zincke H, Farrow GM, Myers RP, et al.: Relationship between grade and stage of adenocarcinoma of the prostate and regional lymph node metastases. J Urol 128:498–501, 1982.

33. Kramer SA, Spahr J, Brendler CB, Glenn JF, Paulson DF: Experience with Gleason's histo-

pathologic grading in prostate cancer. J Urol 124:223–225, 1980.

34. Oesterling JE, Brendler CB, Epstein JI, Kimball AW, Walsh PC: Correlation of clinical stage, serum prostatic acid phosphatase and preoperative Gleason grade with final pathologic stage in 275 patients with clinically localized adenocarcinoma of the prostate. J Urol 138:92–98, 1987.

35. Foster CS, Mostofi FK: Prostate cancer: quo vadis? Hum Pathol 23:402–406, 1992.

36. Epstein JI, Steinberg GD: The significance of low grade prostate cancer on needle biopsy—a radical prostatectomy study of tumor grade, volume and stage of the biopsied and multifocal tumor. Cancer 66:1927–1932, 1990.

37. Mills SE, Fowler JE: Gleason histologic grading of prostatic carcinoma: correlation between biopsy and prostatectomy specimens. Cancer 57:346–349, 1986.

38. Mostofi FK: Grading of prostate cancer, current status. In Bruce AW, Trachtenberg J (eds): Adenocarcinoma of the Prostate. New York: Springer-Verlag, pp 29–46, 1987.

39. Mostofi FK, Sesterhenn IA, Davis CJ: A pathologist's view of prostatic carcinoma. Cancer 71:906–932, 1993.

40. Kovi J: Microscopic differential diagnosis of small acinar adenocarcinoma of the prostate. Pathol Ann 20:157–196, 1985.

41. Srigley JR: Small acinar patterns in the prostatic gland with emphasis on atypical adenomatous hyperplasia and small acinar carcinoma. Semin Diagn Pathol 5:254–272, 1988.

42. Epstein JI: Variants of prostatic adenocarcinoma. In: Prostatic Biopsy Interpretation. New York: Raven Press, pp 169–193, 1989.

43. Remmele W, Weber A, Harding P: Primary signet-ring cell carcinoma of the prostate. Hum Pathol 12:478–480, 1988.

44. Melicow MM, Pachter MR: Endometrial carcinoma of prostatic utricle (uterus masculinus). Cancer 20:1715–1722, 1967.

45. Melicow MM, Tannenbaum M: Endometrial carcinoma of uterus masculinus (prostatic utricle). Report of 6 cases. J Urol 106:892–902, 1971.

46. Nicolaisen GS, Williams RD: Primary transitional cell carcinoma of the prostate. Urology 24:544–549, 1984.

47. Epstein JI: Transitional cell carcinoma. In: Prostatic Biopsy Interpretation, Biopsy Interpretation series. New York: Raven Press, pp 205–217, 1989.

48. di Sant'Agnese PA, de Mesy Jensen KL: Neuroendocrine differentiation in prostatic carcinoma. Hum Pathol 18:849–856, 1987.

49. di Sant'Agnese PA: Neuroendocrine differentiation in human prostatic carcinoma. Hum Pathol 23:287–296, 1992.

50. Tetu B, Ro JY, Ayala AG, Ordonez NG: Small cell carcinoma of the prostate: immunohistochemical and electron microscopic studies of 18 cases. Cancer 59:977–982, 1987.

51. Stratton M, Evans DJ, Lampert IA: Prostate adenocarcinoma evolving into carcinoid: selective effect on hormonal treatment. J Clin Pathol 39:750–756, 1986.

52. Montasser AY, Ong MG, Mehta UT: Carcinoid tumor of the prostate associated with adenocarcinoma. Cancer 44:307–310, 1979.

53. Glezerson G, Cohen RJ: Prognostic value of neuroendocrine cells in prostate adenocarcinoma (abstr). J Urol 145:296, 1991.

54. Cohen RJ, Glezerson G, Haffejee Z, Afrika D: Prostate carcinoma: histological and immunohistochemical factors affecting prognosis. Br J Urol 66:405–410, 1990.

55. di Sant'Agnese PA: Neuroendocrine differentiation in carcinoma of the prostate. Diagnostic, prognostic and therapeutic implications. Cancer 70:254–268, 1992.

56. Sesterhenn IA, Becker RL, Avallone FH, et al.: Image analysis of nucleoli and nucleolar organizing regions in prostate hyperplasia, intraepithelial neoplasia and prostatic carcinoma. J Urogen Pathol 1:61–74, 1991.

57. Tannenbaum M, Tannenbaun S, DeSanctis PN, Olsson CA: Prognostic significance of nucleolar surface area in prostate cancer. Urology 19:546–551, 1982.

58. Diamond DA, Berry SJ, Jewett HJ, Eggleston JC, Coffey DS: A new method to assess metastatic potential of human prostate cancer: relative nuclear roundness. J Urol 128:729–734, 1982.

59. Epstein JI, Berry SJ, Eggleston JC: Nuclear roundness factor. A predictor of progression in untreated stage A2 prostate cancer. Cancer 54:1666–1671, 1984.

60. Clark TD: Nuclear roundness factor: a quantitative approach to grading in prostate cancer, reliability of needle biopsy tissue and effect of tumor stage on usefulness. Prostate 10:199–206, 1987.

61. Deitch AD, deVere White RW: Flow cytometry as a predictive modality in prostate cancer. Hum Pathol 23:352–359, 1992.

62. Tribukait B: Flow cytometry in assessing the clinical aggressiveness of genito-urinary neoplasms. World J Urol 5:108–122, 1987.

63. Tribukait B: Rapid flow cytometry of prostate fine needle aspiration biopsies. In Karr JP, Coffey DS, Gardner Jr W (eds): Prognostic Cytometry and Cytopathology of Prostate Cancer. New York: Elsevier, pp 236–242, 1988.

64. deVere White RW, Deitch AD, Tesluk H, Lamborn KR, Meyers FJ: Prognosis in disseminated prostate cancer as related to tumor ploidy and differentiation. World J Urol 8:47–50, 1990.

65. McIntire TL, Murphy WM, Coon JS, et al.: The prognostic value of DNA ploidy combined with histological substaging for incidental carcinoma of the prostate gland. Am J Clin Pathol 89:370–373, 1988.

66. Montgomery BT, Nativ O, Blute ML, et al.: Stage B prostate adenocarcinoma. Flow cytometric nuclear DNA ploidy analysis. Arch Surg 125:327–331, 1990.

67. Stephenson RA, James BC, Gay H, et al.: Flow cytometry of prostate cancer: relationship of DNA content to survival. Cancer Res 47:2504–2507, 1987.

68. Falkmer UG: Methodologic sources of error in image and flow cytometric DNA assessments of the malignancy potential of prostatic carcinoma. Hum Pathol 23:360–367, 1992.

69. Frankfurt OS, Slocum HK, Rustum YM, et al.: Flow cytometric analysis of DNA aneuploidy in primary and metastatic human solid tumors. Cytometry 5:71–80, 1984.

70. Jones EC, McNeal J, Bruchovsky N, deJong G: DNA content in prostatic adenocarcinoma. A flow cytometric study of the predictive value of aneuploidy for tumor volume, percentage Gleason grade 4 and 5 and lymph node metastases. Cancer 66:752–757, 1990.

71. Smith Jr JA: Management of localized prostate cancer. Cancer 70:302–306, 1992.

72. Nemoto R, Hattori K, Uchida K, et al.: S-phase fraction of human prostate adenocarcinoma studied with in vivo bromodeoxyuridine labelling. Cancer 66:509–514, 1990.

73. Sandberg AA: Chromosomal abnormalities and related events in prostate cancer. Hum Pathol 23:368–380, 1992.

74. Atkin NB, Baker MC: Chromosome study of five cancers of the prostate. Hum Genet 70:359–364, 1985.

75. Atkin NB, Baker MC: Chromosome 10 deletion in carcinoma of the prostate. N Engl J Med 312:315, 1985.

76. Lundgren R, Kristofferson U, Heim S, Mandahl N, Mitelman F: Multiple structural chromosome rearrangements, including del(7q) and del(10q), in an adenocarcinoma of the prostate. Cancer Genet Cytogenet 35:103–108, 1988.

77. Lundgren R, Heim S, Mandahl N, Anderson H, Mitelman F: Chromosome abnormalities are associated with unfavorable outcome in prostate cancer patients. J Urol 147:784–788, 1992.

78. Carter BS, Ewing CM, Ward WS, et al.: Allelic loss of chromosomes 16q and 10q in human prostate cancer. Proc Natl Acad Sci USA 87:8751–8755, 1990.

79. Gleason DF: Histologic grading of prostate cancer: a perspective. Hum Pathol 23:273–279, 1992.

80. McNeal JE: Normal histology of the prostate. Am J Surg Pathol 12:619–633, 1988.

8

Current Research Directions in the Radiation Therapy of Localized Prostate Cancer

Kenneth J. Russell, M.D.

DIVERSE OPTIONS/COMMON CONCERNS

At a recent prostate cancer symposium a medical oncologist delivered a lecture entitled "Rational Choices in the Treatment of Prostate Cancer." Only half in jest, the speaker both began and concluded his remarks by emphasizing the internal contradictions in the speech title. Indeed, to the outside observer, there appears to be little order in the way treatment decisions for localized prostate cancer are reached. There are strong proponents for surgical management, equally dogmatic supporters for radiation therapy, and a growing vocal minority advocating delayed, or so-called "expectant" therapy.

For the patient who has elected to receive radiotherapy, the abundance of treatment options even within this specialized discipline can be baffling. The current radiotherapy armamentarium for the treatment of localized prostate cancer includes a spectrum of technologies both old and new. Treatments vary in their use of atomic entities (neutrons, protons, photons), method of treatment delivery (external beam treatment versus implantation of internal radioactive seed sources), and complexity of treatment planning and delivery ("conformal therapy").

Within each of these broad categories, there are further refinements of machine capabilities, treatment technique, choice of isotope, and other technical aspects that account for substantive differences in treatment outcome. It is imprecise to talk generically about prostate radiotherapy treatment results or complications without specifying which of these alternative modalities and methods one is discussing. Even among the proponents of prostate brachytherapy there is debate as to the relative merits and toxicities of permanent versus temporary implants, implants designed as primary treatment versus those serving as boost treatment, or the value of each of the three commonly implanted radioactive isotopes.

Although a multitude of "new" radiotherapy options is available, they are all conceptually derived from a pair of common concerns: (1) how to improve radiation dose localization to the tumor and minimize the radiation injury to surround-

Prostate Cancer, pages 133–149 © 1994 Wiley-Liss, Inc.

ing normal organs, and (2) how to increase the absolute radiation dose to the tumor over what has been historically achievable with technologically simpler approaches.

These two issues are obviously quite closely related. Although the first concern is somewhat independent of the second, the second concern cannot be met without some success in mastering the first. Depending on clinical circumstances, one priority tends to take precedence over the other. For patients with aggressive tumors, the emphasis has been on achieving higher doses of radiation to the tumor, accepting the possibility of greater side effects in exchange for a more favorable survival outcome. For patients with historically favorable tumors, the emphasis has been less toward dose escalation and more toward dose localization, with the hope of causing less treatment morbidity.

Each of the current research directions in prostate radiotherapy addresses at least one of these two central priorities. Conformal therapy attempts to increase tumor dose through the use of closely tailored radiation fields matching the contours of the tumor volume, while employing complex field arrangements to avoid rectal, bladder, and bowel injury. Clinical trials involving particle irradiation have approached these issues from the perspective of: (1) improved radiation dose localization (protons) or (2) more "cytotoxic" radiation (fast neutrons). Improved dose localization is a driving force behind the renaissance of interest in interstitial prostate brachytherapy. Accordingly, these three different research approaches are reviewed here in reference to their common concerns so as to apply a conceptual framework to what otherwise may appear to be a series of unrelated investigations.

ENDPOINTS: OLD AND NEW

The two major endpoints by which the success of radiotherapy treatment has been historically measured have been patient survival and local tumor control. The historical survival results of conventional external beam photon radiotherapy for localized prostate cancer are well known and have been amply documented. For low-grade, incidentally discovered disease, patient survival following radiotherapy matches that of age-adjusted actuarial life tables for patients without prostate cancer.[1] For patients with organ-confined tumors, the 1987 NIH prostate cancer consensus conference concluded that both radiotherapy and surgery were equivalent treatments in terms of patient survival.[2] Even for patients with locally advanced stage C tumors, the five-year survival and freedom from relapse rates following radiotherapy have been in the range of 64–72% and 46–59%, respectively.[3]

Local control of stage A and B tumors by external beam photon radiotherapy, as measured by digital rectal examination (DRE), has been in the range of 97% and 77%, respectively, and approximately 67% for more bulky and aggressive primary lesions.[3]

These traditional endpoints have been challenged by endpoints involving prostate-specific antigen (PSA) or posttreatment biopsy results. Although patient survival will never be replaced as the ultimate arbiter of treatment success or failure, PSA is rapidly being embraced as a very powerful marker for following patients following radiotherapy, and is being increasingly used as a new yardstick for measuring radiotherapy treatment outcomes.[4,5] As an example of the disparity between old endpoints and new, it is known that the majority of patients with stage D1 tumors are subjectively and clinically well one year after completion of radiotherapy. However, 69% of these patients will have a persistently abnormal PSA at this time after treatment. Clearly these patients have persistent cancer, as the high frequency of subsequent clinical relapse demonstrates.[6]

Whether the PSA data is yielding new information about these patients or simply revealing to investigators what they already knew, albeit sooner after treatment, remains a point of some debate. However, as PSA data accrues on patients treated both with traditional techniques as well as some of the newer modalities, the decision as to whether progress in radiotherapy has been made will need to incorporate endpoints involving PSA.

Similarly, the systematic use of multiple transrectal biopsies to document tumor eradication by radiotherapy has revealed the inaccuracy of DRE for assessing local tumor control, and is rapidly replacing this endpoint as the most rigorous standard for determining local treatment efficacy. For patients with stage C tumors, the customary local tumor control rates (by DRE) of 67% may well be closer to 30% when posttreatment biopsy information is included.[7] The true incidence of postradiotherapy-positive biopsies on a stage-by-stage basis is still unknown, as there has been little uniformity in the process by which patients are selected to undergo biopsy. Nonetheless, progress in radiotherapy toward improved local tumor control will be increasingly judged by this endpoint.

CONFORMAL THERAPY

A primary motivation behind the interest in prostate conformal therapy is to increase the cure rates of patients with bulky primaries. These are the patients with stages B2 and C tumors in whom the 70% incidence of persistently positive biopsies has been documented following conventional radiation doses of 7,000 cGy. Achieving greater histologic tumor clearance will require dose escalation. Dose escalation, in turn, can only be achieved through sophisticated treatment planning and execution with strict attention to controlling normal tissue morbidity.

The potential for increased tumor control with increasing radiation dose is suggested by existing dose-control correlations that have been made for patients with stage C tumors.[8,9] Clearly, increasing the tumor dose beyond 7,000 cGy via conventional radiation fields is an unacceptable approach, as this has resulted in a disproportionate increase in normal tissue (primarily rectal) complications, when the tumor dose has been delivered through these simple portals.[9–11]

At its simplest, conformal therapy is just what it states: prostate radiation fields that conform to the shape of the prostate and seminal vesicles. At its most complex, conformal therapy integrates the disciplines of medical physics, radiation dosimetry, computer science, statistics and probability, radiology, and radiation oncology. How the concept has evolved from its simplest incarnation to its most complex requires a brief review of historical radiation fields as well as the general process of radiotherapy treatment planning and treatment delivery.

Conventional radiotherapy fields for prostate cancer involve standardized portal arrangements and field sizes. Historically, these arrangements were based upon clinical assessment of prostate dimensions by DRE and by the use of standard bony landmarks of the pelvis for the establishment of radiation field borders. Accordingly, a typical prescription for a prostate radiation field directed in an anterior and posterior direction would be to use a 7 × 7 to 8 × 8 cm square portal centered 1 cm superior to the symphysis pubis. For fields directed laterally through the pelvis, such a rectangular field was generally centered on the femoral neck.

Despite the availability of computerized tomography (CT) and more recently magnetic resonance imaging (MRI), these treatment plans are frequently still employed. The limitations of these standardized fields have been made very apparent when imaging studies delineating the volume and location of prostate and seminal vesicles have been superimposed on standard radiation portals. These investigations have demonstrated that patients' prostate volumes routinely exceed the volume that can be adequately treated by the small square radiation boost portals of prior years.[12,13] Even more current "scaled-up" standard prescriptions of field size and arrangement have also proved to be insufficient to adequately encompass the variation in prostatic dimensions for the individual patient.[14] A recent analysis of treatment "misses" has discussed strictly the location of the inferior edge of "standard" prostate field prescriptions relative to the position of the prostate apex. Analyzing just this single field edge, the investigators demonstrated that 25% of routine field prescriptions passed through the prostate apex, resulting in a "geographic miss" of a portion of the tumor.[15]

Traditional dosimetry of prostate radiation involves calculating doses to the prostate and adjacent organs through a single transverse plane of the patient. These doses, produced as a series of curves ("isodose curves") not unlike geographical contour lines on a topographical map, are superimposed on the patient's anatomy obtained from a transverse "slice" of the patient taken at the level of the central axis of the radiation field. The adequacy of coverage of the prostate, as well as the degree of radiation to bladder, rectum, and small bowel, is assessed at this single plane. Such treatment planning is referred to as "two-dimensional", as it ignores the reality of three-dimensional tumor and normal tissue *volumes*, and the variability in organ contours from one level to another.

Conformal therapy therefore differs from traditional treatment fields and dosimetry by: (1) contouring of treatment fields based on accurate delineation of individual patient anatomy and (2) treatment planning based on three-dimensional representations of the entire organ and tumor volumes. These two elements of treatment planning yield a high assurance that the tumor has been fully encompassed, and secondarily permit more customized shielding of adjacent bladder and rectum. An example of a conformal approach is shown in Figure 1, where radiation fields and dose contours are superimposed on coronally reconstructed pelvic CT data at multiple levels. With the state-of-the-art computer capabilities currently available, volumetric anatomy can be more fully reconstructed and displayed, in real time, from any perspective desired. Typically, the perspective chosen is that of the radiation beam's view (the so-called "beam's-eye-view" or BEV). An example of such a treatment display is shown in Figure 2. Such a planning system permits field arrangements to be selected from angles (or planes) that optimize what the physician and dosimetrist wish to accomplish with respect to tumor coverage and sparing of adjacent tissues. Small areas of radiation underdosing or overdosing are easily detected. With such unrestricted planning, some investigators have elected to routinely use six or eight radiation fields per patient as alternatives to more conventional four-field arrangements.

In addition to volumetric reconstructions, one can also now calculate what percentage of any anatomic structure is receiving any given percentage of the delivered radiation dose. One can use the rectum as an example of a dose-limiting organ where detailed information about dose is desired. It is a straightforward matter to determine for a given patient and a given treatment plan what percentage of the rectum has received 100% of tumor dose, what percentage of the rectum has received only 50% of the tumor dose, and so forth. This method of analyzing partial volumes of organs and partial radiation doses generates graphs known as dose–volume histograms (DVHs). These DVHs can be used for deciding between competing radiation

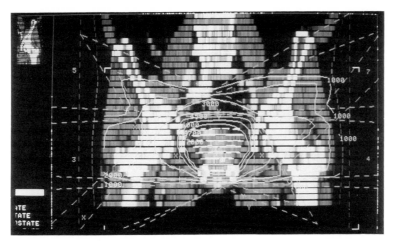

Fig. 1. Conformal radiotherapy dosimetry plan for prostate cancer. The dose contributions of radiation fields (diverging dotted lines) and dose contours (numbered by cGy dose) are superimposed on multiple cuts of coronally reconstructed pelvic CT data. The prostate, represented as a series of stacked "wire-loop" contours, can be seen at the center of the dose contour labeled 7,000 cGy. A total of eight fields were used, directed in three different planes.

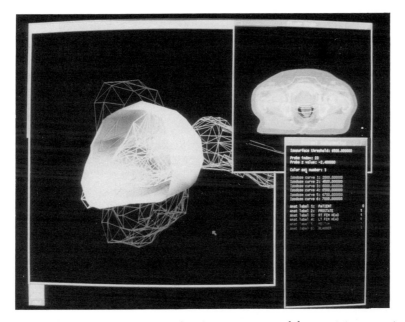

Fig. 2. "PRISM" radiation treatment planning program used for prostate cancer treatment at the University of Washington. The prostate is shown as a "wire-frame" volume, as are bladder (anterior), rectum (posterior), and left femoral head. The volume information is derived from CT imaging. The "eggshell" enclosing the prostate represents the summed doses from multiple radiation fields and is the volume of tissue that will receive 7,000 cGy. Real-time rotation of the perspective allows easy detection of geographic misses of tumor. It can be seen that this radiation plan has not included the entire seminal vesicles in the 7,000 cGy volume. The seminal vesical apex is seen protruding from the dose contour. The upper right panel shows conventional, single-plane transverse dosimetry plan taken through the prostate at the level of the femoral necks.

plans, by choosing the plan that ideally offers the most homogeneous dose profile for the tumor and the lowest dose profile for normal organs. DVH data will eventually permit refinement of mathematical models of radiation normal tissue complication probabilities. Such models exist today but are limited by the current paucity of truly quantitative clinical dose-response data for normal tisssue injury.[16–18]

Also germane to the concept of conformal therapy is the realization that sophisticated treatment planning requires sophisticated treatment delivery. Treatment of patients from oblique angles and planes requires precise positioning of the patient on a daily basis which, in turn, implies patient immobilization. Preliminary data on the use of custom body molds, immobilization "cradles," and similar devices has suggested a diminution in daily treatment variations compared to treatments delivered without such restraints. This results in greater treatment accuracy.[19] Such accuracy is a prerequisite to dose escalation efforts, as the delivery of higher tumor doses will require that the margin of radiation encompassing the tumor be made narrower so as not to deliver excessive dose to surrounding organs.

More recently, conformal therapy investigators have had to accept the reality that the prostate and adjacent rectum and bladder are not static in position. The prostate moves in response to physiological states of distension of both bladder and rectum, and this range of motion varies from patient to patient.[20] The definition of target volume may have to be further individualized based on the dynamics of prostate motion for the individual.

Therefore, a number of theoretical and procedural factors must be controlled in order to test the potential of conformal therapy in prostatic cancer. Some of these elements are within grasp and others remain problematic. This dichotomy is exemplified by the difficulties inherent in simply defining "the target volume." The anatomy of the prostate and seminal vesicles, in static relationship to the adjacent normal organs, is adequately visualized by current imaging modalities. However, the motion of the prostate, in response to the various physiological states described, remains incompletely characterized.

To date, pilot investigations have focused only on individual facets of conformal therapy. Treatment planning has received the most attention, either in the analysis of the above-mentioned uncertainties in target definition,[21] choosing between alternative treatment plans,[22] or in the development of intuitive and streamlined treatment planning systems that are suitable for routine use (as in the current NCI-sponsored Radiotherapy Planning Tools Project).

In terms of dose escalation, preliminary reports suggest that 7,400–8,040 cGy may be delivered to the prostate with minimal increases in normal tissue side effects.[23] To the extent that such doses yield improved local tumor control, this should ultimately translate to gains in patient survival, as local tumor failure has been directly correlated with the subsequent development of distant metastases.[24]

The NCI has recently formed a cooperative clinical research group composed of selected institutions with experience in prostate conformal therapy. The mandate for this group is the design and execution of large-scale phase II and phase III clinical trials exploring both the potential advantages and toxicities of conformal prostate radiotherapy compared with best conventional radiotherapy. This group will likely focus its attentions on the patients with locally advanced tumors, as previously defined.

Although conformal techniques have already demonstrated a favorable impact in diminishing the acute and delayed side effects of *conventional* radiation doses for patients with *favorable* tumors[25,26] its long-term value lies mainly in improving the treatment outcomes for those patients whose tumors have been historically refractory to radiation.

PROSTATE BRACHYTHERAPY

Brachytherapy of localized prostatic cancer is a concept whose popularity has waxed and waned, and is once more an area of active inquiry. The selective delivery of high doses of radiation to prostatic tumors by the implantation of radioactive seeds whose radiation penetrates only short distances has always been an appealing concept. To date, however, the initially high expectations for this treatment approach have not been realized and controversies abound surrounding its indications and success relative to conventional external beam irradiation. Within the radiation oncology community, opinions are sharply divided, largely due to the experience with older implant methods that appeared, at best, to yield comparable results to external beam treatment and, at worst, resulted in less local tumor control. Differences of opinion notwithstanding, there has been a renaissance of interest in brachytherapy due to a number of technological advances that offer the potential for improved results. This topic has recently been reviewed by the author elsewhere,[27] and a condensed synopsis of this review is presented here.

As was the situation with conformal therapy, progress in medical imaging and computer technology have permitted much of the technological gains in brachytherapy to be realized. Current high-resolution CT and real-time biplanar transrectal ultrasound permit a more accurate visualization of the prostate gland than the imaging capabilities of the 1970s, when the original technique of ^{125}I prostatic implantation was developed. The routine availability of these modalities has encouraged the development of transperineal implant techniques which appear to avoid the technical inaccuracies inherent in the traditional implants techniques, which were performed through an open surgical approach.

The sophistication and speed of current computerized radiation dose computations, in conjunction with fixed geometry perineal templates to percutaneously guide the placement of interstitial radioactive sources, now permit a realistic *pre-implant* calculation of doses to tumor and surrounding normal organs, and accurate deposition of the radiation sources in reproducible arrays.

Finally, understanding of the radiobiology of continuous low-dose irradiation has led to investigative use of more rapidly decaying isotopes than ^{125}I for the treatment of faster growing (higher grade) tumors for which iodine may have been a suboptimal radiobiological choice.

The great majority of the historical prostate implants were performed using radioactive iodine (^{125}I), using a technique first popularized at Memorial Sloan-Kettering Cancer Center (MSKCC).[28] This consisted of a formal retropubic exploration, pelvic lymph node sampling, and mobilization of the prostate gland from the deep pelvic fascia. Once the prostate was freed from the surrounding tissues, stainless steel trocars were inserted "freehand" into the gland, with spacing of the needles determined by dosimetry calculations that also specified the implant seed activity and the number of seeds required. ^{125}I seeds were deposited with obturators through the needles and into the prostate tissue at supposedly uniform spacing while the trocars were being withdrawn. This spacing was obtained either by ruler measurements as the needles were removed, or aided by semiautomatic implant devices that stored the seeds in cartridges and were calibrated to withdraw the needles incrementally as seeds were deposited.

The activity of ^{125}I required for an individual prostate gland was calculated by a nomogram also developed at MSKCC, and commonly known as "dimension averaging."[29,30] In this system, the total activity to be implanted was equal to the average of the three dimensions of the proposed implant volume multiplied by a proportionality constant unique to the isotope being used.

Multiple problems were inherent to the traditional implant procedure and the dosimetry of this era. With respect to the placement of the sources, the overwhelming problem was inhomogeneity of the implanted seeds. With respect to dosimetry, the problems related to the overly simplified and idealized nature of the nomogram. The original equation required modifications over time as experience showed that the single numerical constant initially employed to calculate the required amount of implanted activity proved inadequate for larger glands. Additionally, the end result of the dosimetric calculations was the calculation of a dose delivered to an *idealized* ellipsoid volume with the same average dimensions as measured *clinically* for the prostate. Two problems intrinsic to such a calculation were: (1) the actual shape of an individual's prostate rarely conformed to that of the idealized ellipsoid, and (2) the value of the calculated dose did not depend upon actual radiation source distribution. Accordingly, well- and poorly distributed implants could yield the same value for tumor dose.

A consequence of these procedural and dosimetric limitations was the potential for inadequate radiation doses to at least some portion of the tumor. Analogous to the situation with external beam treatment of the day, retrospective CT studies identifying the position of implanted seeds relative to prostatic tissue have confirmed the technical inadequacy of many of the original implants. Reconstruction of implant doses delivered to the prostate have revealed underdosing by as much as 40%.[31] Underdosing of tumors clearly had an adverse

impact on treatment outcomes, as documented in analyses studying the dose-response relationships of these implants.[24,32,33]

A detailed comparison of historical implant results with external beam results of the same era is beyond the scope of this discussion and has been reviewed elsewhere.[34] As a rough generalization, however, it appears that the traditional implant procedures, their procedural limitations notwithstanding, appeared equivalent to the historical results with external beam irradiation (*their* previously mentioned limitations notwithstanding) for low-stage and -grade tumors, but were inferior to external beam for local control of the higher stage and grade tumors.

Contemporary investigations in prostate brachytherapy are attempting to improve on the historical results by increasing the accuracy of source placement, employing modern treatment planning methods, and incorporating recent radiobiologic data. A clearer understanding of radiobiologic and physics principles has been critical in evaluating issues of tumor doubling time, dose-rate effects, and normal tissue toxicity. CT imaging and transrectal ultrasound technology permit accurate preimplantation determination of target volume and precision guidance of trocars percutaneously via the transperineal route without the need for surgical exposure. For permanent implants, these horizons have been further broadened by the availability of new high dose-rate permanent implant sources such as palladium-103 (^{103}Pd) which may be more effective against more rapidly dividing high-grade tumors. For removable implants, approaches using iridium-192 (^{192}Ir) have been aided by the arrival of a new generation of remote afterloading devices capable of precision conformal brachytherapy.

The treatment planning and dosimetry procedures for contemporary prostate brachytherapy are remarkably similar to the process involved in conformal therapy using external beam radiation. CT or trans- rectal ultrasound images of the prostate from base to apex are obtained at 0.5 cm increments and adjacent rectum and blad- der neck are identified. The contours of the prostate target volume, bladder neck, and rectum are entered into the dosimetry computer so that different arrangements of needles and source strengths can be con- sidered. Three-dimensional radiation dose distributions for prostate, rectum, and bladder are generated with the radiation variables adjusted to optimize the tumor dose relative to normal tissues.

The implant itself is done via one or more modifications of a closed procedure of transperineal percutaneous implanta- tion that was originally described in 1983.[35] When permanent sources are to be used, the implant is done on an outpatient basis, most frequently employing spinal anesthesia. Templates of various designs are positioned against the patient's peri- neum to guide the trocars along pre- defined paths. Most approaches employ real-time transrectal ultrasound imaging, which permits direct visualization of the needle position in reference to on-screen coordinates corresponding to the template design in use.

Needles that have been preloaded with alternating sources and absorbable spacers are then introduced through the appropri- ate template holes as dictated by the do- simetry plan. Alternatively, specialized needles unique to specific automated com- mercial applicator devices may be intro- duced in a similar manner. The prostate gland is a surprisingly mobile and distens- ible organ in the intact pelvis. Dynamic, real-time visualization during the needle insertion process is used to recognize and correct cephalad displacement, internal distortion, and rotation of the prostate.

Postimplant confirmatory dosimetry is performed by obtaining 1:1 scale CT im- ages of the prostate at 0.5 cm intervals from base to apex, and approximating the ultrasound volume study. If required, MRI imaging can be performed, as both the io- dine and palladium seed casings are non- ferrous (titanium). Images are scanned with both soft tissue and bone density windows in order to define the prostate volume on the soft tissue images and to accurately count the seeds on the bone density images. Isodose curves are then generated for each CT image, yielding a detailed analysis of implant quality.

As previously mentioned, both theoreti- cal and practical considerations have en- couraged the recent use of isotopes other than ^{125}I. The majority of the transperineal implants still employ ^{125}I because of its commercial availability, ease of handling with respect to personnel radiation expo- sure, and the familiarity with its use. ^{125}I has a half-life of 60 days, and delivers radi- ation at a lower rate relative to other com- mercially available isotopes with a shorter half-life. Concerns have been raised that tumor cells with a potentially shorter dou- bling time may reproduce and repopulate faster than they can be eliminated by such low dose-rate irradiation.[36–39] Accordingly, there has been interest in the use of higher dose-rate isotopes to address these biolog- ical concerns in the tumors of higher histo- logical grade. These isotopes differ in their half-life (decay rate), tissue penetration, and dose rate (cGy/hour) delivered to the tumor. Two additional isotopes that have come into use for prostate implants have been palladium (^{103}Pd) and iridium (^{192}Ir).

Palladium has a half-life of 17 days but a penetration through tissue that is not sig- nificantly different than ^{125}I. Its faster de- cay delivers a greater hourly dose rate to the higher grade tumors for which it is be- ing utilized. Although theoretical consider- ations suggest an advantage of palladium over iodine for faster growing tumors, clinical data directly comparing the results of the two isotopes in terms of tumor con- trol are still not available.

^{192}Ir is a widely used isotope that has been most frequently utilized for intersti- tial implantation of carcinomas of the fe-

TABLE 1. Transperineal Prostate Implants: Recent Results

Reference	No. Pts.	Isotope	Tumor Stages	External Beam	Pos Post-Rx Bx (%)	Local Control (%)	PSA WNL (%)	Follow-up (mos.)
Russell and Blasko[27]	235	125I	A_1–B_3	—	6d	98	90	12–66; median = 36
	78	125I	A_2–C	+	3d	94	85	13–57; median = 32
	42	103PD	A_2–B_3	—	10d	98	93	12–45; median = 25
	41	103PD	A_2–C	+	4d	98	88	12–45; median = 25
Bertermann et al.[54]	103	192IR	A_2–C	+	18	99	94	25 (mean)
Beyer[55]	121	125I	A–B_2	—	NA	NA	88	12–39
Bosch et al.[56]	43	192IR	A_2–C	+	52a	NA	NA	6 (min)
Brindle et al.[57]	51	192IR	C	+	16.5	100	NA	45 (median)
Brosman[58]	88	192IR	C	+	25	83	NA	50 (mean)
Donnelly et al.[59]	170	192IR	A_2–C	+	25	100	NA	6–91
Goffinet[60]	18	192IRb	C	+	NA	89	33	12 (mean)
Iversen et al.[61]	33	125I	A–Bc	+	48	NA	NA	35 (median)
Olson and Kaye[62]	22	125I	A–B_1	—	NA	NA	91	12–24
	32	125I	A–B_3	+	NA	NA	91	12–24
Puthawala et al.[63]	100	192IR	A_2–C	+	11	98	NA	24 (median)
Wallner[34]	20	125I	B	—	NA	100	85	3–24

a 23% A/B; 75% C.
b With interstitial hyperthermia.
c Poorly differentiated.
d All patients not biopsied. Percent of patients with "indeterminate" biopsy result = 26%, 5%, 30%, and 33% for the four cohorts in descending order.
NA = Not available.

male breast. Its penetrating gamma energy mandates its use as a temporary, removable implant, and requires it to be used with attention to personnel exposure. As a relatively high dose-rate isotope (ranging from 50 to 80 cGy/hour), its efficacy compared to the low initial dose-rate of an ^{125}I implant (7–10 cGy/hour) is also unknown. However, the great body of clinical experience with ^{192}Ir has favored its use as a high dose-rate alternative to [125]I.

Results from many investigations are preliminary. Many series using these newer techniques still have short follow-up, and much of the data have been presented only at symposia and clinical meetings and are not as yet published in the peer-reviewed literature. These caveats aside, there is a considerable amount of data available for consideration, which has been reviewed in detail elsewhere.[27]

A summary of much of the current data is shown in Table 1. As can be readily appreciated, a spectrum of different tumor stages has been treated with combinations of implant alone or implant plus external beam irradiation. As a general rule, implants plus external beam have been used for the locally more advanced tumors, while implants alone have been used for the lower stage tumors. Removable implants involving ^{192}Ir have also been used most frequently as a boost treatment for locally advanced tumors, and [103]Pd is being used for the higher grade tumors as well. The largest series of transperineal implants has been accrued at the Northwest Tumor Institute in Seattle, treating patients with ^{125}I or [103]Pd, either alone or in combination with external beam radiation. Preliminary data on 318 patients implanted between 1985–1990 are summarized in this table as well.

Generalizations regarding effectiveness of treatment are hazardous among these experiences involving patients of differing tumor stages and different treatment approaches. However, it appears that the posttreatment biopsy results as well as the percentage of patients with normal PSA levels following implants compares favorably with data from the external beam irradiation literature.[6,40–42]

Complication rates for these implants have varied with the technique, isotope used, and type of implant (permanent versus temporary). As a generalization, more complications have been reported with the use of the highly penetrating (and high dose-rate) [192]Ir implants compared with the less tissue penetrating and lower dose-rate implants.

An analysis of complications has been published for the 274 patients in the Seattle series treated with ^{125}I implantation as a component of the delivered treatment. Overall, 13% of patients had late complications of treatment that required medical or surgical intervention. Eight percent of the patients were felt to have permanent sequelae of treatment. The majority of the complications and sequelae involved the urinary tract. Most common was a 7% incidence of chronic irritative uropathy, which was defined as a degree of urinary frequency, urgency, and discomfort that interfered with the patient's lifestyle and appeared to be permanent. Incontinence occurred in 14 (5%) of the 274 patients with 7/14 patients having stress incontinence only. Incontinence was found to be strongly associated with a transurethral resection of the prostate (TURP), either preexisting or postimplantation. Of the patients with a TURP, 17% (11/66 patients) experienced this complication as compared to 0% (0/130) without a history of TURP.[43]

PARTICLE THERAPY

Radiotherapy using atomic particles rather than conventional photons (X-rays) has been used to treat a variety of solid tumors for upwards of 50 years. The rationale for using particles relates to the physical properties of particles, and how particles deposit ionizing radiation while passing through tissue. Today, the overwhelming majority of particle therapy involves either neutrons or protons. The properties of these particles differ from conventional photons either in how much energy is deposited per unit length of tissue (neutrons), or in the relative pattern of energy deposition (protons).

Modern megavoltage photons deliver their maximum dose of radiation 1 or more centimeters below the skin surface of a patient's body, with gradual attenuation of the dose as the beam is absorbed in its transit through the patient.

Neutrons

Neutrons have the same pattern of dose distribution as photons, but deposit from 20–100 times more ionizing radiation per unit of tissue traversed. Therefore, although neutrons cannot be "aimed" any better than photons, neutrons deliver more potent radiation injury along their path, through a variety of mechanisms. The biological consequences of this high deposition of energy (so-called "high linear energy transfer" or LET) are many.

Cellular sensitivity to neutrons appears to be considerably less affected by certain tumor parameters which often limit photon radiosensitivity. These factors include slow tumor growth kinetics or poor tumor oxygenation. Whereas photon radiosensitivity varies considerably according to cellular position in the cell cycle, this effect is less prominent for neutrons. Slow-growing tumors and poorly oxygenated tumors are typically radioresistant to photons. This resistance is less prominent when such tumors are treated with neutrons. With respect to tumor repair of injury, certain types of cellular mechanisms for repairing radiation DNA injury are less functional following neutron radiation than following photon irradiation.

The net result of these biological differences is that neutrons induce cellular injury that is considerably greater than that produced by an equivalent amount of photon irradiation. The relative biological effectiveness (RBE) of a given dose of neutrons relative to photons varies with the tumor type or organ irradiated, and can vary from a proportionality constant of 3 to approximately 8. To the extent that specific tumors exhibit an *incrementally* greater sensitivity to this high LET radiation than do normal surrounding tissues, a therapeutic gain may be expected. These issues are more fully reviewed elsewhere.[44,45].

A number of institutions worldwide have had favorable pilot experiences treating prostate cancer with neutrons,[46] but only two phase III randomized clinical trials have been performed. Both trials have been carried out in the United States, the first trial under the auspices of the Radiation Therapy Oncology Group (RTOG) and the second by the Neutron Therapy Collaborative Working Group (NTCWG).

In the first trial (RTOG 77-04), 91 analyzable patients with stages C and D_1 tumors were enrolled between the years of 1977–1983,. These patients were randomized to receive either photon radiation or a radiation regimen alternating neutrons and photons in a so-called "mixed-beam" (neutron/photon) schedule. This mixed-beam schedule was composed of three days/week neutron treatment and two days/week photon treatment, resulting in a combined treatment that was approximately 60% neutrons. This combination was chosen for the experimental arm out of concerns about the unknown potential for late tissue complications using neutrons alone. The two patient groups were balanced with respect to the major prognostic variables. Five- and 10-year actuarial results for clinically assessed local control were 86% for the mixed-beam group and 61% for the photon group ($P = 0.03$ at 10 years). The corresponding five- and 10-year cancer-specific survival data were 82% and 46% for the mixed-beam group versus 62% and 29% for the photon group ($P = 0.04$ at 10 years).[47]

Based on these favorable results, a second trial was initiated in 1985 (NTCWG 85-23), in which patients were randomized to receive neutrons alone versus photons alone. Between 1986 and 1990, 172 patients with stages D1, C, and high-grade B2 (summed major and minor Gleason pattern score >7) were randomized and completed treatment. The median patient follow-up is now 4.2 years (range 2.0–6.5 years).

The five-year actuarial "clinical" local/regional control for patients treated with neutrons or photons is 91% versus 70% ($P < 0.01$). Incorporating the results of routine posttreatment prostate biopsies, the resulting "histological" local/regional tumor control rates for neutrons and photons were 82% versus 60% ($P = 0.04$). Eliminating patients with proven stage D_1 disease, the histological local/regional tumor control rates for neutrons and photons were 92% versus 59% ($P < 0.01$). To date, survival rates are the same for both patient cohorts, with an actuarial five-year cancer-specific survival of 89% and 92% for neutrons and photons, respectively ($P =$ n.s.).[48] However, as local/regional tumor control is a determinant of survival, the improved local tumor control achieved by neutrons should lead to a survival advantage for neutron-treated patients as the follow-up data mature.

In this study, late complications of treatment were higher for the neutron-treated patients (11% vs. 1%). Many of the complications were rectal. Interestingly, as might be expected from the prior discussion of conformal therapy, rectal complications from neutron treatment were inversely correlated with the degree of neutron beam shaping available at the participating institutions. When neutron beam shaping capabilities allowed conformal radiation fields, the incidence of severe rectal injury was 0%.[48]

Protons

Protons have the same relative biological effectiveness as photons, but can be "aimed" more selectively because of the way proton energy is distributed along the radiation beam. Protons can penetrate through the superficial body tissues, delivering a relatively low radiation dose, and then deposit a peak of high-dose radiation (the so-called "Bragg peak") prior to completely dissipating. Using appropriate energy proton beams and proper depth of target, one can localize the Bragg peak of energy deposition over the tumor, thus achieving a relative dose-sparing to the surrounding tissues.

The majority of proton radiation research and treatment takes place in the United States at the Massachusetts General Hospital/Harvard Cyclotron Facility in Boston, as well as at the more recently opened facility in Loma Linda, California. Although the author is not aware of any data from phase III trials directly comparing the two modalities for the treatment of prostate cancer, there is single-institution phase II data from the former facility that suggests that using protons rather than photons to boost the prostate after photon pelvic irradiation has been completed permits a 10% increase in tumor dose without any attending increases in normal tissue toxicity.[49] At the time of that report, no survival or local tumor control advantages had been reported for the proton-boosted patients compared with the photon-boosted patients.

RADIOTHERAPY PLUS HORMONES

All of the previously discussed topics have involved one form or another of radiation as a single modality treatment. A brief mention is warranted of the current efforts combining radiation with androgen ablation as primary management of prostate cancer. Contrary to the prior research directions (which have attempted radiation dose escalation or improved dose localization as the investigation approach), this approach is predicated on the assumption that conventional doses of radiation may prove adequate to treat locally advanced tumors if the tumor burdens have been cytoreduced by androgen ablation.

The data for this is somewhat circumstantial, but has precedents in single-institution experiences with adjuvant hormonal therapy following either radical prostatectomy[50] or primary radiotherapy.[51] In these experiences, adjuvant hormonal therapy has been reported to confer a survival advantage over treatment with either surgery or radiotherapy alone. Prospective randomized cooperative group trials are currently in progress to more fully address this question.[52,53]

SUMMARY

The current areas of investigation in the radiotherapy of prostate cancer have been designed to achieve one of two goals: (1) improved survival for patients with locally advanced tumors for which conventional radiotherapy is suboptimal, or (2) equivalent survival as conventional methods but with less side effects of treatment.

For the patient with favorable, organ-confined disease, multiple treatment options exist both within and outside the discipline of radiation oncology. As the success rate of conventional treatment for these patients is already high, one should not assume that any of the treatment methods discussed above will deliver incremental improvements in survival outcome.

For the patient with locally advanced tumors, these efforts are all well-reasoned approaches to increasing tumor cell kill within acceptable levels of patient tolerance. Clearly, however, more follow-up is necessary to gauge the magnitude of progress that has been achieved.

REFERENCES

1. Kaplan ID, Bagshaw MA, Cox CA, Cox RS: External beam radiotherapy for incidental adenocarcinoma of the prostate discovered at transurethral resection. Int J Radiat Oncol Biol Phys 24(3):415–421, 1992.

2. NIH Consensus Development Conference: The management of clinically localized prostate cancer. J Urol 138(6):1369–1375, 1987.

3. Hanks GE: External beam radiation treatment for prostate cancer: still the gold standard. Oncology 6(3):79–89, 1992.

4. Russell KJ, Boileau MA: Current status of prostate specific antigen in the radiotherapeutic management of prostatic cancer. Sem Rad Oncol 3(July):154–168, 1993.

5. Oesterling JE: Prostate specific antigen: a critical assessment of the most useful tumor marker for adenocarcinoma of the prostate. J Urol 145(5):907–923, 1991.

6. Russell KJ, Dunatov C, Haferman MD, Griffeth JT, Polissar L, Pelton J, Cole SB, Taylor EW, Wiens LW, Koh WJ, Austin-Seymour MM, Griffin BR, Russell AH, Laramore GE, Griffin TW: Prostate specific antigen in the management of patients with localized adenocarcinoma of the prostate treated with primary radiation therapy. J Urol 146:1046–1052, 1991.

7. Freiha FS, Bagshaw MA: Carcinoma of the prostate: results of post-irradiation biopsy. Prostate 5:19–25, 1984.

8. Perez CA, Pilepich MV, Garcia D, Simpson JR, Zivnuska F, Hederman MA: Definitive radiation therapy in carcinoma of the prostate: experience at Mallinckrodt Institute of Radiology. NCI Monogr 7:85–94, 1988.

9. Hanks GE, Martz KL, Diamond JJ: The effect of dose on local control of prostate cancer. Int J Radiat Oncol Biol Phys 14:243–248, 1988.

10. Smit WG, Helle PA, van Putten WL, Wijnmallen AJ, Seldenrath JJ, van der Werf Messing BH: Late radiation damage in prostate cancer patients treated by high dose external radiotherapy in relation to rectal dose. Int J Radiat Oncol Biol Phys 1990(1):23–29, 1990.

11. Pilepich MV: Radiation Therapy Oncology Group Studies in carcinoma of the prostate. NCI Monogr 7:61–65, 1988.

12. Asbell SO, Schlager BA, Baker AS: Revision of treatment planning for carcinoma of the prostate. Int J Radiat Oncol Biol Phys 6:861–865, 1980.

13. Ten Haken RK, Perez-Tamayo C, Tesser RJ, McShan DL, Fraass BA, Lichter AS: Boost treatment of the prostate using shaped, fixed fields. Int J Radiat Oncol Biol Phys 16(1):193–200, 1989.

14. Low NN, Vijayakumar S, Rosenberg I, Rubin S, Virudachalam R, Spelbring DR, Chen GT: Beam's eye view based prostate treatment planning: is it useful? Int J Radiat Oncol Biol Phys 19(3):759–768, 1990.

15. Roach M, Pickett B, Holland J, Zapotowski KA, Marsh DL, Tatera BS: The role of the urethrogram during simulation for localized prostate cancer. Int J Radiat Oncol Biol Phys 25(2):299–307, 1993.

16. Emami B, Lyman J, Brown A, Coia L, Goitein M, Munzenrider JE, Shank B, Solin LJ, Wesson M: Tolerance of normal tissue to therapeutic irradiation. Int J Radiat Oncol Biol Phys 21:109–122, 1991.

17. Burman C, Kutcher GJ, Emami B, Goitein M: Fitting of normal tissue tolerance data to an analytic function. Int J Radiat Oncol Biol Phys 21:123–136, 1991.

18. Kutcher GJ, Burman C, Brewster L, Goitein M, Mohan R: Histogram reduction method for calculating complication probabilities for three-dimensional treatment planning evaluations. Int J Radiat Oncol Biol Phys 21:137–146, 1991.

19. Soffen EM, Hanks GE, Hwang CC, Chu JC: Conformal static field therapy for low volume low grade prostate cancer with rigid immobilization. Int J Radiat Oncol Biol Phys 20(1):141–146, 1991.

20. Ten Haken RK, Forman JD, Heimburger DK, Gerhardsson A, McShan DL, Perez TC, Schoeppel SL, Lichter AS: Treatment planning issues related to prostate movement in response to differential filling of the rectum and bladder. Int J Radiat Oncol Biol Phys 20(6):1317–1324, 1991.

21. Urie MM, Goitein M, Doppke K, Kutcher JG, LoSasso T, Mohan R, Munzenrider JE, Sontag M, Wong JW: The role of uncertainty analysis in treatment planning. Int J Radiat Oncol Biol Phys 21:91–107, 1991.

22. Munzenrider JE, Brown AP, Chu JCH, Coia LR, Doppke KP, Emami B, Kutcher GJ, Mohan R, Purdy JA, Shank B, Simpson JR, Solin LJ, Urie MM: Numerical scoring of treatment plans. Int J Radiat Oncol Biol Phys 21:147–163, 1991.

23. Sandler HM, Perez TC, Ten HRK, Lichter AS: Dose escalation for stage C (T3) prostate cancer: minimal rectal toxicity observed using conformal therapy. Radiother Oncol 23(1):53–54, 1992.

24. Fuks Z, Leibel SA, Wallner KE, Begg CB, Fair WR, Anderson LL, Hilaris BS, Whitmore WF: The effect of local control on metastatic dissemination in carcinoma of the prostate: long-term results in patients treated with 125I implantation. Int J Radiat Oncol Biol Phys 21(3):537–547, 1991.

25. Soffen EM, Hanks GE, Hunt MA, Epstein BE: Conformal static field radiation therapy treatment of early prostate cancer versus non-conformal techniques: a reduction in acute morbidity. Int J Radiat Oncol Biol Phys 24(3):485–488, 1992.

26. Vijayakumar S, Awan A, Karrison T, Culbert H, Chan S, Kolker J, Low N, Halpern H, Rubin S, Chen GT, et al.: Acute toxicity during external-beam radiotherapy for localized prostate cancer: comparison of different techniques. Int J Radiat Oncol Biol Phys 25(2):359–371, 1993.

27. Russell KJ, Blasko JC: Recent advances in interstitial brachytherapy for localized prostate cancer. In: Lange PH, Paulson DF (eds): Problems in Urology, Therapeutic Strategies in Prostate Cancer. Hagerstown, MD: J.B. Lippincott, 7(2):260–279, 1993.

28. Whitmore WF, Hilaris B, Grabstald H: Retropubic implantation of iodine 125 in the treatment of prostatic cancer. J Urol 108:918–920, 1972.

29. Henschke UK, Cevc P: Dimension averaging: a simple method for dosimetry of interstitial implants. Rad Biol Ther 9:287–298, 1968.

30. Anderson LL: Dosimetry for interstitial radiation therapy. In: Hilaris BS (ed): Handbook of Interstitial Brachytherapy. Acton, MA: Publishing Sciences Group, pp 87–115, 1975.

31. Stone NN, Forman JD, Sogani PC, et al.: Transrectal ultrasonography and I-125 implantation in patients with prostate cancer. J Urol 139:604A, 1988.

32. Morton JD, Peschel RE: Iodine-125 implants versus external beam therapy for stages A2, B, and C prostate cancer. Int J Radiat Oncol Biol Phys 14(6):1153–1157, 1988.

33. Shipley WU, Kopelson G, Novack DH, et al.: Preoperative irradiation, lymphadenectomy, and ^{125}I implantation for patients with localized prostate carcinoma: a correlation of implant dosimetry with clinical results. J Urol 124:1578–1582, 1980.

34. Wallner K: Iodine 125 brachytherapy for early stage prostate cancer: new techniques may achieve better results. Oncology 5(10):115–122, 1991.

35. Holm HH, Juul N, Pederson JF, et al.: Transperineal 125-iodine seed implantation in prostatic cancer guided by transrectal ultrasonography. J Urol 130:283–286, 1983.

36. Marchese MJ, Hall EJ, Hilaris BS: Encapsulated ^{125}I in radiation oncology. I. Study of the relative biological effectiveness (RBE) using low dose rate irradiation of mammalian cell cultures. Am J Clin Oncol 7:607–611, 1984.

37. Mitchell JB, Bedford JS, Bailey SM: Dose-rate effects on the cell cycle and survival of S3 HeLa and V79 cells. Radiat Res 79:520–536, 1979.

38. Dale RG: Radiobiological assessment of permanent implants using tumor repopulation factors in the linear-quadratic model. Br J Radiol 62:241–244, 1989.

39. Ling CC: Permanent implants using Au-198, Pd-103, and I-125: radiobiological considerations based on the alpha/beta model. Int J Radiat Oncol Biol Phys 23:81–87, 1992.

40. Stamey TA, Kabalin JN, Ferrari M: Prostate specific antigen in the diagnosis and treatment of adenocarcinoma of the prostate. III. Radiation treated patients. J Urol 141:1084–1087, 1989.

41. Landmann C, Hunig R: Prostate-specific antigen as an indicator of response to radiotherapy in prostate cancer. Int J Radiat Oncol Biol Phys 17:1073–1076, 1989.

42. Kaplan I, Prestidge BR, Cox RS, Bagshaw MA: Prostate specific antigen after irradiation for prostatic carcinoma. J Urol 144:1172–1176, 1990.

43. Blasko JC, Ragde H, Grimm PD: Transperineal ultrasound-guided implantation of the prostate: morbidity and complications. Scand J Urol Nephrol (Suppl) 113–118, 1991.

44. Griffin TW: Fast neutron radiation therapy. Crit Rev Oncol Hematol 13(1):17–31, 1992.

45. Griffin TW, Wambersie A, Laramore G, Castro J: International Clinical Trials in Radiation Oncology. High LET: heavy particle trials. Int J Radiat Oncol Biol Phys 1:S83–92, 1988.

46. Russell KJ, Laramore GE, Griffin TW, Parker RG, Maor MH, Davis LW, Krall KM: Fast neutron radiotherapy in the treatment of locally advanced adenocarcinoma of the prostate: clinical experiences and future directions. Am J Clin Oncol 12(4):307–310, 1989.

47. Laramore GE, Krall JM, Thomas FJ, Russell KJ, Maor MH, Hendrickson FR, Martz KL, Griffin TW, Davis LW: Fast neutron radiotherapy for locally advanced prostate cancer. Final report of Radiation Therapy Oncology Group randomized clinical trial. Am J Clin Oncol 16(2):164–167, 1993.

48. Russell KJ, Krall JM, Laramore GE, Burneson M, Maor MH, Taylor ME, Zink S, Davis LW, Griffin TW: Photon versus fast neutron external beam radiotherapy in the treatment of locally advanced prostate cancer: preliminary results of a randomized prospective trial of the neutron therapy collaborative working group. Int J Radiat Oncol Biol Phys 28(1):47–54, 1994.

49. Munzenrider JE, Austin-Seymour M, Blitzer PJ, Gentry R, Goitein M, Gragoudas ES, Johnson K, Koehler AM, McNulty P, Moulton G, et al.: Proton therapy at Harvard. Strahlentherapie 161(12):756–763, 1985.

50. Zincke H: Extended experience with surgical treatment of stage D1 adenocarcinoma of prostate. Significant influences of immediate adjuvant hormonal treatment (orchiectomy) on outcome. Urology 33(5 Suppl):27–36, 1989.

51. Zagars GK, Johnson DE, von Eschenbach AC, Hussey DH: Adjuvant estrogen following radiation therapy for stage C adenocarcinoma of the prostate: long-term results of a prospective randomized study. Int J Radiat Oncol Biol Phys 14(6):1085–1091, 1988.

52. RTOG, RTOG #8531: A phase III study of zoladex adjuvant to radiotherapy in unfavorable prognosis carcinoma of the prostate. Pre-Meeting Report, July 1, 1989, pp 211–214.

53. Pilepich MV, Krall J, Al-Sarraf M, Roach M, Doggett RLS, Sause W, Lawton CA, Abrams RA, Rotman M, Rubin P, Shipley WU, Cox JD: A phase III trial of androgen suppression before and during radiation therapy for locally advanced prostatic carcinoma: preliminary report of RTOG protocol 8610. Proc Am Soc Clin Oncol 12:229 (abstr), 1993.

54. Bertermann H, Hansen J, Wirth B, Loch T, Schultze J, Quirin A, Watzel HJ, Kohr P: Iridium-192: five years experience with interstitial high dose brachy- and external teletherapy in locally confined prostate cancer. Presented at the Pacific N.W. Cancer Foundation Symposium: Prostate Cancer: The Role of Interstitial Implantation. Seattle, Washington, 1991.

55. Beyer D: Early prostate specific antigen response to radioisotope implantation. Endocuriether Hypertherm Oncol (in press).

56. Bosch PC, Forbes KA, Prassvinichai S, Miller JB, Golji H, Martin DC: Preliminary observations on the results of combined temporary 192 iridium implantation and external beam irradiation for carcinoma of the prostate. J Urol 135(4):722–725, 1986.

57. Brindle JS, Martinez A, Schray M, Edmundson G, Benson RC, Zincke H, Diokno A, Gonzalez J: Pelvic lymphadenectomy and transperineal interstitial implantation of IR 192 combined with external beam radiotherapy for bulky stage C prostatic carcinoma. Int J Radiat Oncol Biol Phys 17(5):1063–1066, 1989.

58. Brosman SA: Iridium-192 implants in patients with large stage C prostate cancer. EORTC Genitourinary Group Monograph 10. Urological Oncology: Reconstructive Surgery, Organ Conservation, and Restoration of Function, pp 281–290, 1991.

59. Donnelly BJ, Pedersen JE, Porter AT, McPhee MS: Iridium-192 brachytherapy in the treatment of cancer of the prostate. Urol Clin North Am 18(3):481–483, 1991.

60. Goffinet DR: Iridium-192 removable transperineal interstitial hyperthermia prostate implants. Presented at the Pacific N.W. Cancer Foundation Symposium: Prostate Cancer: The Role of Interstitial Implantation. Seattle, Washington, 1991.

61. Iversen P, Bak M, Juul N, Laursen F, von der Masse H, Nielsen L, Rasmussen F, Torp PS, Holm HH: Ultrasonically guided 125iodine seed implantation with external radiation in management of localized prostatic carcinoma. Urology 34(4):181–186, 1989.

62. Olson D, Kaye K: Minnesota Prostate Center and Twin Cities Urology, Minneapolis (personal communication), 1992.

63. Puthawala AA, Syed AMN, Tansery LA, Shanberg A, Austin PA, McNamara CS: Temporary iridium-192 implant in the management of carcinoma of the prostate. Endocuriether Hypertherm Oncol 1:25–34, 1985.

9

Recent Advances in the Surgical Management of Localized Prostate Cancer

Daniel B. Rukstalis, M.D.

INTRODUCTION

The diagnosis of clinically localized adenocarcinoma of the prostate in men identifies a population of individuals whose malignancies are potentially amenable to curative therapy with surgical extirpation. Historically, 55–65% of patients exhibit clinically localized cancer at the time of their initial presentation.[1,2] The growing enthusiasm for early detection of prostatic cancer coupled with the application of serum prostate-specific antigen (PSA), transrectal ultrasound, and random prostatic biopsy will likely result in a shift in the clinical stage distribution toward patients identified with localized adenocarcinoma at the time of diagnosis.[3] Therefore, physicians will be faced with therapeutic decisions regarding the management of localized adenocarcinoma in an increasing number of patients. The optimal treatment for these individuals remains controversial and is complicated by the variable and unpredictable natural history of this malignancy. Valid arguments may be made for surgical extirpation, external beam radiation therapy, early hormonal ablation, and watchful waiting. The majority of reports in the literature are retrospective with few randomized series, making comparison of these various treatment modalities difficult. Despite these limitations, evidence exists to support the role of surgical extirpation as optimal therapy for patients with locally confined prostate cancer and at least a 10-year life expectancy.

SURGICAL THERAPY FOR LOCALIZED PROSTATIC CANCER

Therapeutic Outcome

Patients treated with radical prostatectomy for cancer limited to the prostate may expect disease-free survival similar to men without cancer. Jewett reported on 447 patients treated with radical perineal prostatectomy between 1909 and 1963.[4] The 15-year survival for patients with stage B cancer was 54%, with an additional 33% of the patients dying without evidence of recurrence. Other investigators have reported series of patients with 5-, 10-, and 15-year follow-up after radical prostatectomy. Overall, disease-free survival rates for organ-confined cancers have ranged from 80–91% at 5 years, 47–63% at 10 years, and 25–50% after 15 years.[5–7] The addition of serum PSA as an indicator of recurrence may result in a reduction in the disease-free survival rates. Frazier et al. demonstrated that 9.8% of patients with organ-

Prostate Cancer, pages 151–164 © 1994 Wiley-Liss, Inc.

confined cancer will exhibit a detectable PSA within three years, while 39.4% of specimen-confined cancers fail with an elevated PSA in this time interval.[8] Despite the concern raised by a postoperative elevation in the serum PSA, the clinical failure rates following surgical extirpation of confined cancer suggest that many such cancers may be cured with a radical procedure.

The disease-free survival rates discussed above support the application of radical prostatectomy in the treatment of clinically localized prostatic adenocarcinoma. However, direct comparison of the results of surgery to other treatment modalities is lacking in the literature. There has been only a single prospectively randomized study comparing external beam radiation therapy to radical prostatectomy. A multi-institutional trial was conducted between 1975 and 1978 on 509 men with newly diagnosed prostatic carcinoma.[9] Patients were evaluated with isotopic bone scanning and open pelvic lymphadenectomy. All patients with evidence of disseminated disease, an occult focal cancer, or clinical stage C cancer were excluded from randomization. Ultimately, 56 patients without evidence of extraprostatic cancer were randomized to external beam radiation, with 41 patients treated with radical prostatectomy. Although this study has been criticized for statistical reasons it did demonstrate an advantage for radical surgery in time to first evidence of treatment failure at 80 months following initial therapy. Certainly, similar trials are required to confirm these observations. Additionally, there is a growing body of literature that suggests that a conservative strategy of watchful waiting with androgen ablation therapy administered to patients with progression may exhibit survival rates similar to surgery. Progression-free survival has been reported at 71.8% after five years and 53.1% following 10 years after initial diagnosis for otherwise untreated individuals

with stage T0–T2 (stage A or B) adenocarcinoma.[10,11] It is therefore of significant importance that a prospective comparison of surgical extirpation to watchful waiting be conducted. However, it is unlikely that a single therapeutic approach will be efficacious for all patients with localized adenocarcinoma of the prostate. It is important to continue efforts to identify prognostic variables that will allow for stratification of patients into various risk groups for which an optimal treatment may be identified.

Anatomic Approach to Radical Retropubic Prostatectomy

If radical surgical therapy is to remain a viable treatment option for patients with prostatic adenocarcinoma, the operative morbidity and mortality must be minimized. The complication rates from several published series of radical retropubic prostatectomy are displayed in Table 1. Historically, radical removal of the prostate has been associated with a high rate of incontinence and erectile dysfunction. Additionally, the procedure often resulted in extensive blood loss due to bleeding from the dorsal venous complex. However, Reiner and Walsh illustrated the surgical anatomy of the deep dorsal vein of the penis and the venous plexus of Santorini in 1979, which provided an operative approach for control of these venous structures.[12] These techniques have reduced the attendant operative blood loss and have facilitated the removal of the prostate in a field free of blood. Consequently, further attention could be directed to other problematic portions of the operation, particularly the apical prostatic dissection. Anatomic studies by Walsh and Donker have delineated the course of the autonomic parasympathetic and sympathetic nerve fibers, which are involved in normal erectile function.[13] The anatomic relationship of the pelvic nerve plexus to the pros-

TABLE 1. Perioperative and Postoperative Complications of Radical Prostatectomy

Author	No. Patients	Mortality (%)	Rectal Injury (%)	Stricture (%)	Incontinence (%)	
					Stress	Severe Stress or Total[a]
Leandri, 1992	620	1 (0.1)	3 (0.5)	3 (0.5)	21 (5.0)[b]	0
Walsh, 1990[63]	593	—	—	—	46 (7.7)	2 (0.3)
Igel, 1987[64]	692	4 (0.6)	9 (1.3)	63 (9.2)	140 (20.2)	39 (5.6)
Crawford, 1983[65]	75	0	0	2 (2.6)	5 (6.6)	1 (1.3)
Middleton, 1981	50	0	1 (2.0)	3 (6.0)	5 (10.0)	2 (4.0)
Frazier, 1992	122[c]	0	—	8 (7.0)	5 (4.0)	—
	51[d]	1 (1.9)	—	4 (8.0)	2 (4.0)	

[a]Defined as incontinence requiring more than two pads per day.
[b]One year follow-up for 398 patients.
[c]Treated with radical perineal prostatectomy.
[d]Radical retropubic prostatectomy.

tate and urethra is depicted in Figure 1. The information provided by these studies has led to the development, by Walsh and others, of a more anatomic approach to the surgical removal of the prostate. The dissection of the prostatic apex in a bloodless field allows for preservation of the nerves to the corpora cavernosa in appropriate patients but also facilitates the proximal urethral dissection in all patients, with an improvement in postoperative continence.

Urinary Incontinence

Urinary incontinence following surgical removal of the prostate in 2.5–87% of men is a serious complication that appears to be related both to external sphincter and bladder dysfunction.[14,15] Although the exact etiology of the high-pressure bladder dysfunction identified in some patients is uncertain, the alterations in sphincteric function may be directly related to the surgical technique. An improved understanding of the surgical anatomy of the prostatic apex and its relationship to the membranous urethra has provided an opportunity for minimizing injury to the external sphincter as well as improvements in the vesico-urethral anastomosis. Several investigators have demonstrated a reduction in postoperative incontinence secondary to incorporation of periurethral tissue into the anastomosis.[16,17] Walsh and coauthors reported on a series of 593 patients followed for at least one year and found that 92% were completely continent and 8% exhibited stress incontinence of variable severity. There was no patient with total incontinence.[17] It also appears that the preservation of the nerves to the corpora cavernosa during a nerve-sparing prostatectomy is associated with improved continence. The pelvic plexus of nerves, which provides innervation to the penis, additionally innervates the intrinsic musculature of the membranous urethra.[13] One study of 34 patients treated with a nerve-sparing radical retropubic prostatectomy demonstrated an increased rate of postoperative urinary control (94% to 70%) relative to patients who had a non-nerve-sparing procedure.[18]

Erectile Dysfunction

The delineation of the autonomic innervation to the pelvic organs, particularly the proximal urethra and corpora cavernosa, has provided the basis for an anatomic approach to the radical retropubic prostatectomy.[13] The parasympathetic efferent fi-

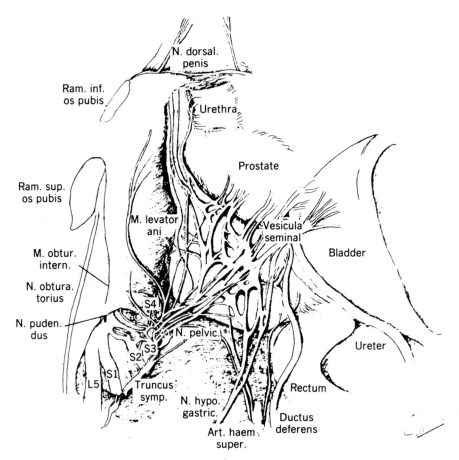

Fig. 1. Dissection of left pelvic plexus in male newborn. Bladder has been retracted to right side. Peritoneum, pelvic vessels, pelvic fascia, and pubic symphysis have been removed. Reprinted from ref. 13 with permission of Williams & Wilkins.

bers arising from S2 to S4 sacral cord levels and the sympathetic fibers from the thoracolumbar cord coalesce in the pelvic plexus and enter the pelvis as the pelvic nerve. The pelvic nerve travels within the endopelvic fascia, ultimately arborizing branches to the prostate, urethra, and corpora cavernosa. These branches are located outside of the prostatic capsule and posterior to Denonvillers' fascia.[19] The position of these microscopic nerve fibers relative to the prostatic capsule provides the opportunity for precise surgical removal of the gland without injury to the innervation to the corpora. The resultant potency-sparing modification of the radical retropubic prostatectomy has greatly reduced the incidence of postprostatectomy erectile dysfunction in appropriately selected patients. Several authors have published reports of large series of patients treated with this surgical modification.[20–22] The rate of preservation of potency from several contemporary series is reported in Table 2. Overall, potency is maintained in approximately 52–91% of the patients with either one or both neurovascular bundles preserved. It appears that the probability of return of potency is greatest in men less than 50 years of age and is reduced in pa-

TABLE 2. Preservation of Erectile Function Following Radical Nerve-Sparing Prostatectomy

Author	No. Patients in Series	Total (%)[a]	Age of Patient (Years)		
			<60 (%)	60–70 (%)	>70 (%)
Leandri, 1992	106	59 (56)	21/33 (64)	38/68 (56)	0/5 (0)
Quilan, 1991	503	342 (68)	217/280 (78)	122/211 (58)	3/12 (25)
Catalona, 1990	112	71 (63)	34/42 (81)	33/58 (57)	4/12 (33)
Petros, 1991	148	91 (61)	—	—	—
Eggleston, 1985	60	42 (70)	—	—	—

[a]Total number of patients with preserved erectile function.
Follow-up at least six months with at least a unilateral nerve-sparing procedure.

tients over the age of 70 irrespective of the number of bundles left intact.

Since the nerve-sparing modification of the radical prostatectomy requires that only a minimal amount of posterolateral extraprostatic tissue be removed with the prostate gland, questions have been raised regarding the impact of this modification upon the complete resection of prostatic cancer. Catalona and Dresner examined 52 patients treated with a nerve-sparing radical retropubic prostatectomy and discovered that the incidence of positive surgical margins (18% for stage A and B1 tumors, 57% for B2) was not statistically different from a group of 25 patients who underwent the standard dissection.[23] Similar findings have been published by Eggleston and Walsh in a series of 100 consecutive nerve-sparing radical operations.[24] In their experience 41% of the specimens demonstrated capsular penetration but only 7% had positive margins. In no patient was tumor identified at the inked margin solely at the site of the nerve-sparing modification.

RADICAL PERINEAL PROSTATECTOMY FOR LOCALIZED PROSTATE CANCER

Although surgical extirpation of the prostate gland can be accomplished through either a radical retropubic or radical perineal approach, the majority of patients treated in the United States receive a retropubic operation. However, there is a growing enthusiasm for the radical perineal approach within the urologic community, largely due to recent advances in laparoscopy. The modern technique for radical perineal prostatectomy may be traced back to Young in 1905[25] and appears to possess several advantages and disadvantages relative to the radical retropubic prostatectomy. The surgical approach to the prostate through a perineal incision allows for removal of the gland with a reduced operative blood loss and a potentially reduced recuperative time.[26] The median length of hospital stay for 46 patients treated with a radical perineal prostatectomy at the University of Chicago was three days.[27] This compares favorably with the 10-day hospitalization for radical retropubic prostatectomy patients reported by Frazier et al.[26] However, the University of Chicago patients underwent the radical perineal prostatectomy without an abdominal incision for a pelvic lymph node dissection and therefore the postoperative morbidity was related to the perineal incision alone. Other authors have reported a 6–12-day hospitalization for radical perineal prostatectomy performed in conjunction with an open pelvic lymph node dissection.[26,28] Additional advantages provided by the perineal approach include a potentially less difficult prostatic apical dissection and bladder neck reconstruction.[29] The perineal dissection proceeds along the anterior wall of the rectum until the rectourethralis muscle and ventral rectal fascia, parenthetically also known as the posterior layer of Denonvilliers' fascia, are encountered. This fascial layer may be incised, to expose the anterior layer of Denonvilliers' fascia and the prostatic capsule, in a horizontal manner as in the standard perineal prostatectomy or in a vertical fashion in a nerve-sparing modification.[28] However, removal of the ventral rectal fascia in continuity with the prostate provides an opportunity for extending the surgical resection in patients with more locally advanced cancers. This wide-field radical perineal prostatectomy may potentially reduce the incidence of positive surgical margins if applied in patients at risk for extracapsular disease.[30]

The disadvantages of radical perineal prostatectomy relative to the retropubic prostatectomy include the potential for an increased incidence of positive surgical margins, predominantly in the anterior portion of the gland. The standard or nerve-sparing modification of the perineal prostatectomy appears to remove the gland with a reduced amount of extra-prostatic soft tissue. It is possible that tumors with capsular penetration into the extracapsular fibroareolar tissue may not be completely removed by a perineal operation. If this argument is correct, then the incidence of positive surgical margins in patients treated with a radical perineal prostatectomy should be increased relative to a similar cohort of patients undergoing a radical retropubic operation. Frazier and coworkers compared 122 patients with clinical stage A or B cancers treated with a perineal procedure to 51 individuals treated by the radical retropubic approach.[26] The incidence of positive margins was 29% and 31%, respectively. This difference was not statistically significant. Additionally, if the radical perineal operation is an inadequate method for surgical extirpation of localized prostatic cancer, then this should be reflected as an increased rate of local recurrence or reduced survival. Although there are few pub-

lished reports that directly compare these two surgical procedures it does appear that the local control and disease-free survival rates are similar.[4,5,8,31]

A second potential disadvantage of the perineal approach is the reduced ability to perform a potency-sparing procedure. The anatomy of the neurovascular bundles, as previously described, requires that these structures be incised or retracted laterally as the prostate is removed. A nerve-sparing modification of the radical perineal prostatectomy has been described by Weldon and Tavel that provides an anatomic rationale for a potency-sparing perineal operation.[28] In a small series of 22 preoperatively-potent men treated with a nerve-sparing perineal prostatectomy, Frazier and coworkers report return of erectile function in 17 or 77.3%.[26] Despite these optimistic results, the probability of potency following a nerve-sparing radical perineal prostatectomy is uncertain and must still be considered inferior to the radical retropubic approach.

Perhaps the most obvious disadvantage of the perineal operation for prostate cancer is the necessity for a separate abdominal incision for examination of the regional pelvic lymph nodes. Nodal evaluation is an important step in the clinical staging of prostatic adenocarcinoma. The presence of microscopic or macroscopic lymphatic metastases has important and severe implications for the ability of a radical prostatic operation to eradicate the cancer. It has been argued that even the presence of one microscopically positive pelvic lymph node eliminates the potential for cure with surgical extirpation or radiation therapy.[32] Although other investigators have suggested that a single positive lymph node may not indicate a worse prognosis,[33] it has generally been accepted that patients with metastatic disease in the regional pelvic lymph nodes exhibit a poor prognosis and require alternative management such as radical prostatectomy coupled with androgen ablation or androgen ablation alone. Given the prognostic significance of lymphatic involvement in patients with prostatic cancers, and the relative inability of radiologic methods to accurately assess these regional nodes, an open lymph node dissection is routinely required in patients undergoing surgical therapy. Nodal evaluation in patients treated with a radical perineal operation necessitates a second abdominal incision, thereby potentially prolonging the operative time and increasing postoperative morbidity.[34]

Recent advances in the technology and instrumentation of minimally invasive laparoscopic surgery, as well as an improved understanding of the predictive ability of a preoperative serum PSA level, have obviated the necessity for a second abdominal incision prior to perineal prostatectomy. A laparoscopic pelvic lymphadenectomy was first performed in animals in 1990[35] and subsequently in men with prostatic adenocarcinoma by several investigators.[36,37] It appears that a laparoscopic dissection of the external iliac and obturator nodal tissue is comparable to that obtained with an open incision.[38,39] Although there is a steep learning curve prior to mastering these techniques, ultimately patient morbidity is reduced relative to the open lymphadenectomy.[40] In a series of over 100 men treated with a laparoscopic pelvic lymph node dissection at the University of Chicago the average length of postoperative hospitalization was 1.6 days. These minimally invasive procedures provide the surgeon with an alternative approach for nodal evaluation with potentially reduced patient morbidity. The indications and complications relative to laparoscopic pelvic lymph node dissection are discussed further in a subsequent section in this chapter.

Pathologic evaluation of the regional pelvic lymphatic tissue alters the management strategy only in patients with metastatic disease to those tissues. The remainder of patients, without evidence of metastases, must shoulder the risk of complications in the absence of benefit. If patients with an increased risk of lymphatic metastases could be identified preoperatively then a lymphadenectomy, either open or laparoscopic, could be performed. Those patients in a favorable category with a reduced risk for distant disease could be spared the potential morbidity of the nodal dissection while receiving a radical perineal prostatectomy for cure of the cancer. The concept of surgical extirpation of the prostate through a perineal operation without a concomitant lymphadenectomy is not new. Despite the absence of a nodal dissection, several reports of patients treated with a radical perineal prostatectomy alone before 1960 have demonstrated survival of patients with pathologic B disease comparable to more modern publications.[4,5]

Recent advances in the understanding of the prognostic value of a preoperative serum PSA level, either alone or in combination with histologic tumor grade and clinical stage, have provided surgeons with the ability to estimate the statistical likelihood of lymphatic metastases prior to surgical resection. Serum prostate-specific antigen levels correlate well with the volume of prostatic malignancy despite a large degree of overlap between PSA values in patients with or without cancer.[41,42] Several authors have further extended the value of a serum PSA in relation to the disease status of the regional lymphatics. Serum PSA values of ≤10 ng/ml with the Yang polyclonal radioimmunoassay or ≤10–20 ng/ml with the Tandem-R PSA immunoradiometric assay identify a patient population at low risk of lymphatic involvement.[42,43] However, since there is significant overlap in the PSA values between patients with lymphatic metastases and those with disease confined to the prostatic fossa, the predictive ability of PSA as a solitary prognostic factor for individual patients is low.[44,45] The predictive accuracy of PSA for nodal involvement may be improved if analyzed in combination with the tumor's histologic grade and clinical stage. In a recent review of 945 patients with prostate cancer, Kleer and colleagues developed nomograms that provided an estimate of the statistical risk of lymphatic disease in relation to PSA, clinical stage, and Mayo Clinic grade.[46] Although the feasibility of orienting the management of patients with prostatic cancer according to preoperative prognostic variables remains to be established through outcome studies, several institutions have begun to offer radical perineal prostatectomy alone without a concomitant pelvic lymphadenectomy to patients with a low risk of lymphatic spread. At the University of Chicago 46 men with clinically localized cancer and a serum PSA ≤20 ng/ml, as well as a Gleason grade ≤7 have undergone a radical perineal prostatectomy alone. After a minimum of three months' follow-up, 98% of the men demonstrated a reduction of the serum PSA to undetectable levels.[47] The single patient with persistently detectable serum PSA postoperatively developed bone lesions after eight months. All other individuals have maintained undetectable PSA levels with a median follow-up of eight months. These results, in addition to published reports demonstrating long-term disease-free survival in patients treated only with perineal prostatectomy, suggest that the perineal prostatectomy without a pelvic lymph node dissection represents a treatment alternative for patients with favorable cancers.

LAPAROSCOPIC PELVIC LYMPHADENECTOMY IN LOCALIZED PROSTATE CANCER

Minimally invasive laparoscopic surgical techniques have rapidly gained acceptance in the urologic and medical oncologic communities. These procedures appear to provide equivalent therapeutic benefit with reduced patient morbidity when compared to traditional open operations. Laparoscopic surgery is primarily efficacious in staging of pelvic malignancies such as prostatic adenocarcinoma. As detailed in the previous sections of this chapter, evaluation of regional lymphatics is an important adjunct in the management of patients with this neoplasm. A laparoscopic dissection of nodal tissue in the primary drainage sites for the prostate, specifically the external iliac and obturator nodes, may be accomplished without difficulty. However, prostate cancer also metastasizes to the hypogastric and presacral lymph nodes, which are not routinely included in a laparoscopic dissection. This raises the potential for understaging if a limited removal of nodal tissue is performed. Fortunately, this question has been previously discussed relative to the extent of an open lymphadenectomy. In a series of 115 patients treated with an extended open pelvic lymphadenectomy, 40% exhibited positive lymph nodes in the obturator–hypogastric region alone, while 23% harbored lymphatic metastases in the external iliac nodes alone.[48] Golimbu and coworkers advocated an extensive node dissection that included the presacral and presciatic nodes.[49] Their results demonstrated that 12 of 15 patients with positive pelvic lymph nodes possessed disease in the presciatic, presacral, or common iliac regions. Despite this elevated percentage, only 2 of 15 (13%) patients would have been understaged with a more limited dissection. It appears that a limited template dissection, as originally advocated by Brendler and Paulson,[50] provides adequate staging accuracy with a reduced rate of complications. The anatomic limits of the modified template dissection include the external iliac vein laterally, the hypogastric artery posteriorly, the obliterated umbilical artery medially, and the bifurcation of the common iliac artery superiorly. Nodal tissue from this template may also be effectively sampled with a laparoscopic procedure. The number of lymph nodes removed laparoscopically is essentially equivalent to that obtained in an open fashion.[39,40] The capacity for accurate nodal evaluation through the laparoscope effectively limits the need for a second abdominal incision in patients in whom a radical perineal prostatectomy is contemplated. Additionally, patients with an elevated risk for lymphatic spread may be treated with a laparoscopic node dissection prior to a radical retropubic prostatectomy with the procedure terminated if frozen-section analysis of the nodes demonstrates cancer.

The complication rate following an open pelvic lymph node dissection ranges from 3.9% to 52.9%.[34] Although the exact morbidity of a laparoscopic lymphadenectomy in a large number of patients is uncertain, several reports suggest that the rate of complications is comparable or reduced relative to an open procedure. In a series of 372 patients compiled from the initial experience with laparoscopic pelvic lymphadenectomy at eight institutions, the overall incidence of complications was 55 of 372 (14.7%). A total of 13 patients required a second open procedure for repair of a laparoscopic injury. There were no deaths associated with the laparoscopic procedure.[51] As urologic surgeons become more facile with these techniques the complication rate will likely diminish, since the overall complication rate from the latter portion of the previous series was 3%.

The advantages of the laparoscopic lymphadenectomy in patients with prostatic cancer appear obvious; however, the indications for such a procedure are less certain. As stated previously, the individuals most likely to benefit from this operation are those with positive lymph nodes whose subsequent treatment is influenced by the identification of metastatic spread. Therefore, only patients with a significant risk of lymphatic involvement, in whom

the radical prostatectomy would be abandoned if the regional nodes contain cancer, should receive a laparoscopic lymph node dissection prior to a radical retropubic prostatectomy. Additionally, patients with unfavorable cancers should undergo a laparoscopic evaluation before a radical perineal prostatectomy. The criteria for laparoscopic lymphadenectomy at the University of Chicago include men with locally confined adenocarcinoma of the prostate with a serum PSA >20 ng/ml or a Gleason grade ≥7. Furthermore, any patient with a clinically advanced cancer, i.e., stage C, is a candidate for laparoscopy if surgical resection or definitive external beam radiation therapy is contemplated.

INDICATIONS FOR SURGICAL EXTIRPATION RELATIVE TO CLINICAL STAGE

Stage A1

Patients diagnosed with well- to moderately well-differentiated adenocarcinoma in less than 5% of the specimen from a transurethral resection of the prostate are candidates for radical prostatectomy if their life expectancy is greater than 15 years. Although the majority of individuals with this stage of cancer will enjoy a prolonged survival without further therapy, approximately 6.8% to 16% will demonstrate progression of their disease.[52,53] This data is complicated by the findings that approximately 30% of patients with stage A1 cancer will possess greater than 1 cc residual tumor volume if treated with radical prostatectomy.[54] The risk of disease progression and death due to prostate cancer must then be evaluated relative to the incidence of surgical morbidity from therapy in patients with stage A1 cancer. The need for nodal evaluation is likely to be quite low in this patient population and could be predicated upon serum PSA, at a reasonable time interval following transurethral resection of the prostate (TURP), and Gleason grade.

Stage A2

The rate of disease progression, extracapsular disease, and lymphatic spread is much increased in patients with stage A2 cancer relative to stage A1. Approximately 90% of these patients will harbor residual cancer at the time of radical prostatectomy, with 52% exhibiting greater than 1 cc in volume.[54] Both radical retropubic and perineal prostatectomy are likely to eradicate the remainder of cancer. However, the previous TURP may increase the difficulty of the perineal prostatectomy by reducing the bulk of the prostate and by obliterating the tissue planes between the prostate and the rectum. Again, the indication for lymphadenectomy should rest upon the prognostic variables of grade and serum PSA. An additional consideration in this stage is the 25–34% incidence of positive surgical margins, particularly in the anterior region of the prostate.[55] The identification of positive surgical margins upon pathologic review of the surgical specimen is associated with a significantly increased 5–10-year progression rate.[8,31,56] If preoperative prognostic factors, such as serum PSA levels, indicate an increased likelihood of local extension, an effort should be made to resect the prostate with wider surgical margins. Therefore, a radical retropubic prostatectomy or a wide-field radical perineal prostatectomy should be considered, particularly if the preoperative PSA is greater than 10–20 ng/ml.

Stage B0

This stage will also be designated T1C when and if the TMN staging system is universally accepted. This category represents a prostatic malignancy diagnosed by routine serum PSA without palpable evidence of a prostatic nodule. The natural history of neoplasms diagnosed in this manner is presently incompletely understood. Although the PSA value corresponds with the volume of cancer there is considerable overlap between patients with organ-confined cancer and those individuals with extracapsular disease. Most men with this clinical stage exhibit a wide range of tumor volumes, potentially resulting in highly variable clinical outcomes. Surgical extirpation with either a radical retropubic or perineal prostatectomy is indicated in these patients. The need for a lymph node dissection prior to the perineal prostatectomy could be predicated upon the PSA value and tumor grade. Additionally, the necessity for a more extended surgical resection should be identified by these preoperative prognostic factors. The majority of men with a serum PSA below 10 ng/ml in one study exhibited organ-confined disease.[57] Conceptually, these individuals would then be candidates for a nerve-sparing procedure.

Stage B1

The identification of a unilateral prostatic nodule less than 1.5 cm in size represents the optimal indication for surgical extirpation with curative intent. The incidence of lymphatic metastases is quite low[58] and as such a radical perineal prostatectomy without concomitant lymphadenectomy may be considered. Additionally, the incidence of positive surgical margins is reduced in comparison to other stages of disease[4,55] so that a nerve-sparing retropubic or perineal approach is feasible.

Stage B2

The presence of a unilateral nodule larger than 1.5 cm or bilateral disease is more often associated with extracapsular extension of the cancer as well as pelvic lymphatic metastases. Approximately 40–66% of men with this stage will exhibit positive surgical margins.[5,55] In these circumstances a more extended surgical resection is indicated, such as a non-nerve-sparing retropubic or wide-field perineal prostatectomy. Additionally, since the incidence of pelvic lymphatic involvement is increased to between 9.7% and 43%,[59] a strong consideration must be given to a laparoscopic lymphadenectomy prior to radical prostatectomy if the removal of the prostate would be abrogated by the finding of positive nodes.

Stage C

The indication for surgical extirpation in patients with clinical evidence of extracapsular extension of the cancer either to the seminal vesicles, bladder neck, or pelvic side wall is controversial. The elevated risk of pelvic lymphatic involvement certainly indicates the need for a laparoscopic lymph node dissection prior to definitive resection of the prostate. Tomlinson and coworkers reported on 24 patients treated with radical prostatectomy compared to 26 patients receiving TURP alone. Androgen ablation therapy was administered to 43% of the radical prostatectomy group and 90% of the TURP group. The five-year survival was 82% in the first group and 69% in the second.[60] Similar findings in favor of radical resection have been reported by other investigators.[61,62] Surgical therapy may therefore be considered for limited stage C cancer in order to improve local control and perhaps in combination with androgen ablation. The extracapsular extent of this stage of disease obviates the potential for a nerve-sparing procedure.

Stage D1

Approximately 5–30% of patients undergoing an attempt at curative surgical resection for clinically localized prostatic adenocarcinoma will be found with metastatic disease in the regional lymph nodes at the time of surgery. Traditional management of these individuals dictates that the radical prostatectomy not be performed.

The patient is then treated with androgen ablation therapy in the form of orchiectomy or luteinizing hormone-releasing hormone (LHRH) analogs. Several investigators have questioned the rationale for this approach and have proceeded with the radical prostatectomy in the presence of microscopic nodal disease. Patients are administered androgen ablation therapy in addition to the prostatectomy. In one series of 631 patients from the Mayo Clinic with stage D1 disease, 251 received a radical prostatectomy and orchiectomy, while 60 received orchiectomy alone following the lymphadenectomy. The remainder of patients received various other treatments and are outlined in the manuscript. Although this report represents the retrospective analysis of this patient group and is subject to all the liabilities of retrospective studies, the results are encouraging. The cause-specific five- and 10-year survival rates for the radical prostatectomy–orchiectomy group were 91% and 78%. The orchiectomy-alone group exhibited rates of 66% and 39%. These differences were statistically significant.[64] Although these results suggest that a subgroup of individuals with stage D1 cancer will benefit from an aggressive surgical approach, the issue remains controversial. Patients should be informed of the various treatment options and the decision to proceed with radical prostatectomy employed selectively.

CONCLUSION

The surgical management of clinically localized prostatic adenocarcinoma continues to be refined. Overall, survival rates for patients with organ-confined malignancies following surgical extirpation are comparable to men without prostate cancer. The application of serum PSA to the diagnosis and staging of this neoplasm will potentially alter the stage distribution at presentation toward organ-confined disease, as well as provide some rationale for the choice of surgical treatment. The advent of the minimally invasive laparoscopic lymphadenectomy has provided an alternative method for nodal evaluation with reduced patient morbidity. Although only a subset of individuals require such a procedure, the availability of laparoscopy has rejuvenated interest in the radical perineal prostatectomy. Men with adenocarcinoma of the prostate may now choose between two methods for surgical extirpation, each with its own attendant advantages and disadvantages. The advantages of both the radical retropubic and radical perineal prostatectomy have become augmented over the past 15 years with the development of an anatomic approach to the dissection. The reduced morbidity of radical surgery has provided the stimulus for aggressive surgical treatment strategies even in patients with pelvic lymphatic metastases. Ultimately, the exact role for surgical removal of locally confined prostate cancer will be defined by randomized clinical trials that incorporate all treatment modalities, including watchful waiting.

REFERENCES

1. Murphy GP, Natarajan N, Pontes JE, Schmitz RL, Smart CR, et al.: The National Survey of Prostate Cancer in the United States by the American College of Surgeons. J Urol 127:928–934, 1982.

2. Catalona WJ, Smith DS, Ratliff TL, Dodds KM, Coplen DE, et al.: Measurement of prostate specific antigen in serum as screening test for prostate cancer. N Engl J Med 324(17):1156–1161, 1991.

3. Gerber GS, Chodak GW: Digital rectal examination in the early detection of prostate cancer. Urol Clin N Am 17(4):739–744, 1990.

4. Jewett HJ: Radical perineal prostatectomy for palpable, clinically localized, non-obstructive cancer: experience at the Johns Hopkins Hospital 1909–1963. J Urol 124:492–494, 1980.

5. Elder JS, Jewett HJ, Walsh PC: Radical perineal prostatectomy for clinical stage B2 carcinoma of the prostate. J Urol 127:704–706, 1982.

6. Smith JA: Management of localized prostate cancer. Cancer 70 (Suppl 1):302–306, 1992.

7. Lepor H, Walsh PC: Long term results of radical prostatectomy in clinically localized prostate cancer: experience at the Johns Hopkins Hospital. NCI Monogr 7:117–122, 1988.

8. Frazier HA, Robertson JE, Humphrey PA, Paulson DF: Is prostate specific antigen of clinical importance in evaluating outcome after radical prostatectomy? J Urol 149:516–518, 1993.

9. Paulson DF: Randomized series of treatment with surgery versus radiation for prostate adenocarcinoma. NCI Monogr 7:127–131, 1988.

10. Johansson JE, Adami HO, Andersson SO, Bergstrom R, Holmberg L, et al.: High 10 year survival rate in patients with early, untreated prostatic cancer. JAMA 267(16):2191–2196, 1992.

11. Johnasson JE, Andersson SO, Krusemo UB, Adami HO, Bergstrom R, et al.: Natural history of localized prostatic cancer. Lancet 1:799–803, 1989.

12. Reiner WB, Walsh PC: An anatomical approach to the surgical management of the dorsal vein and Santorini's plexus during radical retropubic surgery. J Urol 121:198–200, 1979.

13. Walsh PC, Donker PJ: Impotence following radical prostatectomy: insight into etiology and prevention. J Urol 128:492–497, 1982.

14. Presti JC, Schmidt RA, Narayan PA, Carroll PR, Tanagho EA: Pathophysiology of urinary incontinence after radical prostatectomy. J Urol 143:975–978, 1990.

15. Leach GE, Yun SK: Post-prostatectomy incontinence: Part 1. The urodynamic findings in 107 men. Neurourology Urodynamics 11:91–97, 1992.

16. Klein EA: Modified apical dissection for early continence after radical prostatectomy. Prostate 22:217–223, 1993.

17. Walsh PC, Quinlan DM, Morton RA, Steiner MS: Radical retropubic prostatectomy. Improved anastomosis and urinary continence. Urol Clin N Am 17:679–684, 1990.

18. O'Donnell PD, Finan BF: Continence following nerve-sparing radical prostatectomy. J Urol 142:1227–1229, 1989.

19. Lepor H, Gregerman M, Crosby R, Mostofi FK, Walsh PC: Precise localization of the autonomic nerves from the pelvic plexus to the corpora cavernosa: a detailed anatomical study of the male pelvis. J Urol 133:207–212, 1985.

20. Catalona WJ: Patient selection for, results of, and impact on tumor resection of potency-sparing radical prostatectomy. Urol Clinics N Am 17(4):819–826, 1990.

21. Quinlan DM, Epstein JI, Carter BS, Walsh PC: Sexual function following radical prostatectomy: influence of preservation of neurovascular bundles. J Urol 145:998–1002, 1991.

22. Leandri P, Rossignol G, Gautier JR, Ramon J: Radical retropubic prostatectomy: morbidity and quality of life. Experience with 620 consecutive cases. J Urol 147:883–887, 1992.

23. Catalona WJ, Dresner SM: Nerve-sparing radical prostatectomy: extraprostatic tumor extension and preservation of erectile function. J Urol 134:1149–1151, 1985.

24. Eggleston JC, Walsh PC: Radical prostatectomy with preservation of sexual function: pathologic findings in the first 100 cases. J Urol 134:1146–1148, 1985.

25. Young HH: The early diagnosis and radical cure of carcinoma of the prostate: being a study of 40 cases and presentation of a radical operation which was carried out in four cases. Bull Johns Hopkins Hosp 16:315, 1905.

26. Frazier HA, Robertson JE, Paulson DF: Radical prostatectomy: the pros and cons of the perineal versus retropubic approach. J Urol 147:888–890, 1992.

27. Rukstalis, DB, Bales G, Gerber GS, Chodak GW: Radical perineal prostatectomy as monotherapy for localized prostatic cancer. J Urol 149(4):380A, 1993.

28. Weldon VE, Tavel FR: Potency-sparing radical perineal prostatectomy: anatomy, surgical technique and initial results. J Urol 140:559–562, 1988.

29. Paulson DF: Perineal prostatectomy. In Walsh PC, Retik AB, Stamey TA, Vaughan ED (eds): Campbell's Urology, 6th ed, vol 3. Philadelphia: W.B. Saunders Co., pp 2887–2899, 1992.

30. Paulson DF: The Surgical Technique of Radical Perineal Prostatectomy. AUA Update Series, vol 5, no 38, 1986.

31. Paulson DF, Moul JW, Walther PJ: Radical prostatectomy for clinical stage T1-2N0Mo prostatic adenocarcinoma: long-term results. J Urol 144:1180–1184, 1990.

32. Gervasi LA, Mata J, Easley JD, Wilbanks JH, Seale-Hawkins C, et al.: Prognostic significance of lymph nodal metastases in prostate cancer. J Urol 142:332–336, 1989.

33. Prout GR, Heaney JA, Griffin PP, et al.: Nodal involvement as a prognostic indicator in patients with prostatic carcinoma. J Urol 124:226–231, 1980.

34. Paul DB, Loening SA, Narayana AS, Culp DA: Morbidity from pelvic lymphadenectomy in staging carcinoma of the prostate. J Urol 129:1141–1144, 1983.

35. Gershman A, Daykhovsky L, Chandra M, Danoff D, Grundfest WS: Laparoscopic pelvic lymphadenectomy. J Laparoendoscop Surg 1(1):63–68, 1990.

36. Schuessler WW, Vancaillie TG, Reich H, Griffith DP: Transperitoneal endosurgical lymphadenectomy in patients with localized prostate cancer. J Urol 145:988–991, 1991.

37. Parra RO, Andrus C, Boullier J: Staging laparoscopic pelvic lymph node dissection: comparison of results with open pelvic lymphadenectomy. J Urol 147:875–878, 1992.

38. Loughlin KR, Kavoussi LR: Laparoscopic lymphadenectomy in the staging of PCa. Contemporary Urol 4(5):69–82, 1992.

39. Chodak, GW, Levine LA, Gerber GS, Rukstalis DB: Safety and efficacy of laparoscopic lymphadenectomies. J Urol 147(4):126A, 1992.

40. Winfield HN, See WA, Donovan JF, Godet A, Farage YM, et al.: Comparative effectiveness and safety of laparoscopic versus open pelvic lymph node dissection for cancer of the prostate. J Urol 147(4):124A, 1992.

41. Partin AW, Carter HB, Chan DW, Epstein JI, Osterling JE, et al.: Prostate specific antigen in the staging of localized prostate cancer: influence of tumor differentiation, tumor volume and benign hyperplasia. J Urol 143:747–752, 1990.

42. Stamey TA, Kabalin JN, McNeal JE, Johnstone IM, Freiha F, et al.: Prostate specific antigen in the diagnosis and treatment of adenocarcinoma of the prostate. II. Radical prostatectomy treated patients. J Urol 141:1076–1083, 1989.

43. Gerber GS, Rukstalis DB, Chodak GW: Correlation of prostate specific antigen and tumor grade with nodal status in men with clinically localized prostate cancer. J Urol 149(4):448A, 1993.

44. Greskovitch FJ, Johnson DE, Tenney DM, Stephenson RA: Prostate specific antigen in patients with clinical stage C cancer: relation to lymph node status and grade. J Urol 145:798–801, 1991.

45. Hudson MA, Bahnson RR, Catalona WJ: Clinical use of prostate specific antigen in patients with prostate cancer. J Urol 142:1011–1017, 1989.

46. Kleer E, Larson-Keller JJ, Zincke H, Osterling JE: Ability of preoperative serum prostate specific antigen value to predict pathologic stage and DNA ploidy. Urology 41(3):207–216, 1993.

47. Rukstalis DB, Bales GT, Gerber SS, Chodak GW: Radical perineal prostatectomy as monotherapy for localized prostatic cancer. J Urol 149(6):380A, 1993.

48. Fowler JE, Whitmore WF: The incidence and extent of pelvic lymph node metastases in apparently localized prostatic cancer. Cancer 47:2941–2945, 1981.

49. Golimbu M, Morales P, Al-Askari S, Brown J: Extended pelvic lymphadenectomy for prostate cancer. J Urol 121:617–620, 1979.

50. Brendler CB, Cleeve LK, Everett CE, Anderson EE, Paulson DF: Staging pelvic lymphadenectomy in staging carcinoma of the prostate. J Urol 129:1141–1144, 1983.

51. Kavoussi LR, Sosa E, Chandhoke P, Chodak G, Clayman RV, et al.: Complications of laparoscopic pelvic lymph node dissection. J Urol 149:322–325, 1993.

52. Byar DP, and the VACURG: Survival of patients with incidentally found microscopic cancer of the prostate: results of a clinical trial of conservative treatment. J Urol 108:908–913, 1972.

53. Cantrell BB, DeKlerk DP, Eggleston JC, Boitnott JK, Walsh PC: Pathological factors that influence prognosis in stage A prostatic cancer: the influence of extent versus grade. J Urol 125:516–520, 1981.

54. Greene DR, Egawa S, Neerhut G, Flanagan W, Wheeler TM, et al.: The distribution of residual cancer in radical prostatectomy specimens in stage A prostate cancer. J Urol 145:324–329, 1991.

55. Rosen MA, Goldstone L, Lapin S, Wheeler T, Scardino PT: Frequency and location of extracapsular extension and positive surgical margins in radical prostatectomy specimens. J Urol 148:331–337, 1992.

56. Epstein JI, Pizov G, Walsh PC: Correlation of pathologic findings with progression after radical retropubic prostatectomy. Cancer 71(11):3582–3593, 1993.

57. Catalona WJ, Smith DS, Ratliff TL, Dodds KM, Coplen DE, et al.: Measurement of prostate specific antigen in serum as a screening test for prostate cancer. N Engl J Med 324(17):1156–1161, 1991.

58. Petros JA, Catalona WJ: Lower incidence of unsuspected lymph node metastases in 521 consecutive patients with clinically localized prostate cancer. J Urol 147:1574–1575, 1992.

59. Middleton RG, Larsen RH: Selection of patients with stage B prostate cancer for radical prostatectomy. Urol Clin N Am 17(4):779–785, 1990.

60. Tomlinson RL, Currie P, Boyce WH: Radical prostatectomy: palliation for stage C carcinoma of the prostate. J Urol 117:85–87, 1977.

61. Zincke H, Utz DC, Taylor WF: Bilateral pelvic lymphadenectomy and radical prostatectomy for clinical stage C prostatic cancer: role of adjuvant treatment for residual cancer and in disease progression. J Urol 135:1199–1205, 1986.

62. Flocks RH, O'Donoghue EPN, Milleman LA, Culp DA: Management of stage C prostatic carcinoma. Urol Clin N Am 2(1):163–179, 1975.

63. Cheng CW, Bergstralh EJ, Zincke H: Stage D1 prostate cancer: a nonrandomized comparison of conservative treatment options versus radical prostatectomy. Cancer 71(3):996–1004, 1993.

64. Walsh PC, Quinlan DM, Morton RA, Steiner MS: Radical retropubic prostatectomy: improved anastomosis and urinary continence. Urol Clin N Am 17(3):679–684, 1990.

65. Igel TC, Barrett DM, Segura JW, Benson RC, Jr, Rife CC: Perioperative and postoperative complications from bilateral pelvic lymphadenectomy and radical retropubic prostatectomy. J Urol 137:1189–1191, 1987.

66. Crawford ED, Kiker JD: Radical retropubic prostatectomy. J Urol 129:1145–1148, 1982.

10

Alternative Therapies for Local or Locally Recurrent Prostate Cancer

Thomas E. Kingston, M.D., and Barry S. Stein, M.D.

INTRODUCTION

The standard management of men with localized prostatic carcinoma (stages A1, A2, B1, B2) is either radical prostatectomy or external beam radiotherapy. Despite the potential therapeutic benefits of both treatments, alternative forms of treatment are being sought because of the significant morbidity of both. The most significant complications of radical prostatectomy include urinary incontinence and impotence. About 5% of post-radical prostatectomy patients have total incontinence and 15–20% have mild to moderate stress incontinence.[1,2] Historically, impotence after radical prostatectomy exceeded 90% until recent technical modifications by Walsh significantly decreased the rate of erectile dysfunction.[3] Because of this, radical prostatectomy has become a more acceptable therapeutic option; however, it remains a major surgical procedure with its attendant complications and occasionally delayed recovery. Radiation therapy also constitutes a major choice for the treatment of localized prostate carcinoma. Approximately 7,000 rads are delivered to the prostate, usually with 4,500 to 5,000 rads to the prostate and regional lymph nodes and the remainder to the prostate alone.[4] Complications of external beam radiotherapy include cystitis in 10%, inconti-

nence and/or urethral stricture in 5–8%, radiation enteritis in 10% and impotence in 41%.[4–9] Bagshaw reported the 30-year Stanford experience with 900 patients in 1988. The actuarial survival for patients with organ-confined disease was comparable to that of radical prostatectomy.[4,10–16] In addition, postirradiation biopsies have been found to be positive in 24–93% of patients although it remains controversial whether a positive biopsy proves that a tumor is biologically significant. Recent follow-up prostate-specific antigen (PSA) data from the Stanford group raises some concern about the success of radiotherapy in treating prostate cancer.[17] Since both radiation and surgery cause significant morbidity, alternative therapies for localized prostate cancer have been sought. This chapter reviews the status of cryosurgery, hyperthermia, laser treatment, and salvage prostatectomy.

CRYOSURGERY

Cryosurgery, or the use of subzero temperatures to destroy diseased prostatic tissue, was first pioneered by Gonder in 1964.[18] Theoretically, it was felt that this form of therapy could permanently eliminate all primary tumor in the prostate and, thereby, cure localized diseases while preserving the functional and structural integ-

Prostate Cancer, pages 165–174 © 1994 Wiley-Liss, Inc.

rity of surrounding structures. In addition, some early investigators believed cryotherapy might induce a host-protective immune response, but no clinical and little laboratory data support this at present.

The current technique employs real-time transrectal ultrasonic guidance of the treatment. With the patient in the perineal position, prepped and draped, a percutaneous suprapubic tube is placed (Fig. 1). Urethral warming is accomplished by circulating heated water (44°C) through an angioplasty catheter. Real-time transrectal ultrasound (TRUS) is then performed to determine the prostate shape and size. Next, an 18-gauge needle is placed into the prostate and a .038 J-wire is placed through the needle to the prostatic capsule. The tract is then dilated and a 7-mm cryoprobe is inserted. From one to five probes may be used. TRUS is used to monitor correct probe placement. Next, liquid nitrogen is passed into the probes, and the freezing process is observed on TRUS. The treatment proceeds through the prostatic capsule, but short of the rectal wall.[19]

The cryosurgical probe tip achieves a temperature of between −180°C and −190°C and produces tissue destruction by a variety of mechanisms, including crystallization with membrane rupture, intracellular dehydration, protein denaturation, and thermal shock.[20]

While Gonder primarily utilized transurethral cryosurgery, which significantly limited treatment of peripheral zone cancer, Flocks in 1969 utilized a standard perineal exposure for controlled application of cryotherapy under direct vision.[21] Therapy was utilized hoping to shrink metastases, as Soanes had reported three cases of regression of metastatic lesions within several months of transuretheral cryotherapy.[22]

O'Donoghue and associates reported on transperineal cryosurgical treatment of 154 patients for metastatic disease and found that 75% had pain relief, but only one had regression of a metastatic lesion.[23] They noted the major benefit to be destruction of the local lesion, unfortunately associated with a 14% incidence of ureterocuta-

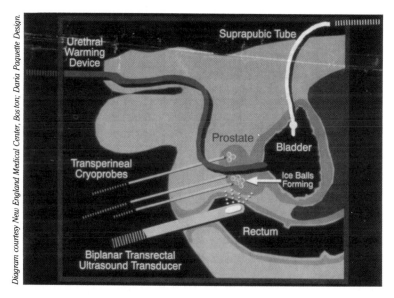

Diagram courtesy New England Medical Center, Boston; Daria Paquette Design.

Fig. 1. Transperineal cryosurgery treatment with transectal ultrasonic guidance. (Reprinted with permission from Lipner M: Prostate cancer '93: new advances in early detection, treatment, and patient selection. Oncology Times, July 1993.)

neous fistula. Gursel found improvement in bone pain in 8 of 11 patients after cryosurgery.[24]

In 1982, Bonney and associates utilized an open transperineal approach with visual monitoring of prostate freezing.[25] In 229 patients, the use of direct vision only made it difficult to determine the freezing in relation to the rectum and urethra as well as the margins of the tumor. Among the 229 patients were 69 stage C patients, 10 stage B_2 patients, and 14 stage A or B patients (remainder were stage D_1 and D_2 patients). At five-year follow-up, they noted stage survival probability equal to radical prostatectomy, both of which were higher than other forms of treatment (radiation therapy, endocrine therapy). They reported a urethrorectal fistula rate of 1.4%, urethrocutaneous fistula rate of 10.7%, and erectile dysfunction in 7.4%, all of which were attributed to the inability to properly monitor the freezing process. In 1983, Bonney et al. further reported on the efficacy of cryosurgery in controlling the primary tumor.[26] He reported that in 66% of cases all palpable tumor was eliminated following therapy, but 41% suffered recurrent disease. At least 50% of the patients received concomitant endocrine therapy and a significantly great proportion of the non-hormonally treated group (61%) had local recurrence. The complications included 15% of patients with stress or total urinary incontinence.

Most recently, Onik and associates reported on the use of transrectal ultrasound guided percutaneous transperineal cryosurgery on the prostates of six dogs.[27] They were able to follow the complete freezing process successfully and avoid any injury to the rectum or urethra. Thermocoupling devices connected to Foley catheters to monitor intraurethral temperature are presently under investigation. Following their successful work on animal models, Onik et al. published their preliminary results on 55 patients undergoing this procedure.[19] Only 23 of these men had

even reached their three-month follow-up examinations by the time this study was published. The technique utilized was as described in the beginning of this section. Patients selected for this treatment were determined to have intraprostatic cancer, and no evidence of metastasis. Pelvic lymph node dissections were performed for PSA values of >10 ng/ml. Exclusion criteria included bleeding disorders and active urinary tract infection. Hormone therapy, if initiated previously, was discontinued postoperatively. Two techniques were utilized. Group 1 consisted of eight patients who underwent treatment with two probes placed in multiple areas, and group 2 consisted of patients treated with a newer machine capable of supporting five probes simultaneously. Of the eight patients in group 1, three (37.5%) had residual disease found by the three-month posttreatment biopsy. The only patient in this group who had prior radiotherapy was among the failures. In group 2, only 1 of the 15 patients had a positive biopsy by three months (6.7%). Two patients in this group were radiotherapy failures, and both had negative biopsies.

Complications were reported on the entire group of 55 men. In four, freezing of the rectum occurred, leading to urethral–rectal fistulas in two, and sloughing of the prostatic urethral tissue in three. Of the patients followed to three months, 65% of those who were potent pre-op were impotent following treatment, indicating potential freezing of the cavernosal nerves.

Von Eschenbach and associates at M.D. Anderson reported on 12 patients treated with cryosurgery using transrectal guidance.[28] All men were initially stage B or C, and had been previously treated with external beam radiotherapy (N = 11) or gold seeds (N = 1). The treatment was tolerated well. Follow-up is too short for conclusions.

With the use of ultrasound and more precise freezing techniques, cryosurgery may hold significant promise for local control of disease or potential cure in a select group of patients who have large inoperable prostate carcinomas or are generally a poor anesthesia risk. To date, however, the lack of real follow-up in the TRUS-guided cryosurgery treatments should temper enthusiasm. Prostate cancer is a slowly progressive disease, and three-month follow-up biopsies do not a cure make. This is a feasible treatment with acceptable morbidity. The results must stand the test of time. Cryosurgery also appears feasible in postirradiation therapy failures. Again, long-term data will tell the tale.

HYPERTHERMIA

Hyperthermia has been long known to cause destruction of tissues, and the cytotoxic effects of hyperthermia on tumor cells both in vitro and in vivo have been demonstrated by many investigators.[29,30] Interest in the use of hyperthermia to treat cancer can be traced back as far as 1917 but for some reason interest declined between 1930 and 1960. During the past 15 years, however, a renewed interest in the use of heat for the treatment of malignant diseases has developed. Several factors have emerged that may explain why hyperthermia might be useful in the treatment of cancer both by itself and in conjunction with other forms of therapy. Most importantly, tumor vascularity does not dilate in the presence of heat like normal tissue does, and this renders the tumor more susceptible to heat damage.[31,32] In addition, neoplastic cells appear to be intrinsically more sensitive to heat than normal cells[33,34] and cells in S phase or hypoxic cells tend to be resistant to radiotherapy but sensitive to heat, so that the two treatments might complement each other.[35]

It has been shown that at temperatures above 45°C both normal and malignant cells are killed by heat and that at temperatures below 40°C both normal and tumor cells survive.[36] Further, it appears that sub-

lethal heating of tumor tissue may actually confer resistance to further heat treatment.[37] Ideally, therefore, according to one author, the tissue temperature should be raised to 43°C for 1 hour to achieve the most pronounced differential in heat sensitivity.[36]

Investigation into the effects of hyperthemia on neoplastic prostate tissue has been limited. Yerushalmi et al. were the first to report on the use of deep microwave hyperthermia delivered transrectally for the treatment of local or locally advanced prostate carcinoma.[38] In his series of 15 patients, 10 were stage C, 1 was stage B, and 4 were stage D. All but one had severe local symptoms (pain, dysuria, urinary retention), and each was given 6–9 treatments lasting an average of 60 minutes at 42–43°C. All patients were treated on an outpatient basis without anesthesia or sedation. Some patients were given posttreatment radiotherapy (6,200 cGy), and some were treated with DES (3 mg per day) or orchiectomy 3–4 weeks prior to hyperthemia treatment. Four patients treated with hyperthemia alone had recurrent symptoms within six months and five patients treated with radiotherapy immediately after hyperthermia developed marked diarrhea and frequency after only small doses of radiation. The six patients given hormonal therapy prior to hyperthermia all had marked improvement in symptoms. They report minimal complications except as noted above and attributed the above complications to radiotherapy. Follow-up was short. Given the variety of adjunctive therapies these patients received with hyperthermia, it appears difficult to sort out how much benefit can actually be attributed to the hyperthermia effects. Yerushalmi et al. followed this report in 1986 with a further report of 32 patients treated similarly with adjunctive radiation or hormonal therapy.[39] In this report, the few patients treated with hyperthermia alone had objective tumor regression but again they relapsed after six months. The best results were obtained in 20 patients (stage C) treated with combined radiotherapy and hyperthermia.

Montorosi et al. treated 46 patients with D_1 or D_2 disease who developed bladder outlet obstruction, urinary retention, or severe pelvic or perineal pain after total androgen blockage.[40] The hyperthemia was delivered transrectally through a specially designed device composed of a rectal heat applicator with microwave source, three thermocouples, for determination of rectal temperatures, a cooling system for the anterior rectal wall, and a specially designed 18°F urethral catheter with three thermocouples to monitor prostatic uretheral temperature. Patients underwent 10 60-minute sessions delivered over five weeks with a calculated intraprostatic temperature of $43.5 \pm 0.5°C$. They reported significant improvement in obstructive symptoms and 50% of patients in urinary retention were catheter-free immediately (38% at two years). They reported minimal complications.

Most recently, Servadio and Leib reported on 44 patients treated with transrectal hyperthemia in combination with radiotherapy or hormonal therapy.[41] Twenty-seven of these patients had locally advanced disease and all had severe local obstruction and irritative symptoms or urinary retention. They noted no complications attributable to hyperthemia and significant improvement in symptoms was noted in the majority of patients. Two of twenty-seven patients had progression of disease at four-year follow-up, and 9 of 11 cases who underwent follow-up biopsy were negative.

Sorensen et al. from Windsor, Ontario, reported on 12 patients undergoing transurethral microwave thermotherapy using hyperthermia (Prostatron).[42] All patients underwent radical prostatectomy 6 to 19 days post-microwave treatment. The depth of effective injury was 1.0 to 1.5 cm, with a well-demarcated line. Tumors located posteriorly were not affected by the treatment, however.

Tucker et al. recently used the Dunning prostate tumor model with interstitial seeds placed into the prostate followed with an external oscillating magnetic field to create intraprostatic hyperthemia.[43] They found that although a single treatment of 2 hours' duration did not delay tumor growth, two treatments separated by 48 hours or more did. The authors felt that in the future this technique could be used alone or in combination with radiotherapy seeds.

Clearly the use of microwave hyperthemia is in its nascent stage but may demonstrate some benefit for the treatment of local or locally advanced prostate cancer. Its use adjunctively with radiotherapy appears logical theoretically, but well-controlled studies with adequate follow-up are lacking. The issue of thermotolerance, as well as treatment length, frequency, and duration, are all questions that will need to be answered in the future.

LASER

Laser in the treatment of localized carcinoma of the prostate has also been explored. Lasers transform light energy into heat within the prostatic tissue, resulting in a temperature above 60°C for a few seconds. Rapid protein denaturation and necrosis results. The depth of penetration of light and, therefore, the volume of affected tissue is dependent on the wavelength of the applied laser.[44-46] The power density can be extremely variable in biologic tissue because of the oblique angle of application of laser energy usually required when using endoscopes with 0-degree lens systems. With the recent advent of the right-angle laser fiber, more precise application of laser energy to the prostate can be given.

Sander and Beisland pioneered the use

of the Nd:YAG laser for the treatment of localized prostate cancer.[47] Nd:YAG laser irradiation produced a homogenous coagulation to a depth of 3–4 mm without removal of the tissue. The necrosis gradually changed into fibrotic scar tissue with only minor shrinkage. They treated over 100 patients between 1981 and 1986 with localized lesions (stage T_1–T_3) with transurethral and/or suprapubic access to the gland (trocar cystoscope). The trocar cystostomy was utilized to access all capsular areas of the prostate not treatable with the laser fiber transurethrally, since they used a bare fiber. All patients initially underwent "extended transurethal resection of the prostate (TURP)" exposing capsular fibers throughout the extent of the resection. Three to five weeks later, a thorough lasering of the prostatic capsular bed was performed using 40–50 w applied in bursts of 1–4 seconds for a total of 7,000–21,000 joules. The transformation of tissue into a gray-white mass by visual inspection was used as an endpoint for adequate treatment in a given area of the prostate. All patients were given spinal anesthesia and the procedure duration was approximately 30 minutes. They reported no bleeding complications or problems from the suprapubic insertion of the trocar cystostomy, and postoperatively reported one case each of acute cystitis, acute epididymitis, and spinal headache. They generally left a 16F Foley catheter overnight and reported no incontinence or strictures. No rectal injuries were encountered since the temperature in the rectum never exceeded 52°C. Urethrocystoscopy was performed three to six months after laser treatment, and all patients had smoothly epithelialized and open prostatic cavities without ulcerations or protrusions suspicious for tumor. At two years follow-up, 56 of the original 63 patients were deemed disease free and seven cases were treatment failures. The failures occurred in patients in whom only the transurethral approach was utilized.[48]

Samdal and Brevik reported similar results in 26 patients with stages T_0–T_2 prostate cancer.[49] All patients underwent extended TURP followed in six weeks by Nd:YAG laser treatment at 45 w in 3-second pulses for a total of 11,000–35,000 joules. They reported minimal perioperative complications but did report eight late complications: four patients developed bladder neck contractures, two developed stress incontinence, one developed erectile dysfunction, one had meatal stenosis, and one developed bilateral hydronephrosis secondary to fibrosis. They stress the importance of thermistor monitoring of the rectal temperature (not to exceed 60°C). To date, they report 22 disease-free survivors (6–42 month follow-up). Because of the multifocal nature of prostate carcinoma, effective ablation of all tumor-bearing tissue involves effective ablation of the entire prostate. Follow-up PSA as a reflection of complete ablation has demonstrated a generalized decrease in PSA levels, but none have decreased to zero or undetectable.

Littrup and associates have reported on the percutaneous placement of needles into the prostate in order to insert a Nd:YAG laser fiber.[50] A study in dogs demonstrated focal areas of necrosis and coagulation extending up to 14 mm. Although needles could be placed accurately using ultrasound, the laser treatment was imprecise and penetration depth variable.

At Brown University, we have been studying the laser as a treatment for radiotherapy failure patients.[51] Vigorous transurethral prostatectomy (TURP) or endocrine therapy may be necessary to downsize the tumor. Right-angle laser fiber allows for more accurate treatments, followed with real-time transrectal ultrasound (Fig. 2). Results are too preliminary to comment.

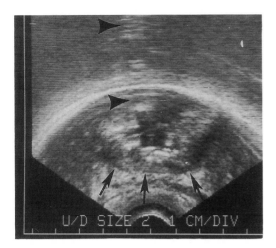

Fig. 2. Laser treatment of recurrent prostate cancer in progress as followed on transrectal ultrasound. Arrows point to prostatic capsule; arrowheads point to evolution of smoke and heat. Central cavitation is prostatic fossa.

The use of laser for treatment of localized prostate cancer shows promise, particularly with the advent of the right-angle laser fiber. Complications appear minimal and hospital stays are brief. Long-term follow-up studies are required, however, to determine the effectiveness of total ablation.

SALVAGE PROSTATECTOMY

In stage A or B disease, up to 36% of patients treated with definitive external beam radiotherapy or interstitial radiotherapy may have tumor recurrence or persistence at 10 years.[52] If a patient has a life expectancy of 10–15 years at the time radiation failure is detected, salvage radical prostatectomy may be considered. Several studies have been reported on small numbers of patients treated with salvage prostatectomy. Neerhut et al. reported on 16 patients who had failed definitive radiotherapy. Strict criteria for eligibility included an excellent performance status, projected life expectancy of at least 10 years, and a thorough negative evaluation for metastases.[53] They reported a number

of major complications, including rectal injury in 19%, anastomotic stricture in 25%, and total incontinence in 25%. Additionally, 37.5% had positive surgical margins, with the majority being at the apex. Follow-up was short, so survival figures were not meaningful, and PSA levels were not reported. Rainwater and Zincke reported a similar significant complication rate in their series of 30 salvage prostatectomies, with total incontinence in 10% and bladder neck contracture in 17%.[54] In addition, eight patients were upstaged to D_1 disease. In a follow-up paper, Zincke reported on 62 patients undergoing radical prostatectomy or exenteration for recurrent disease after radiotherapy.[55] Morbidity in the radical prostatectomy group included urinary leakage, rectal injury, and incontinence. In spite of the fact that more than 50% of the men had hormone therapy as well, results were not encouraging overall. Patients undergoing extensive surgical procedures (i.e., anterior or total exenteration) did not fare well, with a 45% progression rate and 30% cancer death rate by five years. Men with tumors small enough to allow for radical prostatectomy only did significantly better than those men requiring more involved operations. Thus, only in men with small glands does radical prostatectomy with hormone therapy represent an option. Moul and Paulson reported on 12 patients who underwent radical prostatectomy (N = 4) or cystoprostatectomy (N = 8) for recurrent disease postradiotherapy.[56] Complications were considered minimal (largely sepsis, wound infection, or leaks), but 7 of 12 men suffered some complication. Only 25% had residual disease confined to the prostate with negative capsular margin, and only 4 of 12 had no evidence of disease with a mean follow-up of 49 months. The authors conclude that this approach may be of benefit to selected patients but must be considered as palliative or for local control. Ahlerling and associates reported similar findings in 34 patients undergoing salvage resection. Of the 34 patients, 11 underwent radical prostatectomy only (one surgeon) and 23 underwent cystoprostatectomy (two other surgeons). The latter group included one patient requiring colon resection for tumor invasion, and one patient requiring total exenteration. Twenty-seven of the 34 patients had hormone therapy as well. Incontinence rates were 40% after external beam radiotherapy and 83% following interstitial radiotherapy. Combining both groups, 65% were alive with no detectable PSA levels with a mean postoperative follow-up of 53 months. The authors concluded that surgical debulking plus hormone therapy may be of value.

Stein et al. reported on 13 patients undergoing radical surgery after radiation failure.[57] Two of the 13 underwent cystoprostatectomy due to bladder neck extension of the tumor. Six of the 13 patients suffered complications (urinary leaks, strictures, or rectal injury). On pathologic examination, 6 of the 13 had seminal vesical involvement, 2 had positive surgical margins, and 2 had positive lymph nodes. With limited follow-up, 3 of the 13 have had tumor progression.

Overall, it is obvious that radical cystoprostatectomy or exenteration performed for larger tumor volumes is overall an exercise in futility in these patients. Survival rates do not appear to be greater than would be anticipated with hormone therapy alone. In carefully selected patients, with small tumors, who are amenable to radical prostatectomy, there may be some increase in survival benefit. Patients should accept the increased risk of complications such as prolonged urinary leak, rectal injury, impotence, or incontinence.

REFERENCES

1. Smith JA, Middletown RG: Radical prostatectomy for stage B2 prostatic cancer. J Urol 127:702–703, 1982.

2. Boxer RJ, Kaufman JJ, Goodwin WE: Radical prostatectomy for carcinoma of the prostate, 1951–1976: a review of 329 patients. J Urol 117:208–213, 1977.

3. Walsh PC, Lepor H, Eggleston JC: Radical prostatectomy with preservation of sexual function: anatomic and pathologic considerations. Prostate 4(5):473–485, 1983.

4. Bagshaw MA: Radiation therapy for cancer of the prostate. In Skinner DG, Luskovsky G (eds): Diagnosis and Management of Genitourinary Cancer. Philadelphia: W.B. Saunders, pp 425–445, 1988.

5. Ray GR, Cassady R, Bagshaw MA: Definitive radiation therapy of carcinoma of the prostate: a report on 15 years of experience. Radiology 106:407–418, 1973.

6. McGowan DG: Radiation therapy in the management of localized carcinoma of the prostate: a preliminary report. Cancer 39:98–103, 1977.

7. Perez CA, Bauer W, Garza R: Radiation therapy in the definitive treatment of localized carcinoma of the prostate. Cancer 40(40):1425–1433, 1977.

8. Loh ES, Brown HE, Berler DD: Radiotherapy of carcinoma of the prostate: a preliminary report. J Urol 106:906–909, 1971.

9. Green N, Trenble D, Wallack H: Prostate cancer: post-irradiation incontinence. J Urol 144:307–309, 1990.

10. Hafermann MD: External radiotherapy. Urology 17(Suppl):15–23, 1981.

11. Kabalin JN, Hodge KK, McNeal JE, Freiha KS, Stamey T: Identification of residual cancer in the prostate following radiotherapy: role of transrectal ultrasound guided biopsy and prostate specific antigen. J Urol 142:326–331, 1989.

12. Paulson DF, Lin GH, Hinshaw W, et al.: Radical surgery vs. radiotherapy for stage A₂ and stage B (T₁₋₂NoMo) adenocarcinoma of the prostate. J Urol 128:502–504, 1982.

13. Paulson DF: Treatment selections in organ-confined disease. Prob Urol 1:53–68, 1987.

14. Smith JA, Jr, Haynes TH, Middleton RG: Impact of external irradiation on local symptoms and survival free of disease in patients with pelvic lymph node metastasis from adenocarcinoma of the prostate. J Urol 131:705–707, 1984.

15. Hanks GE: External beam radiation therapy for clinically localized prostate cancer: patterns of care studies in the United States. NCI Monogr 7:75–94, 1988.

16. Shipley WU, Prout GR, Jr, Coachman NM, et

al.: Radiation therapy for localized prostate carcinoma: experience at the Massachusetts General Hospital (1973–1981). NCI Monogr 7:67–74, 1988.

17. Kaplan ID, Cox RS, Bagshaw MA: Prostate specific antigen after external beam radiotherapy for prostatic cancer: followup. J Urol 149:519–522, 1993.

18. Gonder MH, Soanes WA, Smith V: Experimental prostate cryosurgery. Invest Urol 1:610–618, 1964.

19. Onik GM, Cohen JK, Reyes GD, Rubinsky B, Chang Z, Baust J: Transrectal ultrasound-guided percutaneous radical cryosurgical ablation of the prostate. Cancer 72 (4):1291–1299, 1993.

20. Loening S, Lubaroff D: Cryosurgery and immunotherapy for prostatic cancer. Urol Clin N Am 11(2):327–336, 1984.

21. Flocks TH, Nelson CMK, Boatman CL: Perineal cryosurgery for prostatic carcinoma. J Urol 108: 933–935, 1972.

22. Soanes WA, Ablin RJ, Gonder MJ: Remission of metastatic lesions following cryosurgery in prostate cancer. J Urol 104:154–159, 1970.

23. O'Donoghue EP, Milleman N, Flocks LA, et al.: Cryosurgery for carcinoma of prostate. Urology 5(3):308–316, 1975.

24. Gursel EW, Roberts M, Veenema RJ: Regression of prostatic cancer following sequential cryotherapy in the prostate. J Urol 108:928–932, 1972.

25. Bonney WW, Platz CE, Fallon B, Rose EF, et al.: Cryosurgery in prostatic cancer: survival. Urology 19:37–42, 1982.

26. Bonney WW, Fallen B, Gerber WL, Hawtrey CE, Loening SA, Narayana AS, Platz CE, Rose EF, Sall JC, Schmidt JD, and Culp DA: Cryosurgery in prostate cancer: elimination of the local lesion. Urology 22:8–15, 1983.

27. Onik G, Porterfield B, Rubinsky B, et al.: Percutaneous transperineal prostate cryosurgery using transrectal ultrasound guidance: animal model. Urology 37 (3):277–281, 1991.

28. von Eschenbach AC, Johnson DE, Babaian RJ, et al.: Ultrasound-guided cryoablation of recurrent prostate cancer following radiation therapy. J Urol 149:232A, 1993.

29. Storm FK: Hyperthermia in Cancer Therapy. Boston: G.K. Hall, 1983.

30. Oleson JR: Hyperthermia. In DeVita VT, Hellman S, Rosenberg SA (eds): Cancer Principles and Practice of Oncology, 3rd ed. Philadelphia: J.B. Lippincott, p 2426, 1989.

31. Field SB, Bleehan NM: Hyperthermia in the treatment of cancer. Cancer Treat Rev 6:63–94, 1979.

32. Sone CW: Effect of hyperthermia on vascular functions of normal tissues and experimental tumors. J Natl Cancer Inst 60(1):711–718, 1978.

33. Chen TT, Heidelberger C: Quantitative studies on the malignant transformation of mouse prostate by carcinogenic hydrocarbons in vitro. Int J Cancer 4:166–173, 1969.

34. Giovanella BC, Stehlen JS, Morgan AC: Selective lethal effect of supranormal temperatures on human neoplastic cells. Cancer Res 36:3944–3950, 1976.

35. Westra A, Dewey WC: Variations in sensitivity to heat shock during the cell-cycle of Chinese hamster cells in vitro. Int J Radiat Biol 19:467–477, 1971.

36. Servadio C, Leib Z: Hyperthermia in the treatment of prostate cancer. Prostate 5(2):205–211, 1984.

37. Harisiadis L, Sung D, Hall EJ: Thermal tolerance and repair of thermal damage by cultured cells. Radiology 123:505–509, 1977.

38. Yerushalmi A, Servadio C, Leib C, et al.: Local hyperthemia for treatment of carcinoma of the prostate: a preliminary report. Prostate 3:623–629, 1982.

39. Yerushalmi A, Shani A, Fishelovitz Y, et al.: Local microwave hyperthermia in the treatment of carcinoma of the prostate. Oncology 43:299–305, 1986.

40. Montorsi F, Guazzoni G, Colombo R, Galli L, et al.: Transrectal microwave hyperthermia for advanced prostate cancer: long-term clinical results. J Urol 148:342–345, 1992.

41. Servadio C, Leib Z: Local hyperthermia for prostate cancer. Urology 38:307–309, 1991.

42. Sorensen RB, McGarragle MP, Grignon DJ, Dietrich M, Mongeau R: I. Transurethral microwave thermotherapy (TUMT) using the Prostatron: a histopathological evaluation of the thermal effects on carcinoma of the prostate. J Urol 149:232A, 1993.

43. Tucker R, Loening S, Landas S, et al.: The effect of interstitial hyperthermia on the Dunning prostate tumor model. J Urol 147:1129–1133, 1992.

44. Stein BS, Kendall AR: Lasers in urology: I. Laser physics and safety. Urology 23(5):405–411, 1984.

45. Hofstetter A, Stahler G, Weiberg W, Kerditsch E: Risk of intestinal damage from endoscopic neodymium-YAG laser irradiation of bladder tumors. Urologe A 20:305–308, 1981.

46. Halldorsson T: Biophysical fundamentals and

instrumentation of the endovesical Nd:YAG laser application. Urologe A 20:293–299, 1981.

47. Sander S, Beisland HO: Laser in the treatment of localized prostatic cancer. J Urol 132:280–281, 1984.

48. Beisland HO, Sander S: First clinical experiences on neodymium-YAG laser irradiation of localized prostatic cancer. Scand J Urol Nephrol 20(2):113–117, 1986.

49. Samdal F, Brevik B: Laser combined with TURP in the treatment of localized prostatic cancer. Scand J Urol Nephrol 24:175–181, 1990.

50. Littrup PJ, Lee F, Borlaza GS, et al.: Percutaneous ablation of canine prostate using transrectal ultrasound guidance absolute ethanol and Nd:YAG laser. Invest Radiol 23:734–739, 1988.

51. Stein BS: Personal communication, 1993.

52. Scardino PT, Wheeler TM: Local control of prostate cancer with radiotherapy: frequency and prognostic significance of positive results of post-irradiation prostate biopsy. NCI Monogr 7:95–100, 1988.

53. Neerhut GJ, Wheeler T, Cantini M, et al.: Salvage radical prostatectomy for radical recurrent adenocarcinoma of the prostate. J Urol 140:544–549, 1988.

54. Rainwater LM, Zincke H: Radical prostatectomy after radiation therapy for cancer of the prostate; feasibility and prognosis. J Urol 140:1455–1459, 1988.

55. Zincke H: Radical prostatectomy and exenterative procedures for local failure after radiotherapy with curative intent: comparison of outcomes. J Urol 147:894–899, 1992.

56. Moul JW, Paulson DF: The role of radical surgery in the management of radiation recurrent and large volume prostate cancer. Cancer 68(6):1265–1271, 1991.

57. Stein A, Smith RB, deKernion JB: Salvage radical prostatectomy after failure of curative radiotherapy for adenocarcinoma of prostate. Urology 40(3):197–200, 1992.

11

Neoadjuvant Androgen Deprivation Before Radical Prostatectomy: Current Status and Trial Design

Michael L. Cher, M.D., Peter R. Carroll, M.D., Eric J. Small, M.D., and Katsuto Shinohara, M.D.

INTRODUCTION

The sensitivity of prostatic cancer to androgen deprivation has been well established. However, the impact of such therapy has generally been investigated only in those with regional lymphatic spread or distant metastatic disease (stages D1 and D2; N+, M+). More recently, several investigators have begun to use androgen withdrawal in patients with clinically localized disease (stages A–C; T1–4, NX, M0) as neoadjuvant therapy before planned radical prostatectomy. The objectives of such therapy include decreasing the morbidity of surgery (as assessed by blood loss, operating times, urinary continence rates, etc.), reducing the rates of positive surgical margins, and truly "downstaging" locally advanced disease. If either of the latter are possible, it is hoped that local recurrence rates would decrease. The perceived need for other forms of adjuvant therapy such as radiation or long-term androgen deprivation would also be reduced. Finally, another theoretical goal is improvement in long-term survival.

The concept of neoadjuvant androgen deprivation is not new. In 1964, Scott evaluated the impact of androgen deprivation in 31 patients with clinical stage C prostatic cancer.[1] Sixteen or 51.6% survived 10 years free of disease. However, only those who responded well to initial endocrine therapy were offered radical prostatectomy and 90% of the patients who underwent radical prostatectomy had well- or moderately well-differentiated cancers. Since androgen deprivation was permanent (castration), the contribution of it alone is difficult to quantify. Furthermore, this highly select group of patients was treated in an era where local staging was imperfect and prostate-specific antigen (PSA) testing was not available for long-term follow-up. Nonetheless there has been renewed enthusiasm for such therapy, although it remains investigational and its impact on outcome, if any, is a matter of much current debate.

GENERAL CONSIDERATIONS

Androgen Deprivation and the Development of Androgen-Independent Growth

Prostatic cancers are androgen dependent and institution of androgen deprivation results in profound volume decreases in both primary and metastatic cancers in at least 80% of patients. Androgen with-

Prostate Cancer, pages 175–183 © 1994 Wiley-Liss, Inc.

drawal induces a characteristic series of events termed programmed cell death or apoptosis. This is a selective process resulting in death of those cells entering into the apoptotic pathway. It is characterized by endonuclease activation leading to chromatin cleavage and a characteristic ladder of DNA fragments seen in agarose gel electrophoresis of genomic DNA. Cells undergoing apoptosis have a characteristic morphologic appearance as well, although these changes are often transient and not always discernible by routine light microscopy.

Nevertheless, complete eradication of cancer, even in animal models, is rarely, if ever, achieved. Steenbrugge and colleagues transplanted an androgen-dependent, prostate cancer cell line (PC-82) subcutaneously in nude mice.[2] These transplanted tumors regressed to nonpalpable states after castration. However, residual cancer cells remained and reinstitution of circulating androgens resulted in tumor recurrence with doubling times similar to that before castration. In addition, an androgen-independent state occurred even after complete androgen blockade (castration and addition of an antiandrogen).

The mechanisms of androgen independence have been studied by several investigators. Isaacs and colleagues demonstrated that the development of an androgen-independent state was a product of clonal selection: androgen-dependent and -independent populations exist initially and, after androgen withdrawal, the latter population grows selectively.[3] Bruchovsky and colleagues investigated the effects of androgen suppression on the Shinogi mouse mammary cancer, an androgen-dependent cancer that can give rise to recurrent androgen-independent cancer after hormonal withdrawal.[4] These investigators recorded the levels of dihydrotestosterone, nuclear androgen receptor, and 5-α-reductase in parent, regressing, and recurrent cancers as well as the

number of stem cells in each. Androgen receptor concentration and 5-α-reductase activity were low and undetectable, respectively, in the recurrent cancers, consistent with the conclusion that recurrent growth occurred in an androgen-free state and was not due to reflexively elevated dihydrotestosterone. Importantly, androgen deprivation resulted in significant changes in the stem-cell populations. The parent cancer had approximately 1 stem cell per 4,000 parent tumor cells. There was a 20-fold increase in stem cells in the recurrent cancer (approximately 1 in 200). Interestingly, when the stem-cell populations of the regressed tumors were assessed, the stem-cell population had decreased substantially (approximately 1 in 70,000) compared to the parent cancer. Although the origin of androgen-independent cells after androgen deprivation is incompletely understood, the experiments of Bruchovsky and associates suggest that use of androgen deprivation in a neoadjuvant fashion may result in a regressed cancer with fewer stem cells if it is not allowed to achieve an androgen-independent status. This has important implications for patients who opt for neoadjuvant androgen withdrawal. Radical prostatectomy should be timed to coincide with the maximum tumor volume decrease. On theoretical grounds, one should not wait until clonal selection pressures allow androgen-independent cells to predominate.

Androgen withdrawal leads to characteristic pathological changes in the primary tumor. Involutional changes such as cytoplasmic clearing, loss of glandular architecture, and nuclear pyknosis and fragmentation are common, as is a prominent stromal response (Fig. 1).[5] The response of the primary tumor to androgen deprivation may be more durable than that seen in metastatic sites. Carpentier and Schroeder used transrectal ultrasound to monitor the primary tumor of patients with metastatic disease who were treated with androgen

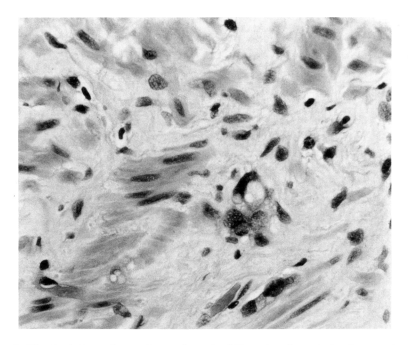

Fig. 1. Histological specimen of a moderately differentiated prostatic adenocarcinoma after treatment with three months of androgen deprivation. Note the prominent clearing of cytoplasm, nuclear pyknosis, and stromal response.

deprivation. They found that progression was frequent in metastatic sites even when the volume of the primary tumor remained small.[6]

Suitable Endpoints for Analysis

The goal of neoadjuvant androgen deprivation should be to improve cause-specific survival rates. Only a long-term analysis of a properly conducted, randomized trial will provide the data to determine if survival can be improved. In the interim, surrogate endpoints may be analyzed, including the impact of such treatment on surgical margins and final pathological stage. Also, perioperative morbidity (operating times, blood loss, postoperative potency and continences rates, etc.) may be analyzed. However, such surrogate endpoints cannot be substituted for cure rates when analyzing this form of therapy. In addition, the powerful impact of adjuvant therapy such as irradiation or continued androgen deprivation must be considered. The impact of neoadjuvant androgen deprivation cannot be reliably evaluated, at least early, in those trials routinely incorporating postoperative adjuvant radiotherapy with continued androgen deprivation given the powerful impact of these treatments on initial outcome regimens. For instance, Belt and Schroeder demonstrated that adjuvant androgen deprivation after radical prostatectomy had an apparent benefit on survival at five years, but no beneficial effect at 10 and 15 years after surgery.[7] In the absence of long-term follow-up, postoperative PSA levels may give preliminary and important insight into the effectiveness of neoadjuvant androgen deprivation, as PSA levels may predict clinical relapse months to years before it is recognized clinically.

The Timing and Type of Neoadjuvant Therapy

Various methods of androgen deprivation have been used as neoadjuvant therapy, including low-dose diethylstilbesterol (1 mg), a luteinizing hormone-releasing hormone (LHRH) analog administered alone, and the combination of an LHRH analog and an antiandrogen. Unlike orchiectomy, these are all reversible forms of androgen deprivation, as libido and erectile function should be preserved in this patient population. Orchiectomy can be performed at a later date if disease status warrants permanent androgen ablation. Currently, most trials use combined androgen deprivation, theorizing that a more rapid and profound reduction in cancer volume may be achieved with this form of therapy compared to monotherapy.[8]

The length of time necessary to ensure maximal response of the primary tumor to androgen deprivation has not been determined. Carroll and associates recorded serial changes in PSA levels as well as total prostatic volumes and prostatic cancer volumes as determined by transrectal ultrasound in patients with stage C (T3) adenocarcinoma of the prostate treated with androgen deprivation before radical prostatectomy (Fig. 2). The majority of the changes recorded occurred during the first two months of therapy. Others have shown that similar changes in volume occur within the first three months of therapy.[9] The magnitude of the PSA reduction has been consistently high, approximately 98%, in trials of neoadjuvant hormonal therapy reported to date. Prostatic volume decreased (35%–52%), as did cancer volume (49%–91%) when serial transrectal sonography was used to monitor response (Fig. 3A,B).

Selection of Patients

Radical prostatectomy alone has been demonstrated to offer excellent long-term disease-free survival in patients with localized prostate cancer. The risk of either local or distant relapse is related to tumor stage and grade. Although androgen deprivation produces impressive changes in both benign and malignant prostatic volume, these effects, even though they may be prolonged, are never permanent. If the objective of neoadjuvant androgen withdrawal followed by radical prostatectomy is to cure cancer, such therapy should be offered to patients at high likelihood of having regionally confined, and therefore

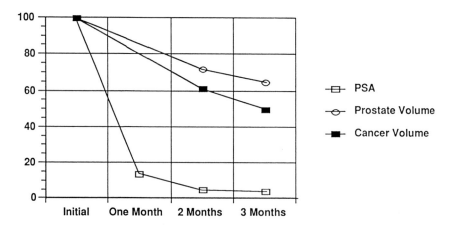

Fig. 2. Serial changes (in percent) of serum PSA and whole prostate and prostate cancer volume during androgen deprivation.

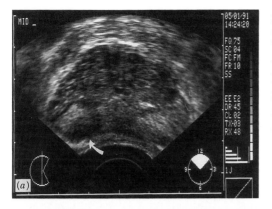

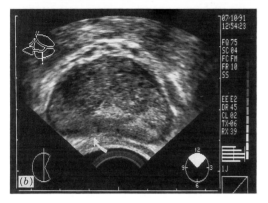

Fig. 3. Transverse, transrectal ultrasound image before androgen deprivation **(a)** and after three months of such therapy **(b)**.

excisable, disease. Neoadjuvant hormonal withdrawal followed by radical prostatectomy is not likely to cure patients with occult metastatic disease.

The frequency of positive surgical mar-

gins has been reported to be quite high (22%–57%) in series of patients with stage B prostatic cancer treated by radical prostatectomy.[10-12] Such patients are commonly offered adjuvant radiation, which may improve local control rates, but is costly, may not influence distant relapse rates, and may be associated with additional morbidity.[13] An examination of relapse patterns after radical prostatectomy alone offers insight into which patients are at risk of local recurrence in the absence of distant relapse and thus are potential candidates for neoadjuvant androgen deprivation (Table 1). Thus, patients with clinical stages A2, B2, and C1 disease would appear to have relapse patterns that would justify consideration of neoadjuvant therapy. Although neoadjuvant therapy may improve local control rates for higher stage disease, such patients are at a considerable risk of distant relapse, which might be delayed but not eliminated by preoperative androgen withdrawal.

Patient selection may be difficult, as the accuracy of clinical staging is generally poor, and reports of a beneficial effect of neoadjuvant androgen deprivation may, in fact, be due to clinical understaging of the primary tumor. Bosch and associates studied pathological specimens from 48 men who underwent radical prostatectomy for presumed stage C prostatic cancer and identified an overstaging error of 24%, a rate remarkably similar to the downstag-

TABLE 1. Local and Distant Recurrence Rates After Radical Prostatectomy Alone[a]

P Stage	Local Recurrence (%)	Distant Recurrence (%)	Distant and Local Recurrence (%)	Elevated PSA
Organ confined	2	1	0	3
Specimen confined	8	1	1	16
Positive margins	25	4	6	13
Positive seminal vesicles	9	23	14	30
Positive lymph nodes	3	22	8	84

[a]See ref. 19.

ing rate reported in many current trials of neoadjuvant therapy.[14] These results indicate that true downstaging may be rare. Both magnetic resonance imaging and transrectal ultrasound suffer from considerable lack of specificity and sensitivity in staging clinically localized prostate cancer.[15,16]

INITIAL CLINICAL RESULTS

Despite the theoretical advantages of neoadjuvant androgen deprivation and enthusiasm for this form of therapy, little clinical data is presently available to support its widespread application. Only limited numbers of patients have been treated, often from multiple institutions. Selection criteria for such treatment has varied, as has the application of adjuvant therapy, making it difficult to compare results. Several investigators have applied such therapy to patients with clinical stage C carcinoma of the prostate in an attempt to improve results over radical prostatectomy alone. Preliminary results from such trials are summarized in Table 2. The results suggest that few patients are "downstaged." In fact, more advanced cancer is commonly encountered, reflecting the extent of clinical understaging. The degree of upstaging is more apparent if one includes those patients thought to have capsular

penetration alone (C1) on clinical evaluation, but are found to have seminal vesicle invasion (pC2) at pathological review. Such a distinction is important, as the risk of distant relapse is much more likely in those patients with seminal invasion compared to those with capsular penetration alone. Epstein recently confirmed that, in the absence of lymph node metastases, seminal vesicle invasion was associated with a substantially greater risk of tumor progression than was capsular penetration.[17] Interestingly, Gleason grade and surgical margins were independent predictors along with seminal vesicle invasion in a multivariant analysis. There was a trend for positive surgical margin rate to predict progression even in those with seminal vesicle invasion. Whether neoadjuvant hormonal therapy could improve progression rates by decreasing the surgical margin rate in such patients is unknown. In addition, approximately 20% of all patients with stage C prostatic cancer treated with neoadjuvant hormonal withdrawal will be found to have lymph node metastases.

Neoadjuvant therapy is being applied to lower stage disease (stages B and C1) as well. In one of the first published trials, Oesterling et al. compared pathological staging in 22 patients with stages B and C prostate cancer who underwent preopera-

TABLE 2. Preoperative Androgen Deprivation Before Radical Prostatectomy in Patients with Clinical Stage C Prostatic Cancer

Reference	Patients	Downstage	No Change	Upstage	Positive Lymph Nodes
Kennedy et al.[20]	7	2	3	2	2
Vapnek and Carroll[21]	26	4	12	10[a]	6[b]
MacFarlane et al.[22]	12	3	5	4	4
Daneshgari et al.[23]	44	13	25	6	6[c]
Mottrie et al.[24]	45	6	28	11	11
Total	134	28 (21%)	73 (54%)	33 (25%)	

[a]Includes upstaging on the basis of a clinical C1 being found to be a pathological C2.
[b]Twenty-nine patients underwent lymph node dissection.
[c]Includes D0 and D1 disease.

TABLE 3. Positive Surgical Margin Rates After Neoadjuvant Androgen Deprivation

			Positive Surgical Margin Rates	
Reference	Number	Stage	Preoperative Therapy (%)	No Preoperative Therapy (%)
Oesterling et al.[18]	22	B2,C	86	38
Daneshgari et al.[23]	44	C1–C3	70[a]	N.S.[c]
Mottrie et al.[24]	45	C	86[a]	N.S.
Fair[25]	55	B	8	13
Labrie et al.[26b]	114	B,C1	13.6	29.2

[a]Stage C, D-0, or D-1.
[b]Randomized trial.
[c]N.S. = Not stated.

tive androgen deprivation to a control group of patients matched for preoperative PSA levels and clinical stage.[18] Although the median decrease in the PSA in treated patients was 98.5%, there was no difference between the groups with respect to pathological stage, maximum tumor dimension, and DNA content. In fact, the incidence of positive surgical margins was greater in those receiving preoperative hormonal therapy. However, Fair[25] and Labrie et al.[26] both noted an improvement in surgical margin rates in patients treated preoperatively with androgen deprivation therapy compared to those who have not received such therapy (Table 3). The reason for the discrepancy between the latter two series and those reported by Oestering et al.,[18] Daneshgari et al.,[23] and Mottrie et al.[24] is unclear. Higher stage patients were included in those series and they were not randomized trials. A possibility remains that a surgeon may compromise the surgical margin if a cancer has regressed substantially in size. Although Oesterling and colleagues do not mention this as a reason for the high positive margin rate in their series, it is important that the surgical approach to areas of presumed extracapsular disease be such as to maximize the likelihood of complete cancer excision, even in those tumors whose volume markedly decreased during the neoadjuvant treatment period.

Interestingly, the rates of lymph node metastases in the series reported by Fair did not differ significantly between those who received preoperative therapy (7%) and those who did not (10%), suggesting that the improvement in surgical margins may be real and not a result of the failure to detect cancer cells at the periphery of the primary tumor due to the effects of androgen withdrawal. Unfortunately, other important endpoints for evaluation, including relapse rates, have not been reported routinely in such series. Even in those patients who have impressive tumor volume and PSA changes, long-term benefit is not guaranteed. In our own series of 26 patients with stage C prostate cancer who received combined therapy (LHRH analog and antiandrogen), specimen-confined disease was noted in 64%. However, at a mean of 18 months of follow-up, 18% have failed locally, 18% distantly, and 41% have detectable PSA levels. These results suggest that patients with stage C disease are at significant risk of disease recurrence despite such aggressive local therapy, that many patients harbor occult metastases, and that neoadjuvant androgen deprivation may be better suited for lower stage cancers.

Although some authors have reported decreased morbidity in those receiving preoperative therapy (i.e., shorter operating times, less blood loss, etc.), this has not been substantiated by the experience of others, including our own.

SUMMARY AND FUTURE PROSPECTS

Neoadjuvant androgen deprivation before radical prostatectomy remains investigational. Although it is well tolerated by patients and there is no evidence of an adverse effect on tumor growth when given for a short period of time, its impact on long-term, disease-free survival is unknown. However, preliminary evidence reported by a variety of investigators suggests that it may be beneficial in selected patients. Patients most likely to benefit would be those with potentially high local recurrence rates with lower stage disease in whom the likelihood of occult distant disease is low (clinical stages A, B, and C1). Only a properly conducted, prospective, randomized trial will determine whether neoadjuvant androgen deprivation before radical prostatectomy is of immediate or long-term benefit to patients. A multicenter randomized trial is currently underway for patients with clinical stage B2 prostate cancer. Three hundred patients will be entered; half will receive combined neoadjuvant androgen ablation prior to radical prostatectomy. The principal endpoints will be pathological staging, surgical complications, time to progression (including PSA increase), and median survival. Until this study and others like it are completed, neoadjuvant androgen ablation should be considered investigational and should not serve as a substitute for good surgical technique.

REFERENCES

1. Scott WW: An evaluation of endocrine therapy plus radical prostatectomy in the treatment of advanced carcinoma of the prostate. J Urol 91:97, 1964.

2. Steenbrugge GJ, Groen M, Romjin JC, Schroeder FH: Biological effects of hormonal treatment regimens on a transplantable human prostatic tumor line (PC-82). J Urol 131:812–817, 1984.

3. Isaacs JT, Coffey DS: Adaptation versus selection as the mechanism responsible for the relapse of prostatic cancer to androgen ablation therapy as studied in the Dunning R-3327-H adenocarcinoma. Cancer Res 41:5070, 1981.

4. Bruchovsky N, Rennie PS, Coldman AJ, Goldenberg SL, To M, Lawson D: Effects of androgen withdrawal on the stem cell composition of the Shionogi carcinoma. Cancer Res 50:2275–2282, 1990.

5. Armas OA, Aprikian AG, Melamed J, Cohen D, Cordon-Cardo C, Fair WR, Reuter VE: Clinical and pathobiological effects of total androgen ablation on clinically localized prostatic carcinoma. J Urol 149:347A, 1993.

6. Carpentier PJ, Schroeder FH: Transrectal ultrasonography in the followup of prostatic carcinoma patients: a new prognostic parameter? J Urol 131:903, 1984.

7. Belt E, Schroeder FH: Total perineal prostatectomy for carcinoma of the prostate. J Urol 107:91–96, 1972.

8. McLeod DG, Crawford ED, Blumenstein BA, Eisenberger MA, Dorr FA: Controversies in the treatment of metastatic prostate cancer. Cancer (Suppl) 70:324–323, 1992.

9. Pinault S, Tetu B, Gagnon J, Monfette G, Dupont A, Labrie F: Transrectal ultrasound evaluation of local prostate cancer in patients treated with LHRH agonist and in combination with flutamide. Urology 34:254, 1992.

10. Rosen MA, Goldstone L, Lapin S, Wheeler T, Scardino PT: Frequency and location of extracapsular extension and positive surgical margins in radical prostatectomy specimens. J Urol 148:331–337, 1992.

11. Catalona WJ, Biggs SW: Nerve-sparing radical prostatectomy: evaluation of results after 250 patients. J Urol 143:538, 1990.

12. Stamey TA, Villers AA, McNeal JE, Link PC, Freiha FS: Positive surgical margins at radical prostatectomy: importance of the apical dissection. J Urol 143:1166–1173, 1990.

13. Anscher MS, Prosnitz LR: Postoperative radiotherapy for patients with carcinoma of the prostate undergoing radical prostatectomy with positive surgical margins, seminal vesicle involvement and/or penetration through the capsule. J Urol 138:1407, 1987.

14. Bosch RJLH, Kurth KH, Schroeder FH: Surgi-

cal treatment of locally advanced (T3) prostatic carcinoma: early results. J Urol 138:816, 1987.

15. Lorentzen T, Nerstrom H, Iversen P, Torp-Pedersen ST: Local staging of prostate cancer with transrectal ultrasound: a literature review. Prostate (Suppl) 4:11–16, 1992.

16. Rifkin MD, Zerhouni EA, Gatsonis CA, Quint LE, et al.: Comparison of magnetic resonance imaging and ultrasonography in staging early prostate cancer—results of a multi-institutional cooperative trial. N Engl J Med 323:621–626, 1990.

17. Epstein J, Carmichael N, Walsh PC: Adenocarcinoma of the prostate invading the seminal vesicles: definition and relation of tumor volume, grade and margin of resection to prognosis. J Urol 149:1040–1045, 1993.

18. Oesterling J, Andrews PE, Suman VJ, Zincke H, Myers RP: Preoperative androgen deprivation therapy: artificial lowering of serum prostate specific antigen without downstaging the tumor. J Urol 149:779–782, 1993.

19. Morton RA, Steiner MS, Walsh PC: Cancer control following anatomical radical prostatectomy: an interim report. J Urol 145:1197–1200, 1991.

20. Kennedy TJ, Sonneland AM, Marlett MM, Troup RH: Luteinizing hormone-releasing hormone downstaging of clinical stage C prostate cancer. J Urol 147:891–893, 1992.

21. Vapnek JM, Carroll PR: Neoadjuvant hormonal downsizing of clinical stage C carcinoma of the prostate. J Urol 147:247A, 1992.

22. MacFarlane MT, Abi-Aad A, Stein A, Danella J, Belldegrun A, deKernion J: Neoadjuvant hormonal deprivation in patients with locally advanced prostate cancer. J Urol 147:246A, 1992.

23. Daneshgari F, Crawford ED, Andros E; Austenfeld M, Stanley B, Williams R, Ross G, Pickard L, Schoborg T: Neoadjuvant hormonal therapy of patients with clinical stage C prostate cancer. J Urol 149:348A, 1993.

24. Mottrie AM, Mappes C, Stockle M, Muller S, Voges G: Neoadjuvant hormonal treatment in clinical stage C prostate cancer. J Urol 149:347A, 1993.

25. Fair W: Pre-op hormonal downstaging of prostatic cancer: fact or fantasy. Special lecture, American Urological Association, San Antonio, 1993.

26. Labrie F, Dupont A, Gomez JL, Fradette Y, Koutsileris M, Lemay M, Tetu B, Diamond P, Cusan L, Suburu ER: Beneficial effect of combination therapy administered prior to radical prostatectomy. J Urol 149:348A, 1993.

12

Observation as a Treatment Option Among Men with Clinically Localized Prostate Cancer

Peter C. Albertsen, M.D., John H. Wasson, M.D., and Michael J. Barry, M.D.

INTRODUCTION

The appropriate treatment of newly diagnosed, clinically localized prostate cancer remains extraordinarily controversial. Many physicians recommend aggressive treatments such as radical prostatectomy and radiation therapy, while others suggest a more conservative approach consisting of either immediate hormonal therapy or observation followed by hormonal therapy should symptomatic metastatic disease develop. The controversy reflects both a fundamental lack of knowledge concerning the natural history of newly diagnosed prostate cancer and the philosophical diversity among physicians concerning the value of different treatment modalities.

Patients are rarely identified with localized prostate cancer because of clinical symptoms. Instead, prostate cancer is diagnosed either as an incidental finding following transurethral resection or following a prostate biopsy performed because of an elevated prostate-specific antigen (PSA) or a palpable prostate abnormality. As a result, the decision to treat localized prostate cancer is not based on the need to relieve current symptoms but rather on the belief that treatment now will prevent the development of symptomatic disease in the future. A physician and patient, therefore, must assess the likelihood that the patient will develop symptomatic disease and whether treatment now will alter the progression of the disease. Furthermore, if they choose treatment, they must weigh the relative benefits of different treatment alternatives against the potential harms.

This chapter reviews the critical factors that affect the probability of developing metastatic disease and assists the reader in determining whether observation as a treatment option is appropriate for some men with clinically localized prostate cancer. Only by carefully weighing the risks of disease progression and the benefits and harms of various treatment alternatives can patients, with the help of their physicians, decide upon the treatment that is right for them.

RISK FACTORS THAT PREDICT THE DEVELOPMENT OF SYMPTOMATIC PROSTATE CANCER

Unlike many other cancers where death from disease is a virtual certainty in the absence of treatment, many men live normal lives with prostate cancer. The disease

Prostate Cancer, pages 185–196 © 1994 Wiley-Liss, Inc.

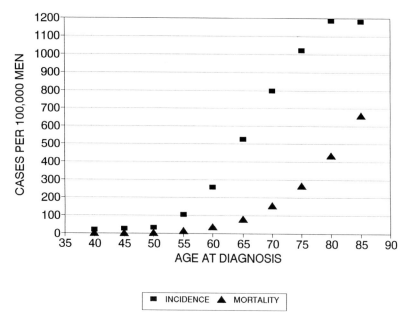

Fig. 1. Age-specific incidence and mortality from prostate cancer for all U.S. men, based on SEER data from 1985–1989 (cases per 100,000 man-years; from 1992).

is relatively rare before age 50 years, but the incidence rises dramatically with each decade, so that by age 80 nearly half of all men will have histologic evidence of prostate cancer (Fig.1).[1] Although physicians have long known that many men older than 50 years have prostate cancer, they are also aware of the striking difference between the incidence and mortality rates from this disease. When adjusted for age and race, the incidence of prostate cancer has risen steadily since the 1970s, but the mortality rate has remained essentially unchanged (Fig. 2). These data suggest an increasing ability to diagnose prostate cancer but an inability to substantially alter the natural course of the disease.

Although prostate cancer is now the most common serious malignancy among American men, accounting for 165,000 new cases and 35,000 deaths in 1993,[2] the potential pool of patients with prostate cancer is much larger. Scardino has estimated that only 1% of the total population reservoir of prostate cancer reaches clinical

diagnosis in any year, and that the annual mortality is only 0.31% of men with histologic evidence of disease.[3]

Prostate cancer has become a more visible public health problem in part because prevention and treatment have reduced other competing disease hazards, particularly cardiovascular disease and stroke. As a consequence, American men are living longer and are therefore at a higher risk for succumbing to prostate cancer. Fortunately, only a relatively small percentage of men will develop clinically significant prostate cancer. Recent statistics compiled by the Surveillance, Epidemiology and End Results (SEER) Program of the National Cancer Institute show that American men now face an 8.7% probability at birth of developing prostate cancer, but only a 2.6% probability of dying from this disease.[4]

Several risk factors have been identified that predict the likelihood of developing symptomatic prostate cancer among men with histologic cancers. Some of these fac-

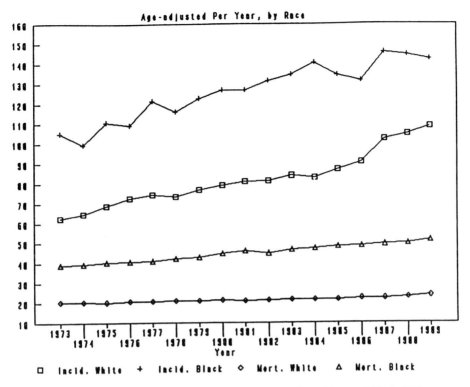

Fig. 2. Incidence and mortality from prostate cancer for white and black U.S. men, 1973–1989. (Reproduced with permission from Surveillance, Epidemiology, and End Results. Incidence and mortality data. Bethesda, MD: Natl Cancer Inst Monogr 22, 1992.)

tors are tumor dependent, such as histologic grade and tumor volume, while others are patient dependent, such as the age of the patient at diagnosis and other competing medical comorbidities. We review each of these factors to assess their ability to predict whether a patient will ultimately die *with* his cancer or *from* his cancer.

TUMOR FACTORS

Histologic Grade

Numerous reports over the past 50 years have documented a strong correlation between the histologic appearance of newly diagnosed prostate cancer and the malignant behavior of the disease.[5,6] Poorly differentiated tumors progress rapidly, well-differentiated tumors progress slowly, and moderately differentiated tumors

fall in between. The most common grading system utilized in the United States is the Gleason score, which assigns a grade from 1 to 5 to each of the two predominant histologic patterns of a pathologic specimen. Lower grades are assigned to well-differentiated tumors, while higher grades reflect poorly differentiated disease. A Gleason score ranging from 2–10 is calculated by summing the grades of the two predominant patterns.

The Gleason system evolved from the Veterans Administration Cooperative Urological Research Group (VACURG) studies that were conducted between 1960 and 1975. These prospective, clinical, randomized trials of the treatment of prostate cancer provided a large database for evaluating the ability of a grading system to predict survival. Nine histologic patterns were identified by their unique appearance, without preconceived ranking.

Correlation of survival data with histologic patterns showed that several of the nine patterns demonstrated similar results. Accordingly, three sets of related patterns and two distinct patterns were arranged into five grades, which were numbered in order of increasing biological malignancy. Even after consolidating the nine patterns into five grades, roughly half of the tumors contained more than one histologic grade. Further analysis demonstrated that patients with two different grades had mortality rates that were intermediate between those of the groups with single-pattern tumors. Accordingly, the two grades were averaged by summing the scores to create the Gleason score. The correlation with mortality rates is shown in Figure 3. A careful review of this graph demonstrates that patients with poorly differentiated cancers (Gleason grades 7–10) have a high probability of dying from their disease, while men with well-differentiated disease (Gleason grades 2–5, and possibly 6) have a very low probability of dying from their disease.

Tumor Volume

McNeal and his colleagues have documented the importance of tumor volume in predicting death from prostate cancer.[7] They have shown that tumors of less than 0.5 cc commonly occur in older men, but are rarely associated with capsular penetration or metastasis. As tumor volume increases to above 1.0 cc, capsular penetration begins to occur, and tumors larger than 3.0 cc frequently demonstrate seminal vesicle invasion. Overt metastases rarely appear before tumors reach 4 cc. Loss of histologic differentiation frequently occurs with increasing tumor volume. In McNeal's large autopsy series, only tumors harboring Gleason patterns 4 and/or 5 developed to a sufficient size to metastasize (Fig. 4). Accordingly, older men

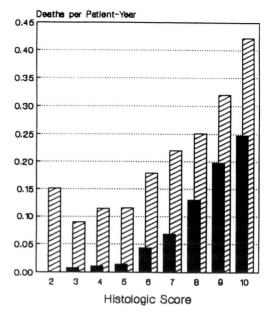

Fig. 3. Mortality rates versus histologic scores (VACURG data; n = 2,911). Solid bars indicate cancer deaths; hatched bars indicate all deaths. (Reproduced with permission from Gleason DF: Histologic grading of prostate cancer: a perspective. Hum Pathol 23:273–279, 1992.)

with small, well- to moderately differentiated tumors (Gleason grades 2–6) appear to be excellent candidates for observation.

Tumor volume can also be assessed indirectly by serum PSA.[8-10] Stamey et al. have shown that serum PSA levels are correlated with tumor volume (Fig. 5). Three PSA assays currently are available for clinical use: two based upon a monoclonal antibody probe (Hybritech's Tandem-R PSA assay and Abbott's IMx PSA assay), and one using a polyclonal antibody probe (Yang's Pros-Check PSA assay). The levels measured by the two monoclonal assays appear roughly similar, while the values associated with the polyclonal assay run about 1.6 times higher[11,12] (see also Chapter 6 for a full discussion of PSA and its uses in clinical settings).

Many researchers discourage the use of PSA as a screening test because of its relatively low sensitivity and specificity in this

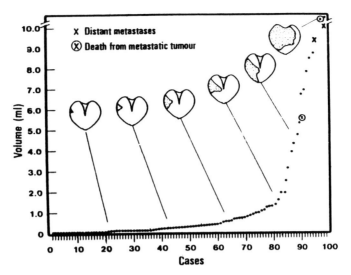

Fig. 4. Volume distribution of 100 prostate tumors in rank order. (Reproduced with permission from McNeal JE, et al.: Patterns of progression in prostate cancer. Lancet 11:60–63, 1986.)

setting. However, for men who have been diagnosed with clinically localized prostate cancer, serum PSA provides valuable information concerning the tumor burden. Catalona et al. have recently described a series of over 10,000 men aged 50 years and older who participated in a screening program for prostate cancer using serum PSA.[13] They found that among the men diagnosed with prostate cancer whose initial PSA screening value was greater than 10 μg/L (Tandem-E assay) and who elected

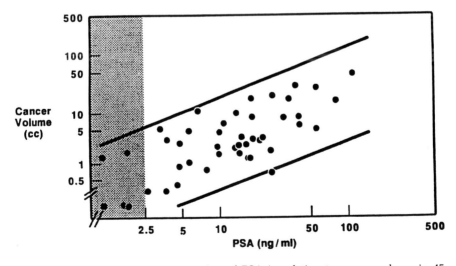

Fig. 5. Preoperative serum concentration of PSA in relation to cancer volume in 45 patients undergoing consecutive radical prostatectomy (log-log plot). (Reproduced with permission from Stamey TA, et. al.: Prostate-specific antigen as a serum marker for adenocarcinoma of the prostate. N Engl. J Med 317:909–916, 1987.)

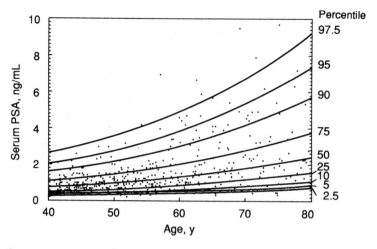

Fig. 6. Serum prostate-specific antigen (PSA) concentration as a function of patient age. Scattergram of the individual serum PSA values for all 471 men, with the nomogram demonstrating the 2.5th, 5th, 10th, 25th, 50th, 75th, 90th, 95th, and 97.5th percentiles for serum PSA according to age. (Reproduced with permission from Oesterling JE, et al.: Serum prostate-specific antigen in a community-based population of healthy men. JAMA 270:860–864, 1993.)

to undergo surgery, only 45% had disease localized to the prostate. Men undergoing surgery who presented with PSA values of less than 10 μg/L had a much higher probability of organ-confined disease.

From these studies, we can conclude that men with a substantially elevated serum PSA have a high probability of tumor extension beyond the confines of the prostate, and are unlikely to benefit from aggressive therapy. Conversely, men with a low serum PSA frequently have a low tumor volume. These men may benefit from aggressive therapy, but only if they have a sufficiently long life expectancy to be at risk for clinical progression.

Carter et al. recently suggested that changes in serum PSA may also be helpful to predict tumor progression. In a retrospective analysis of blood sera from a small number of men who participated in the Baltimore Longitudinal Study on Aging, they found that men who developed clinically significant prostate cancer had an annual increase of approximately 0.75 μg/L in their serum PSA values.[14] Oesterling et

al. have recently shown that serum PSA levels rise as a normal part of aging (Fig. 6).[15] Therefore, it remains to be determined whether rising serum PSA levels identify those men who will develop clinically significant prostate cancer.

HOST FACTORS

Host factors play an equally important role in predicting whether a patient is likely to develop clinically symptomatic prostate cancer. Patient age at diagnosis and other coexistent medical diseases all contribute to whether a patient will ultimately develop treatment-resistant symptomatic disease.

Age

Figure 1 demonstrates the strong correlation between age and the incidence and mortality rate from prostate cancer. Despite the high incidence of prostate cancer among older men, some physicians have argued against diagnosing and treating men who have a life expectancy of un-

TABLE 1. Expectation of Life at Single Years of Age: Male, All Races[a]

Age	Life Expectancy
65	14.6
66	13.9
67	13.3
68	12.7
69	12.1
70	11.6
71	11.0
72	10.5
73	10.0
74	9.5
75	9.0
76	8.6
77	8.1
78	7.7
79	7.3
80	6.9
81	6.5
82	6.1
83	5.8
84	5.5
85	5.2

[a]Source: U.S. Vital Statistics.

der 10 years, because these men are also more likely to die of other causes besides prostate cancer.[16,17] Based upon the 1984 life expectancy for American men age 65 to 85 years (Table 1), this threshold occurs around age 73 for men in average health. Men older than their mid-seventies with newly diagnosed, localized prostate cancer carry a low probability of dying from their cancer and, in general, are good candidates for observational therapy.

Patient Comorbidities

Although many authors have suggested the need to consider the severity of comorbid illness when choosing treatment for localized prostate cancer, explicit assessment of coexistent disease is uncommon in the urologic literature. In a recently published structured review of the prostate cancer treatment literature, Wasson et al. found essentially no studies that adequately controlled for competing disease hazards.[18] Albertsen and colleagues are currently analyzing the survival of over 700 men treated conservatively for newly diagnosed, localized prostate cancer in Connecticut during the 1970s. They have found that comorbidity is equivalent to tumor grade in the ability to predict overall patient survival. Mameghan et al. also have shown that comorbidity is a significant confounder in a series of patients receiving radiation therapy.[19]

Instruments specifically designed to predict health care outcomes among patients with chronic diseases have been developed by several authors, including Charlson et al.,[20] Greenfield et al.,[21] and Kaplan and Feinstein.[22] Each of these instruments categorizes patients into one of four comorbidity classifications. An analysis of the Connecticut series described above showed that men over age 65 in the two highest comorbidity classifications carried a low risk of dying from prostate cancer, succumbing instead to other disease hazards.

OBSERVATION AS A TREATMENT OPTION: BENEFITS AND HARMS

Counseling patients regarding the appropriate treatment of newly diagnosed, clinically localized prostate cancer is as difficult today as it was for Dr. Willet Whitmore at the Memorial Hospital in 1963.[23] Thirty years ago, he wrote that "available evidence does not prove that such surgery (radical prostatectomy) is useful, nor does it prove that such surgery is useless; it merely leaves the question open." This statement about surgery and radiation therapy is as true today as it was then.

Observation as a treatment option is a commonly used treatment strategy for clinically localized prostate cancer in many countries worldwide. Even in the United States, where treatment of localized prostate cancer is much more aggressive than in Europe, a recent commission of the American College of Surgeons found that 66% of stage A cancers remained untreated, compared with only 17% of stage B cancers.[24] Relatively few American investigators have published clinical series of patients managed expectantly,[25,26] but a number of case series have been reported from around the world. In the structured literature review and synthesis reported by Wasson et al., men in 23 of the case series managed with immediate or delayed hormonal therapy analyzed had a median prostate cancer death rate of 0.009 deaths per person-year, compared with a rate of 0.060 for all-cause mortality.[18] These rates are not different from the published series of men treated with radical prostatectomy (Table 2). However, comparisons between series are extraordinarily difficult to make, since results are often confounded by factors such as age at presentation, tumor grade, and patient comorbidities.

One large series reported by Johansson and colleagues deserves particular comment, since this study is community based, has a long duration of follow-up, and has been widely quoted in the medical literature.[27] In this prospective Swedish study, men who had clinically localized prostate cancer and resided in a defined geographic region were enrolled during the 1977 to 1984 period. Men with moderately or poorly differentiated cancer were excluded during the first two years, but were included thereafter. Among the 223 patients followed for an average of 12.5 years, there were 23 prostate cancer deaths (10%) and 148 deaths (66%) from other causes. Ten-year, metastasis-free survival corrected for deaths from other causes was 83%. Tumor grade was the dominant predictor of prognosis among this group of patients with a mean age of 72 years.

Although these results have been criticized because the study enrolled a large number of older men with low-volume disease, they have been supported by other authors. Chodak et al. recently reported the results of an individual-patient level meta-analysis of 762 men from six centers who were managed expectantly.[28] Ten-year adjusted prostate cancer-specific survival among men with well-differentiated disease was 87%, for men with moderately differentiated disease, it was 86%, and for men with poorly differentiated disease,

TABLE 2. Patient Characteristics and Outcomes of Treatment for Clinically Localized Prostate Cancer[a]

	Watchful Waiting		Radiation Therapy		Radical Surgery	
	Median (CI)[b]	n[c]	Median (CI)	n	Median (CI)	n
Patient Characteristics						
Age	71 (69–73)	27	66 (64–66)	49	63 (61–64)	33
Percent High Grade	7 (6–11)	19	21 (13–24)	45	11 (6–25)	22
Outcomes						
Annual Mortality Rate						
All Cause	.060 (.050–.104)	27	.045 (.040–.052)	45	.032 (.020–.044)	27
Cancer-Specific	.009 (.006–.012)	23	.023 (.010–.030)	22	.009 (.007–.013)	23
Metastatic Rate	.017 (.011–.043)	15	.050 (.030–.095)	17	.023 (.014–.025)	18

[a]Source: Wasson et al.: A structured literature review of treatment for localized prostate cancer. Arch Fam Med 2:487–493, 1993.
[b]CI = 95% confidence interval.
[c]n = number of studies, which vary since not all studies supply all variables.

23%. Similarly, Kolon and Albertsen reported on their preliminary analysis of men diagnosed with localized prostate cancer within the state of Connecticut during the 1970s.[29] For men over age 65 at presentation, 15-year, cause-specific survival ranged from 82–93% for men with well-differentiated disease, 67–78% for men with moderately differentiated disease, and 46–53% for men with poorly differentiated disease.

The major risks of observation as a treatment option consist of local tumor progression and the development of metastatic disease that is resistant to hormonal control. Since these risks are also shared by patients selecting radical surgery and radiation therapy, the critical question concerns the additional risk of developing hormone-resistant metastatic disease for patients selecting observation as a treatment option. Unfortunately, the magnitude of this additional risk, if any, has not been quantified.

Fleming et al. recently published an article in which the authors attempted to predict clinical outcomes for different groups of patients using a structured decision analysis.[30] They reviewed the same three strategies that Dr. Whitmore has discussed with his patients for the past 30 years. Specifically, they modeled the clinical outcomes of treatment following radical prostatectomy, radiation therapy, and "watchful waiting" (also referred to as deferred therapy or delayed hormonal therapy).

The decision analysis assumed that both active treatment strategies were beneficial and incorporated estimates of treatment efficacy and complications that were based upon Medicare claims data and a review of the recent medical literature. The analysis also explicitly stratified patients on two significant variables: age at presentation, and the histologic grade of their tumor. The major benefit of treatment was assumed to be a reduction in the chance of death or disutility from metastatic disease, while the risks of treatment were assumed to be the morbidity and mortality directly attributable to interventions.

Several important conclusions can be drawn from the analysis. Patients over age 60 with well-differentiated tumors clinically localized to the prostate appear to have a very low risk of disease progression. Accordingly, aggressive treatment options such as radical prostatectomy or radiation therapy at best offer limited benefit and may result in net harm to the patient. Patients over age 60 with moderate and, especially, poorly differentiated disease have a significantly higher risk of disease progression, and therefore potentially can benefit from aggressive intervention. However, this potential benefit is not shared by patients older than age 70 at the time of diagnosis, since the risk of dying from prostate cancer diminishes in favor of other disease hazards. Furthermore, Catalona has shown that in his large series of men screened for prostate cancer, 43% of the men over age 70 had extracapsular extension of their disease despite the fact that their serum PSA levels were less than 10 µg/L.[13]

The Fleming et al. article concluded by stating that radical prostatectomy and radiation therapy may benefit selected groups of patients with prostate cancer, particularly younger patients with more poorly differentiated tumors. In most cases, however, the model showed that the potential benefits of therapy were small enough that the choice of therapy was sensitive to a patient's treatment preferences.

These recommendations are remarkably similar to those suggested by Dr. Whitmore in 1963.[23] In his article, he recommended that patients with stage A disease and whose general life expectancy due to other comorbidities was less than 15 years would be best served by a conservative, nonsurgical course. For patients with stage B lesions whose anticipated life expectancy due to other disease hazards was less than 10 years, he also recommended a conservative, nonsurgical approach. For patients with stage C and stage D disease, he concluded that aggressive intervention was, at best, experimental.

The Fleming model assumed that watchful waiting would be followed by hormonal therapy should clinically significant metastatic disease develop. This was based upon the fact that "there is no convincing evidence that endocrine therapy applied early in the course of the disease has a greater effect on total life prolongation than when it is applied late in the course of the disease," a comment made by Dr. Whitmore in his 1963 article and still shared by many practitioners.[31]

SUMMARY

Men with newly diagnosed, clinically localized prostate cancer face a difficult treatment decision. Although many physicians strongly encourage the selection of aggressive treatment options such as radical surgery or radiation therapy, no randomized trials have yet been conducted to support the superiority of these treatment options over observation followed by hormonal therapy for those patients who develop symptomatic metastatic disease.

We do know that the vast majority of men with histologic evidence of prostate cancer will never develop clinically significant disease. As a result of screening with PSA, large numbers of asymptomatic men are undergoing rectal ultrasound and prostate biopsy. Once a cancer is diagnosed, both the patient and his physician face a dilemma: will this cancer become clinically significant, or will it remain asymptomatic throughout the patient's lifetime? The safest approach from the clinician's perspective is to recommend ag-

gressive therapy. If the therapy fails, he or she has done "everything possible." If the therapy succeeds, he or she has "cured" the patient.

Unfortunately, neither radical surgery nor radiation therapy has been shown to be effective in controlling disease among patients who are at the highest risk of dying from their disease: those patients with poorly differentiated tumors. Long-term follow-up among men with well-differentiated tumors receiving minimal treatment shows that very few die from their disease.

Who may particularly benefit from more aggressive treatment? Younger patients with minimal comorbidities and a high risk of developing clinically significant disease may have the most to gain from radical surgery or radiation therapy. Older patients, especially those patients with significant comorbidities, may conclude that observation as a treatment option carries the lowest risks and affords an equivalent probability of disease control when compared with more aggressive options.

ACKNOWLEDGMENTS

This work was supported in part by grants HS-06770 and HS-06336 from the Agency for Health Care Policy and Research. Dr. Barry is a Henry J. Kaiser Family Foundation Faculty Scholar in the Department of General Internal Medicine.

REFERENCES

1. Gaynor EP: Zur frage des prostatakrebes virchows. Arch Pathol Anat 301:602–652, 1938.
2. Boring CC, Squires TS, Tong T: Cancer statistics, 1993. CA Cancer J Clin 43:7–26, 1993.
3. Scardino PT: Early detection of prostate cancer. Urol Clin North Am 16:635–655, 1989.
4. Seidman H, Mushinski MH, Gelb SK, Silverberg E: Probabilities of eventually developing or dying of cancer—United States, 1985. CA Cancer J Clin 35:39–54, 1985.

5. Gleason DF, Mellinger G, The Veterans Administration Cooperative Urologic Research Group: Prediction of prognosis for prostatic adenocarcinoma by combined histologic grading and clinical staging. J Urol 111:58–64, 1974.

6. Gaeta JF, Englander LC, Murphy GP: Comparative evaluation of National Prostatic Cancer Treatment Group and Gleason systems for pathologic grading of primary prostate cancer. Urology 27:306–308, 1986.

7. McNeal JE, Bostwick DG, Kindrachuk RA, Redwine EA, Freiha FS, Stamey TA: Patterns of progression in prostate cancer. Lancet 11:60–63, 1986.

8. Stamey TA, Yang N, Hay AR, McNeal JE, Freiha FS, Redwine E: Prostate specific antigen as a serum marker for adenocarcinoma of the prostate. N Engl J Med 317:909–916, 1987.

9. Oesterling JE: Prostate specific antigen: a critical assessment of the most useful tumor marker for adenocarcinoma of the prostate. J Urol 145:907–923, 1991.

10. Cupp MR, Oesterling JE: Prostate-specific antigen, digital rectal examination, and transrectal ultrasonography: their roles in diagnosing early prostate cancer. Mayo Clin Proc 68:297–306, 1993.

11. Vessella RL, Noteboom J, Lange PH: Evaluation of the Abbott IMx automated immunoassay of prostate-specific antigen. Clin Chem 38:2044–2054, 1992.

12. Graves HCB, Wehner N, Stamey TA: Comparison of a polyclonal and monoclonal immunoassay for PSA: need for an international antigen standard. J Urol 144:1516–1521, 1990.

13. Catalona WJ, Smith SS, Ratliff TL, Basler JW: Detection of organ-confined prostate cancer is increased through prostate-specific antigen-based testing. JAMA 270:948–954, 1993.

14. Carter HB, Pearson JD, Metter EJ, Brant LJ, Chan DW, Andres R, Fozard JL, Walsh PC: Longitudinal evaluation of prostate-specific antigen levels in men with and without prostate disease. JAMA 267:2215–2220, 1992.

15. Oesterling JE, Jacobsen SJ, Chute CG, Guess HA, Girman CJ, Panser LA, Lieber MM: Serum prostate-specific antigen in a community-based population of healthy men. JAMA 270:860–864, 1993.

16. Brendler CB, Walsh PC: The role of radical prostatectomy in the treatment of prostate cancer. CA Cancer J Clin 42:212–222, 1992.

17. Lange PH: The next era for prostate cancer: controlled clinical trials. JAMA 269:95–96, 1993.

18. Wasson J, Cushman CC, Bruskewitz RB: A structured literature review of treatment for localized prostate cancer. Arch Fam Med 2:487–493, 1993.

19. Mameghan H, Fisher R, Watt WH, Meagher MJ, Rosen M, Farnsworth RH, Tynan A, Mameghan J: Results of radiotherapy for localized prostatic carcinoma treated at the Prince of Wales Hospital, Sydney. Med J Aust 154:317–326, 1991.

20. Charlson ME, Pompei P, Ales KL, MacKenzi CR: A new method of classifying prognostic co-morbidity in longitudinal studies: development and validation. J Chron Dis 40:373–383, 1987.

21. Greenfield S, Apolone G, McNeil BJ, Cleary PD: The importance of co-existent disease in the occurrence of postoperative complications and one-year recovery in patients undergoing total hip replacement. Med Care 31:141–154, 1993.

22. Kaplan MH, Feinstein AR: The importance of classifying initial co-morbidity in evaluating the outcomes of diabetes mellitus. J Chron Dis 27:387–404, 1974.

23. Whitmore WF: The rationale and results of ablative surgery for prostatic cancer. Cancer 16:1119–1132, 1963.

24. Mettlin C, Jones GW, Murphy GP: Trends in prostate cancer care in the United States, 1974–1990: Observations from the patient care evaluation studies of the American College of Surgeons Commission on Cancer. CA Cancer J Clin 43:83–91, 1993.

25. Whitmore W, Warner J, Thompson I: Expectant management of localized prostatic cancer. Cancer 57:1091–1096, 1991.

26. Jones GW: Prospective, conservative management of localized prostate cancer. Cancer 70 (Suppl):307–310, 1992.

27. Johansson JE, Adami HO, Andersson SO: High 10-year survival rate in patients with early untreated prostatic cancer. JAMA 267:2191–2196, 1992.

28. Chodak GW, Thisted R, Gerber G, Adolfsson J, Johansson JE, Warner J, Chisholm G, Moskovitz B, Jones G: Multi-variate analysis of outcome following observation/delayed therapy of clinically localized prostate cancer (Abstr). J Urol 149:396A, 1993.

29. Kolon TF, Albertsen PC: Conservative treatment of clinically localized prostate cancer: Fifteen year survival analysis stratified by age and histologic grade at presentation (Abstr). J Urol 149:303A, 1993.

30. Fleming C, Wasson JH, Albertsen PC, Barry MJ, Wennberg JE for the Prostate Patient Outcomes Research Team: A decision analysis of alternative treatment strategies for clinically localized prostate cancer. JAMA 269:2650–2658, 1993.

31. Smith PH: The case for no initial treatment for localized prostate cancer. Urol Clin North Am 17:827–834, 1990.

13

Optimal Management of Stage D1 Prostate Cancer

Gregory S. Grose, M.D., and Edward M. Messing, M.D.

INTRODUCTION

Cancer of the prostate is the most common noncutaneous malignancy in men in the United States. Historically, 25% to 40% of patients have presented with stage D disease,[1,2] and clinical understaging has been the rule. Donohue and associates[3] summarized the incidence of positive pelvic lymph nodes (stage D1) by clinical stage in 4,492 patients; the overall incidence was 27%. Based on several large series in the 1970s and early 1980s, up to 30% of clinical stage A and B patients and at least 50% of clinical stage C patients had positive lymph nodes.[4,5]

Recently, however, efforts at earlier detection employing prostate-specific antigen (PSA), digital rectal exam (DRE), and transrectal ultrasound (TRUS)-guided biopsies in widespread formal or *ad lib* screening programs have influenced these statistics considerably. A much lower proportion of patients undergoing surgical exploration for radical prostatectomy have been found to have nodal metastases. In several large series reported since 1992, only 5–7% of surgically staged men with clinically localized prostate cancer, and roughly 25% with clinical stage C tumors, have had stage D1 disease.[1,6,7] These data might indicate that early detection is truly

being accomplished.[8] However, the lower incidence of unsuspected positive pelvic nodes is offset by the recent fivefold increase in the number of radical prostatectomies performed,[9] and the same number of stage D1 patients are probably still being found.

As with other stages of prostate cancer, no unanimity as to ideal management of stage D1 disease exists.[2,10–14] Suggestions have ranged from observation with delayed hormonal therapy upon local or distant progression[15] to aggressive multimodality approaches[16–18] directed at both local/regional and systemic control. However, compelling evidence to support any given approach has all too often depended upon short-term analysis with projected outcomes and comparisons with differently managed nonprospectively randomized controls. Furthermore, many of these studies occurred before the use of PSA to detect recurrent or progressing disease, which has likely altered the timing of "delayed" endocrine or "local" therapies to earlier in the disease course than had previously been done.

Despite intervention, up to 70% of patients will eventually die of their malignancy.[5,19] Conversely, and fortunately, many patients with stage D1 disease survive 10 years or longer after their diagnosis.

Prostate Cancer, pages 197–213 © 1994 Wiley-Liss, Inc.

This chapter reviews the diagnosis and prognosis of stage D1 prostate cancer, and suggests a management regimen based on available data.

CLINICAL STAGING

Despite improved early detection with PSA and TRUS, clinical staging of prostate cancer remains imprecise. Evaluation of the primary tumor with DRE, TRUS, magnetic resonance imaging (MRI), and biopsy is limited by the inability of these modalities to detect microscopic extension. Histological appearance (e.g., Gleason score), serum PSA, enzymatic prostatic acid phosphatase (PAP), and tumor DNA ploidy status (by flow cytometry) are useful staging tools but, with the possible exception of PAP, are sufficiently limited that individual abnormalities can rarely be independently utilized in making clinical decisions about staging or management. Evaluation of the regional lymph nodes with these modalities similarly is less than perfect, and has led to significant clinical understaging.

Imaging the Primary Tumor and Determining Volume

Stamey and associates noted that tumor volume was directly related to the probability of metastasis to pelvic nodes. In a series of 102 men, the mean volume of the primary tumor in stage D1 disease was 17.3 cc,[20] and tumors larger than 4 cc were often locally advanced or metastatic. In a series of 205 radical prostatectomy cases, Villers and associates[21] found only 1% of primary tumors smaller than 4 cc were associated with nodal metastases, compared to 13% of those from 4 to 12 cc and 46% of those larger than 12 cc. Bostwick and colleagues[22] summarized published data from nine pathological studies correlating tumor volume with stage. There was approximately a 50% probability of metastases (not specified as to regional or wide-spread) with a primary tumor volume of 13 cc. They concluded that primary tumor volume was an important predictor of stage, and with improved modalities for estimating volume (e.g., MRI and TRUS), clinical staging accuracy may be improved.

Unfortunately, there is no modality yet that reliably measures intraprostatic tumor volume. DRE provides only a crude estimate of size: if less than 50% of a lobe is involved with palpable tumor, there is a high probability that the volume is less than 4 cc.[23] TRUS accurately estimates prostate gland volume, but the correlation with histologic cancer specimens is only about 0.8.[22] Ultrasound rarely detects lesions of less than 0.2 cc (tumor size 7–8 mm),[24] and often over- or underestimates actual tumor volume. Terris and associates[25] estimated cancer volume in 110 patients preoperatively with TRUS, and despite the use of step-section planimetry, 86% of tumors were underestimated. Furthermore, the cancer was not visualized sonographically in 18% of patients.

Computed tomography (CT) is less useful than TRUS or MRI in assessing tumor volume. Compared with these modalities, it poorly delineates the internal architecture of the gland and local extension.[24]

Magnetic resonance imaging has been promoted as a potentially useful staging tool for prostate cancer, both for the evaluation of the primary tumor and the regional lymph nodes. In a multicenter trial, of 194 patients with clinically localized cancer who underwent MRI and TRUS of the primary tumor followed by radical prostatectomy, 35% of tumors smaller than 1 cm on pathologic step-sectioning were not visualized preoperatively with either modality.[26] Although the volume accuracy was not reported, the staging accuracy of MRI was 69%, which was comparable with TRUS. The authors concluded that the current technology was inadequate for staging; however, endorectal surface imaging, noise reduction, and fat suppression may improve the accuracy in the future. In fact, the use of a balloon-mounted endorectal surface coil has considerably improved the resolution and allows visualization of the prostatic capsule and neurovascular bundles.[24]

The combination of any of these modalities, particularly TRUS, with visually guided biopsy of the periprostatic tissue may improve the preoperative assessment of extraprostatic extension, and indirectly (by inference) may improve the current understaging of nodal metastases.

Gleason Histologic Grade

Gleason pathology score of the primary tumor[5] obtained from biopsy specimens can be an important variable in predicting the presence of pelvic lymph node metastases. In patients with a low score (2–4), the risk of positive regional nodes is 0–13%, while those with a score of 8–10 have a 47–100% risk.[27,28] However, the majority of patients with newly diagnosed prostate cancer will have intermediate scores of 5–7, and in this range, Gleason score is a poor predictor of nodal status.[27]

Moreover, with more contemporary data accrued primarily from patients diagnosed through *de facto* screening, Danella and associates[6] recently reported the positive predictive value (for nodal metastases) of a Gleason score of 7 or greater as only 10%. This probably reflects the low incidence of pelvic nodal metastases (5.7%) in their series.

When quantitative tumor volume is considered together with the percentage of poorly differentiated cancer (Gleason pattern 4–5), predictive value is enhanced. In McNeal and associates'[29] series of 209 patients undergoing radical prostatectomy for clinical stage A and B cancer, positive pelvic lymph nodes were present in 22 of 38 carcinomas (58%) with more than 3.2 cc of poorly differentiated carcinoma, compared to only 1 of 171 tumors with less

than 3.2 cc of poorly differentiated cancer. Unfortunately, prostatic needle biopsies (or transurethral resection of the prostate [TURP]) will often fail to demonstrate the extent of a given Gleason grade in a tumor, contributing to the inaccuracies of non-surgical staging.

DNA Ploidy

The finding of aneuploidy in prostatic cancers predicts tumor aggressiveness, and is more common with increasing tumor grade, stage, and volume. For example, higher Gleason score tumors (7–10) have a higher probability of aneuploidy (80%)[23] and aneuploidy is relatively unlikely for tumors smaller than 4 cc. However, up to one-third of tumors remain diploid at higher stages.[5] Moreover, sampling artifacts and the heterogeneity of ploidy within the same cancer reduce the utility of this technique as a preoperative staging modality. Despite these shortcomings, Mayo Clinic investigations have demonstrated that ploidy analysis of primary tumors after radical prostatectomy has predicted disease progression—and possibly hormonal responsiveness—in men with stage D1 disease.[11]

This group reported on 91 stage D1 patients who had undergone radical prostatectomy and pelvic lymph node dissection (PLND) and were followed for five years or until disease progression.[30] Patients with nondiploid tumors showed progression in 75% of cases (median time 39 months) compared to 15% of diploid tumors (median time 53 months). Similar findings have been reported by deVere White and associates.[31]

Prostatic Acid Phosphatase

There are many reports on the use of PAP measurements in staging known prostate cancer. Heller[32] has summarized data from seven studies that compared PAP to pathologic stage. Various assays were utilized, and PAP was elevated in 10% of patients with intracapsular prostate cancer (although this probably included some stage C tumors), 32% with positive regional nodes, and 73% with skeletal metastases. However, if solid-phase immunofluorescent assays and counterimmunoelectrophoresis were eliminated, most patients with clinically confined cancer and elevated PAP (enzymatic or RIA) had positive pelvic lymph nodes.

The interpretation of PAP results in patients with clinically localized prostate cancer is complicated by the different substrates used, the 24-hour variability of the PAP, the instability of the assays at room temperature, and the lack of specificity for prostatic tissue. Additionally, prostates with large amounts of benign prostatic hyperplasia (BPH; i.e., greater than 40 g) can cause an elevated PAP.[5] Several studies have demonstrated the superior sensitivity (roughly twofold) of PSA over PAP in diagnosis and staging of prostate cancer,[5,33,34] and some authors maintain that PAP adds no unique information in the staging process.[5,35]

Prostate-Specific Antigen

Serum PSA levels have been correlated with the clinical stage of prostate cancer, rising proportionally with increasing tumor burden at approximately 3.5 ng/ml (Yang assay) per gram of intracapsular cancer.[20] The majority of patients with clinically important prostate cancer have an elevated PSA, but among each clinical stage, there is considerable overlap of serum levels. PSA cannot be relied upon to distinguish patients with organ-confined cancer from those with extracapsular spread. Oesterling reported[34] the false-positive rate in predicting cancer beyond the capsule in men undergoing radical prostatectomy with clinically organ-confined disease to be 74% and 65% for cut-off levels of 4 and 10 ng/ml, respectively.

Just as PSA is limited in predicting ex-tracapsular extension, it cannot reliably predict nodal status. In two large studies correlating preoperative PSA levels with pathological stage after radical prostatectomy for clinically localized disease, stage D1 prostatic carcinoma was associated with PSA levels greater than or equal to 10 ng/ml (Tandem-R) in only 41% of patients in one group,[36] but in 100% of patients (Yang assay) in the other.[20] The latter group may have had more extensive local tumor as evidenced by a mean primary tumor volume of 17.3 cc, and PAP elevation in 12 of the 13 patients. Thus, a PSA value less than 10 ng/ml does not preclude the existence of stage D1 disease. Alternatively, preoperative PSA values of 10–20 ng/ml (Yang assay), 20–50 ng/ml, and greater than 50 ng/ml have been associated with pelvic lymph node metastases in 9%, 13%, and 45% of clinical stage A and B prostate cancers, respectively.[5]

These results suggest that the degree of elevation of PSA, although not specific for advanced disease, might be useful in guiding the clinician to consider additional staging studies to evaluate the pelvic nodes in the patient with clinical stage A or B prostate cancer.

Assessment of Regional Lymph Nodes

Lymphangiography, CT, and MRI have been used to evaluate pelvic lymph nodes. Lymphangiography is unique in that it may identify intranodal metastases as small as 5 mm[27] and detects metastases in 50–60% of patients who have them.[4] However, it doesn't consistently opacify the obturator and internal iliac drainage routes when administered by bilateral pedal injections, and is limited by a false-negative rate of 22–50%.[28,37] Additionally, it is an invasive procedure with its own attendant morbidity and requires considerable technical expertise.

In comparison with lymphangiography, CT does not show the internal nodal architecture. The limit of resolution is 1 cm;

nodes larger than this are suspicious for malignancy, and those greater than 1.5 cm are considered malignant.[4,24,27] Most studies suggest a sensitivity of 50–75% and specificity of up to 80%.[24,37]

The initial hope that MRI might improve staging accuracy by allowing superior imaging of the pelvic nodes has not been substantiated. Rifkin and associates[26] reported that MRI correctly identified 155 of 162 patients without pelvic lymph node involvement (96% specificity), but detected only 1 of 23 pathologically positive nodes (4% sensitivity, 12.5% positive predictive value). These parameters are not significantly better than that of CT, although there are potential advantages of MRI: contrast agents are not necessary, and imaging in patients with hip prostheses is superior. Additionally, differentiation of postoperative fibrosis from recurrent tumor mass is possible with MRI.[24]

The addition of percutaneous fine needle aspiration or biopsy to any of these radiologic procedures can unequivocally establish a diagnosis of metastatic disease, but is applicable relatively rarely for clinical stage B or small stage C patients (those who might be candidates for "curative" treatment) because only radiologically positive nodes can be biopsied, and a negative histologic/cytologic study does not exclude metastases.

Pelvic Lymph Node Dissection

Because of inaccuracies in predicting the status of pelvic nodes, PLND remains the gold standard in evaluating regional nodes; it permits histologic inspection of most (if not all) of the primary and secondary drainage sites of prostate cancer. It is routinely performed as the final staging procedure in patients with normal PAPs and negative bone scans prior to radical prostatectomy, and formerly was done prior to radiotherapy.[3]

Various techniques of open dissection have been described,[38] with the modified

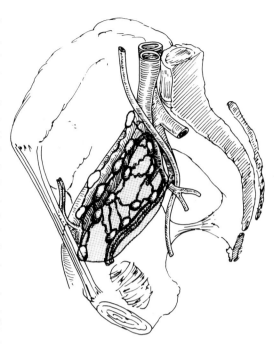

Fig. 1. The limits of an adequate pelvic lymph node dissection are shaded. Reprinted with permission.[39]

staging lymphadenectomy as described by Paulson[28] being most popular because of lessened morbidity and equivalent results in detecting node-positive disease.[4,28,37] An adequate dissection (Fig. 1)[39] will remove all tissue anterior, medial, and posterior to the external iliac artery, extending from the iliac bifurcation superiorly to the crossing of the circumflex iliac vein distally, leaving a strip of tissue on the anterolateral and lateral surfaces of the artery to avoid postoperative lymphedema of the lower extremity. *En bloc* removal of tissue will continue around the external iliac vein for the same distance and also remove, in continuity, the obturator fat pad—skeletonizing the obturator nerve—and anteromedial tissue from the hypogastric artery from the iliac bifurcation cephaladly to the first anterior division distally. Despite this being a relatively straightforward and simple procedure for most experienced surgeons, and rarely taking more than 15–20 minutes per side (including obtaining surgical exposure), there has been a tendency in the recent past for urologists to reduce the scope of the dissection further, which may also be contributing to the lower proportion of node-positive patients in recent studies.

It is recognized that regional lymphadenectomy (in addition to resection of the primary tumor) can play a curative role in penile,[40] many testicular, and some bladder malignancies.[19] However, most urologists believe that in prostate cancer, lymphadenectomy is of prognostic and not therapeutic value.[5,19,28,41] This view is based upon the high percentage of progression and cause-specific mortality discussed earlier.

When is PLND indicated as a separate procedure? When results will influence the treatment rendered, and the suspicion for metastatic disease is high despite a negative staging work-up. This might include patients with stage D0 (elevated PAP, negative bone scan) cancer, poorly differentiated tumor on biopsy (Gleason score 7 or higher), markedly elevated PSA (greater than 20–30), or bulky bilateral primary tumor (including stage C disease). Additionally, patients undergoing a radical perineal prostatectomy would be candidates.[4,23,42]

Recently, laparoscopic pelvic lymphadenectomy (LPLND) has been used to evaluate patients with prostate cancer. Even in experienced hands, compared to open PLND it is more time-consuming, costly, and potentially risky. However, this is offset by the shorter hospitalization (one day) and convalescence (72 hours).[37] A cost analysis by Fulgham and Feagins[42] determined that approximately 50% of patients undergoing the procedure must have positive nodes to justify the additional cost. With the contemporary lower proportion of patients having positive pelvic lymph nodes in clinically localized cancer, the vast majority of patients undergoing radical prostatectomy probably would not be appropriate candidates for LPLND.[6]

LPLND has been promoted as a reliable method of sampling the lymph nodes when compared to open surgery. In Fulgham and Feagins's[42] series, LPLND was immediately followed by open PLND in 47 patients, and 77–90% of the nodes were found to have been removed laparoscopically. No positive nodes were removed by open surgery that had been missed laparoscopically; however, no patient actually had positive nodes. In a smaller series reported by Parra and colleagues,[37] the number of nodes removed laparoscopically in 12 patients was not different from the number removed with open PLND in 12 controls. Nodal metastases were found in 3 of 12 LPLND patients and 1 of 12 open PLND patients; however, the laparoscopic group had more advanced disease on the basis of preoperative PSA and Gleason scores. Of the nine LPLND patients with negative nodes who subsequently underwent radical retropubic prostatectomy, completeness of the endoscopic dissection was verified by intraoperative examination of the pelvis, and no additional nodal tissue was obtained.

Based upon these studies, laparoscopic and open pelvic lymphadenectomies cannot be regarded as equivalent. No patient in Fulgham and Feagins's[42] study actually had positive nodes, and the chance of finding positive nodes in Parra and associates'[37] study was favored by the more advanced cancer in the laparoscopic group. Larger series[43,44] have suggested that open and laparoscopic PLND may be equivalent because of the similar number of nodes removed and the similar incidence of positive nodes detected by the two techniques. Fulgham and Feagins[42] commented on the substantial learning curve with laparoscopy, and Rukstalis et al.[43] reported the need for 15 cases to reliably remove the pelvic nodes with equivalence to an open dissection.

Additional concerns with laparoscopy are the ability to remove the nodal packets *en bloc*, the potential of seeding the trochar tracts or peritoneum with tumor, and the complications unique to laparoscopy. A review of 329 LPLNDs performed in seven institutions reported a complication rate of 15%. Of these, 20% required open laparotomy to resolve the problem.[45] Despite these drawbacks, LPLND does hold promise as a useful technique in staging prostate cancer, particularly in patients at high risk for nodal metastases (high Gleason score, high PSA) and in those undergoing a perineal prostatectomy.

PROGNOSIS IN STAGE D1 PROSTATE CANCER

Even a single microscopically positive lymph node signifies metastatic prostate cancer, and patient survival and time to recurrence are substantially worsened. However, in part because of the long natural history of prostate cancer, 5- and 10-year actuarial survival rates of 68–93% and 34–77%, respectively, have been reported.[11,19,46] The most optimistic percentages were reported by Mayo Clinic investigators[11] in which 62 stage D1 patients were followed for a mean 11.1 years following radical prostatectomy with or without early endocrine therapy. Other series with long-term follow-up have reported significantly lower survival rates.[19]

The stage and grade of the primary tumor have prognostic value in predicting which prostate cancers will metastasize to the pelvic lymph nodes. However, once the diagnosis of stage D1 cancer has been made, it is not clear that the same parameters are as useful in predicting the course of the disease. Brawn and associates[47] found that the histologic pattern of metastases to pelvic nodes in the majority of 82 patients with stage D1 cancer was similar to that of the primary tumor. Most of the nodes harbored moderately differentiated tumors, which portended a significantly better survival than those with poorly differentiated tumors. Only three patients had well-differentiated metastases, which

was consistent with other studies reporting a rarity of such nodes. They concluded that there is a strong relationship between the histologic appearance of lymph node metastases and survival. Others have suggested that increasing Gleason score and elevated acid phosphatase have not been statistically significant prognostic variables.[48]

The prognostic importance of the actual number—or percentage—of positive lymph nodes at PLND is controversial. Schmidt et al.[49] reported that patients with less than 20% of nodes involved had a significantly better progression-free survival (PFS) than those with more extensive pelvic adenopathy. This was based upon 212 patients with surgically confirmed stage D1 prostate cancer who were randomized to chemotherapy (estramustine phosphate or cyclophosphamide) or observation after definitive radiation or surgery. Neither the actual number of positive nodes nor their anatomical distribution had prognostic significance. Long-term follow-up of this group of patients was recently published,[50] and median PFS for radiated patients with limited nodal metastases was longer (39.9 months), regardless of adjuvant therapy, compared to patients with extensive adenopathy (20.7 months). However, in those patients treated surgically, there were no such differences.

Other studies have shown the actual number of positive nodes to be of limited prognostic significance.[19,46] Gervasi and associates[19] followed 152 surgically staged D1 patients after radioactive gold seed implantation and full pelvis external beam irradiation for a mean of 8.6 years. The patients were stratified according to nodal status: N1 patients (n = 37) had a single microscopic positive node, N2 (n = 86) had multiple microscopic positive nodes, and N3 (n = 29) had grossly positive or juxtaregional nodes. N1 patients had a pattern of progression similar to that of N2 and N3 patients, and at 10 years, 80% had distant metastases. The risk of dying of prostate cancer at 10 years was 40% for N1, 66% for N2, and 58% for N3. They concluded that the finding of a single microscopic focus of cancer in a pelvic node indicates systemic disease with a prognosis similar to that of multiple positive nodes. Kramer and associates[51] reported similar findings in smaller groups of patients regardless of the therapeutic modality used.

Steinberg and coworkers[46] claimed that several parameters were useful for predicting survival, progression-free survival, and probability of symptomatic local recurrence. In 120 consecutive patients with stage D1 cancer, these were: (1) microscopic versus macroscopic lymph node metastases, (2) falsely negative frozen section diagnosis (implying a smaller volume of cancer), and (3) percentage of nodes sampled that were positive. Preoperative Gleason grade of the primary tumor, clinical stage, or actual number of positive nodes were not predictors. However, all of the predictors affected the decision to proceed with radical prostatectomy and hence had a direct bearing on symptomatic local recurrence. Moreover, in view of the relatively brief follow-up (mean 48 months), it is not surprising that each parameter, a reflection of metastatic burden, influenced time to progression, rather than the likelihood of progression ultimately occurring. Thus available data support the contention that even a single focus of nodal metastasis indicates the presence of systemic disease.

MANAGEMENT

Despite the curability of some urologic malignancies with regional nodal involvement, most authors agree that stage D1 prostatic carcinoma remains incurable by any current treatment. Therefore, the primary goal of current therapy should be to prolong the cancer-specific and actual survival periods while trying to minimize both disease-related and treatment-related morbidity. Because most patients with

stage D1 disease are asymptomatic (or nearly so) at the time of diagnosis, reducing disease-related morbidity is ultimately dependent upon either preventing or controlling (stabilizing or reversing) disease progression. Systemic disease progression may be a manifestation of pre-existing microscopic metastases, or of continuous metastatic seeding from an incompletely eradicated tumor focus—either in a metastatic or primary tumor site. Local tumor progression reflects incomplete local therapy and may be symptomatic, asymptomatic—but obvious based on physical exam—or clinically silent and only detected by chemical tests (e.g., PSA detectability or elevation) or invasive procedures (e.g., biopsy). Each of these forms of local persistence is a rough reflection of local tumor volume, but whether the capacity for continued disease dissemination is proportional to the local tumor volume is uncertain. With these issues in mind we will discuss available information about the impact of current therapies, and the timing of their administration on survival and disease-related morbidity.

Advocates of aggressive local therapy (radical prostatectomy or definitive radiotherapy) argue that local morbidity is significant in conservatively treated patients, and that by reducing or eliminating the primary tumor burden, the likelihood and/or speed of tumor dissemination is reduced. The former contention would appear logical since up to 90% of D1 patients treated with radical prostatectomy have extracapsular spread of the local tumor.[52] In addition to providing better local control, irradiation or surgery "debulks" the primary tumor prior to the immediate or delayed administration of hormonal therapy.[11,14] However, the benefits of these local therapies in preventing *symptomatic* local progression, without[15] or with concomitant hormonal therapy,[53] is controversial. Furthermore, evidence to support a salutary effect of these local therapies on preventing subsequent metastatic seeding is nonexistent, and those few studies that have claimed such have been hindered by brief follow-ups, use of early hormonal therapy, and lack of suitable controls.[11,54]

Single Modality Therapy

Radiotherapy. Several studies have reported the use of radiotherapy to treat stage D1 prostate cancer (Table 1). In one review, Stein and deKernion[12] reported the median interval to progression for external beam irradiation as 11 to 23 months, with five-year nonprogression rates of 9% to 22%. Similar results were reported for brachytherapy, with or without external beam radiation. The largest series[19] of 152 patients who were treated with combined interstitial radioactive gold and external beam radiation therapy, and followed for 8.6 years, demonstrated an 83% 10-year risk of systemic metastatic disease.

Bagshaw's data[55] have been widely quoted; in 61 stage D1 patients treated with whole pelvis irradiation, the survival rate at 10 years was 20%. Recent reviews of this study noted the inclusion of patients with para-aortic nodal involvement and the use of split-course irradiation, which may be less effective than continuous treatment.[54]

Some of the most impressive results obtained with external beam irradiation for stage D1 disease were reported by Lawton et al.[54] Fifty-six patients who received definitive whole pelvis irradiation were followed for a median 9.3 years, and the 5- and 10-year actuarial survival was 76% and 33%, respectively. Progression-free survival was 61% at 5 years and 48% at 10 years, and local recurrence was reported as 9%. These results are weakened by several factors, however: only 41% of patients had biopsy-proven nodal involvement (the remainder had radiographically documented lymphadenopathy by CT scan and/or bipedal lymphangiography), patients were not routinely followed with posttreatment bone scans, and the method of documenting the local recurrence is not mentioned. This is a notable omission since other series have reported a significantly higher local recurrence rate (24–51%).[15,46] Furthermore, 15 patients received hormonal treatment—12 at time of first recurrence, and three immediately after irradiation—and they are included in the statistical analyses with the patients who were not so treated.

Pelvic irradiation has been compared to hormonal therapy in small series. Steinberg and associates[46] reported on 120 consecutive patients with stage D1 prostate cancer, of whom 21 were treated with external beam radiation to the pelvis and prostate. In comparison to expectant hormonal therapy in 35 patients, local symp-

TABLE 1. Actuarial Survival and Time to Progression for Stage D1 Prostate Cancer Patients Following External Beam Irradiation with or without Au¹⁹⁸ Brachytherapy

Author(s)	No.	Treatment	5-Year Survival (%)	10-Year Survival (%)	Median Months Progress
Smith et al.[15]	47	E.B.	60		<60
Gervasi et al.[19]	152	Comb.	75	43	<36
Steinberg et al.[46]	21	E.B.	68	30	
Kramer et al.[51]	20	E.B.			16
Lawton et al.[54]	56	E.B.	76	33	
Bagshaw[55]	61	E.B.		20	
Paulson et al.[56]	41	E.B.			24

E.B. = external beam irradiation; Comb. = combined Au¹⁹⁸ brachytherapy and external beam irradiation.

tomatic or distant progression-free survival was not significantly different, and
irradiation was associated with significant
side effects (10% total urinary incontinence, 5% fecal incontinence, and 14%
chronic cystitis).

These results are contrary to those reported by Paulson et al.,[56] in which 77 patients with histologically confirmed stage
D1 prostate cancer after staging pelvic
lymphadenectomy were randomized to receive delayed androgen ablation or immediate extended-field megavoltage irradiation. The group of 41 radiated patients
demonstrated better median actual survival (44 versus 34 months) and longer median time to treatment failure (24 versus 12
months). The actual survival advantage
demonstrated in the radiated group was
maintained out to about four years, after
which both groups had similar survival.
These data suggest that irradiation delays
disease progression compared to observation alone, and although a short-term survival advantage is seen, equivalent survival rates are reached at five years. These
data may also be interpreted as indicating
that while disseminated metastases already exist at the time stage D1 disease is
discovered, continued seeding from the local lesion occurs, which may hasten the
patient's demise.

Radical prostatectomy. Until recently,
radical surgery had been recommended as
treatment for only clinically localized prostate cancer. Currently, disappointed by
high progression rates with nonsurgical
modalities, some urologists have begun to
recommend radical prostatectomy for
stage C and D1 disease. The rationale for
"debulking" the primary tumor prior to
hormonal treatment and managing local
disease is debatable; approximately 30% of
D1 patients treated only with hormonal
therapy will eventually require a transurethral resection for local control.[53] This
compares to a 3% to 9% incidence of local
recurrence requiring intervention after

radical prostatectomy for stage D1 disease.[46,52] Comparing the morbidity of a
TURP in 30% of conservatively managed
patients to that of a radical prostatectomy
in 100% of aggressively managed ones reduces the clinical importance of the difference in symptomatic local failure in men
treated with hormonal therapy versus radical prostatectomy.

Although controversial, there are some
stage D1 patients with minimal nodal involvement (i.e., falsely negative frozen
sections) who may have a better prognosis
and benefit from radical prostatectomy.[8,46]
However, in the Mayo Clinic eight-year
follow-up of 33 patients who underwent
radical prostatectomy alone for single
node-positive disease, 100% of the patients demonstrated progression.[57]

Radical prostatectomy has been combined with adjuvant whole-pelvis irradiation for stage D1 cancer with favorable results. Lange et al.[16] reported a five-year
disease-free survival and actuarial survival
of 69% and 74%, respectively, in 36 patients so treated. These were better results
than reported in previous studies that employed either radiation or radical prostatectomy alone. However, the median
follow-up was only 48 months, there were
no controls, and the authors admitted that
the efficacy of adjuvant radiation therapy
was unproved.

Hormonal therapy. In recognition of
the metastatic nature of stage D1 prostate
cancer, hormonal therapy is now commonly used both alone and in combination
with radical surgery (and to a lesser degree
with radiation). The benefits of the latter
treatment strategies are controversial, as is
the timing of hormonal intervention following surgery or diagnosis of stage D1
cancer.

Bilateral orchiectomy and luteinizing
hormone-releasing hormone (LHRH)
agonist therapy have been the standards
of androgen deprivation. More recently,
maximal androgen ablation (orchiectomy

or LHRH agonist in combination with an antiandrogen) has been compared to LHRH agonists or orchiectomy alone in patients with stage D2 prostate cancer.[5,10,58–61] Although these studies have not specifically addressed stage D1 prostate cancer (which may reflect physicians' policies of withholding therapy until the patient is symptomatic), subset analysis of patients with minimal distant metastases in the National Cancer Institute Intergroup study showed significantly better progression-free survival with leuprolide and flutamide than with leuprolide and placebo. At 60 months, median progression-free survival had not been reached in those men treated with combined therapy.[59,61]

Early versus late hormonal therapy.
Many urologists have waited until late in the course of metastatic prostate cancer, with onset of symptoms, to institute hormonal therapy. The results of the Veterans Administration Cooperative Urological Research Group (VACURG) studies may be responsible for this philosophy. VACURG Study I randomized patients with clinical evidence of extraprostatic disease to immediate hormonal treatment or placebo with delayed hormonal treatment once symptoms developed. The authors found no difference in the survival rates, and because of the toxicity of the estrogen dose used, recommended withholding hormonal treatment until patients became symptomatic.[62]

The weaknesses (primarily early crossover from the delayed treatment arm) and possibly erroneous conclusions of the VACURG studies have been described in depth,[10,63] and Sarosdy[2] suggested that the studies were not designed to determine the optimal timing of hormonal intervention.

Since that time, many investigators have reported results favoring early hormonal treatment for stage D1 prostate cancer. In theory, earlier intervention treats a smaller volume of tumor that is composed of a greater percentage of androgen-sensitive cells.[10] In practice, early androgen deprivation (at the time of staging laparotomy or radical prostatectomy) extends the time to disease progression compared to delayed hormonal therapy; however, it does not prolong survival.[5,10,11] Multiple studies comparing early and late treatment have been published; however, none are randomized or prospective, the sample sizes are small, and the authors frequently use Kaplan-Meier projections to predict survival and progression before medians of either are reached.[5]

For example, van Aubel and associates[13] reported retrospectively on 30 patients with clinically localized cancer found to have positive lymph nodes at the time of PLND. All were treated with immediate bilateral orchiectomy alone, and only 46% were projected to have failed treatment by 45 months using Kaplan-Meier projections. However, there was no control group, the mean follow-up was only 34 months, and only three patients who were 45 months out from treatment were still alive.

Controlled, randomized, prospective studies are clearly needed to address the potential benefit of early hormonal treatment in stage D1 prostate cancer. Such studies have been designed and initiated by the European Organization of Research and Treatment of Cancer (EORTC) and the Eastern Cooperative Oncology Group (ECOG). In both the EORTC and one of the ECOG trials, patients believed to have clinical stage A and B disease—found at PLND to have positive nodes—were randomized to immediate hormonal monotherapy (bilateral orchiectomy or LHRH agonist) or observation until disease progression was documented. None of these patients underwent definitive treatment to the prostate (radical prostatectomy or radiotherapy). While the latter trial has been discontinued owing to poor accrual, the former will eventually be completed and should provide critical information in this area.

Combination Therapy

Radical prostatectomy and androgen ablation.

Multiple studies have suggested that early hormonal therapy for stage D1 cancer diagnosed at the time of radical prostatectomy prolongs the time to tumor recurrence. In a retrospective, nonrandomized study, Kramolowsky[64] found a significant delay in median interval to progression of disease in 30 stage D1 patients who underwent radical prostatectomy and received early hormonal treatment (100 months) compared to those 38 patients treated expectantly (43 months). However, the median survival was not statistically different between the groups. DeKernion and associates[65] reported similar results in their retrospective, nonrandomized study of 56 stage D1 patients treated in the same manner.

Zincke and associates, in a series of nonrandomized, retrospective studies from the Mayo Clinic, have assessed the impact of PLND, radical prostatectomy, and adjuvant treatment (hormonal ± radiation) on 380 stage D1 patients.[14,17,18,52] Although they suggest a dramatic improvement in outcome for patients treated with radical prostatectomy and immediate hormonal ablation (especially for those with DNA diploid primary tumors), the lack of randomization, choice of treatment by physician, and use of Kaplan-Meier projections put their conclusions in question.

Myers and associates[11] recently reported on the long-term follow-up of 62 of these Mayo Clinic stage D1 patients who underwent PLND and radical prostatectomy with or without early antiandrogen therapy. Median follow-up was 10 years. There was a significant delay in time to progression of disease in the early treatment group; however, no survival benefit was demonstrated (Fig. 2).[11] The authors noted that the subset of 14 patients with

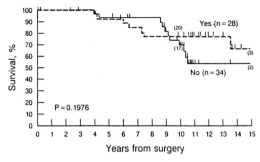

Fig. 2. Actuarial survival for 62 stage D1 prostate cancer patients who underwent radical prostatectomy according to whether patient received early endocrine therapy. Reprinted with permission.[11]

DNA diploid primary tumors who underwent early antiandrogen therapy did remarkably well. The 10-year cause-specific survival was 100% (five men dead of nonprostate cancer causes, no men dead from prostate cancer, nine alive) compared to 67% for the nine diploid cases without early therapy (three men dead of nonprostate cancer causes, two dead from prostate cancer, four alive). However, even for this "responsive" group with diploid tumors, the all-cause and cancer-specific survival benefits were marginal. Furthermore, the data presented failed to address whether radical prostatectomy conferred any survival advantage.

A prospective, randomized, controlled trial carried out by ECOG and the Southwest Oncology Group (SWOG) (EST3886) specifically testing the benefit of immediate versus deferred hormone therapy (either bilateral orchiectomy or goserelin per patient choice) in 100 patients with stage D1 disease who have undergone PLND and radical prostatectomy has recently closed—results will not be available for some time. Hopefully, by comparing the results of this study with the EORTC trial of hormonal therapy in stage D1 patients who have not undergone radical prostatectomy, the benefits of this operation in the face of nodal metastases can be assessed.

Radiation and hormonal therapy.
There is little written about combining
these two treatment modalities in prostate
cancer.[5] Currently, the Radiation Therapy
Oncology Group (RTOG) has two large
phase III trials of primary irradiation plus
androgen deprivation therapy for local
and extensive local disease underway.[54]
The preliminary results of RTOG protocol
8610 (randomization to goserelin and flutamide before and during radiotherapy versus radiotherapy alone for large T_2B, T_3,
and T_4 tumors) have been reported.[66] Although nodal status is not specified, with a
median observation period of 28 months,
more than 50% of patients receiving hormonal and radiation therapies have evidence of progression based upon PSA.
Furthermore, overall survival is not significantly different between the two groups. It
seems likely that the results of this trial
will be similar to those reported in surgical
trials.

**Definitive local therapy and adjuvant
chemotherapy.** The inevitable progression of metastatic prostate cancer with hormonally independent cells has spawned
an extensive search for effective chemotherapeutic agents. Unfortunately, no effective treatment has been found,[5] and little has been written about chemotherapy
in stage D1 disease.

Small nonrandomized studies have suggested that adjuvant chemotherapy in low-
volume stage D1 disease may improve outcome. In a series of 37 stage D1 patients
treated with either radical prostatectomy
or brachytherapy with iodine[125], deVere
White[48] treated 12 men with adjuvant cyclophosphamide and doxorubicin hydro-
chloride over a six-month period (the remaining 25 men were observed). With
follow-up of 12 to 36 months, 12 patients
(48%) in the observation arm had progressed (average time 11.6 months) compared to four patients (33%) in the treatment arm (average time 15 months).
Formal statistical analysis was not pre-

sented, follow-up was short, and patients
were not initially randomized or treated
equivalently (surgery versus radiation).
These shortcomings make it difficult to in-
terpret the results. Other small studies suffer from similar limitations.[67,68]

Schmidt and associates[49,50] reported the
results of two prospective studies designed by the National Prostatic Cancer
Treatment Group (NPCTG) to evaluate adjuvant therapy after radical prostatectomy
(Protocol 900) or radiotherapy (Protocol
1,000) for clinically localized prostate cancer. All patients underwent staging pelvic
lymphadenectomy, and nodal involvement was found in 29% of patients in Protocol 900 and 63% in Protocol 1,000. After
recovery from the primary therapy, patients were randomized to receive intravenous cyclophosphamide (1 g/m² every
three weeks), oral estramustine phosphate
(600 mg/m² daily), or observation. Drug
treatment was delivered for a maximum of
two years, and patients were followed for
a mean of 10 years (range 80–160 months)
with DRE, acid phosphatase, chest radio-
graph, and radionuclide bone scan every
six months.

Of the 48 stage D1 patients in Protocol
900, recurrent disease was detected in
56%, with no significant difference between the assigned adjuvant treatments
or between adjuvant and observation
groups. Median PFS in the observation
group was 57.7 months (n = 14). Of the
146 stage D1 patients in Protocol 1,000,
tumor recurrence occurred in 77% and the
median PFS in the observation group (n =
52) was 20.9 months. The longest median
PFS was 37.3 months in patients receiving
estramustine phosphate (n = 42), but this
was not a statistically significant difference.

When the *degree* of lymph node metastases was considered, the median PFS for
patients in Protocol 1,000 with limited disease (less than 20% nodal involvement)
was significantly longer than that for pa-

tients with more extensive disease (39.9 months versus 20.7 months), regardless of the adjuvant therapy. Moreover, in the group of patients with extensive disease, those receiving adjuvant estramustine phosphate had a significantly longer median PFS (32.8 months) than the cyclophosphamide (22.7 months) or observation (12.9 months) groups.

The difference between median PFS in patients with limited and extensive nodal metastases in Protocol 1,000 was not observed in Protocol 900. This may reflect better control of the primary tumor with radical prostatectomy, or a selection bias to treat patients with lower-stage disease surgically. The authors concluded that there was no apparent benefit of adjuvant therapy with estramustine phosphate or cyclophosphamide in surgically treated stage D1 patients, or in radiated patients with less than 20% pelvic lymph node involvement.[50]

The role of chemotherapy in the management of stage D1 prostate cancer remains undefined, and additional randomized, prospective trials are needed. Newer agents such as suramin are under investigation in treatment of hormone refractory metastatic prostate cancer, but trials in treatment of stage D1 disease are lacking.

SUMMARY

Histologically confirmed stage D1 prostate cancer is metastatic disease. Despite earlier detection efforts and far more surgically staged patients on a national level,[9] it is not clear that the actual number of stage D1 patients is diminishing. With hormonal treatment withheld until disseminated progression occurs, despite extensive local and regional therapies, even the most optimistic series report that over 50% of patients have expired by 10 years.[11,54] Moreover, based primarily on single-arm retrospective studies, the administration of immediate hormone therapy, while de-

laying progression, has not been found to significantly prolong survival when compared with delayed hormonal therapy. Two important cooperative group trials should ultimately identify the role of early hormone therapy—and possibly aggressive local treatment—in affecting cancer-specific survival and disease-related morbidity, but results from these are unlikely to be available for years. Additional questions besides the role of "prophylactic" local therapy and timing of hormonal therapy include whether total androgen ablation and/or systemic nonhormonal therapy will be beneficial. Finally, with further study, individual tumor characteristics or molecular markers may be able to predict subsets of stage D1 patients who are particularly likely (or not likely) to benefit from specific therapies.

As it stands currently, however, there is no compelling evidence that either aggressive local treatment or immediate hormonal therapy will significantly delay death from prostate cancer or will prevent symptoms (from either local or metastatic disease) from developing that cannot usually be managed effectively by standard, relatively nonmorbid means (e.g., hormonal therapy, TURP, etc). As such, a policy of delayed hormonal therapy would seem as effective as more aggressive approaches in the management of patients with stage D1 prostate cancer.

REFERENCES

1. Petros JA, Catalona WJ: Lower incidence of unsuspected lymph node metastases in 521 consecutive patients with clinically localized prostate cancer. J Urol 147:1574, 1992.

2. Sarosdy MF: Do we have a rational treatment plan for stage D-1 carcinoma of the prostate? World J Urol 8:27, 1990.

3. Donohue RE, Mani JH, Whitesel JA, et al.: Intraoperative and early complications of staging pelvic lymph node dissection in prostatic adenocarcinoma. Urology 35:223, 1990.

4. Catalona WJ: Pelvic lymphadenectomy is essential to staging accuracy in most patients

with stages A-2 and B prostate cancer before radical prostatectomy. Sem Urol 1(3):212, 1983.

5. Stamey TA, McNeal JE: Adenocarcinoma of the prostate. In Walsh PC, et al. (eds): Campbell's Urology, 6th ed. Philadelphia: W.B. Saunders, p 1159, 1992.

6. Danella JF, deKernion JB, Smith RB, Steckel J: The contemporary incidence of lymph node metastases in prostate cancer: implications for laparoscopic lymph node dissection. J Urol 149:1488, 1993.

7. Epstein JI, Carmichael M, Partin AW, Walsh PC: Is tumor volume an independent predictor of progression following radical prostatectomy? A multivariate analysis of 185 clinical stage B adenocarcinomas of the prostate with 5 years of followup. J Urol 149:1478, 1993.

8. Hanks GE: The challenge of treating node-positive prostate cancer. Cancer 71:1014, 1993.

9. Lu-Yao GL, McLerran D, Wasson J, Wennberg JE: An assessment of radical prostatectomy: time trends, geographic variation, and outcomes. JAMA 269(20):2633, 1993.

10. Kozlowski JM, Ellis WJ, Grayhack JT: Advanced prostatic carcinoma: early versus late endocrine therapy. Urol Clin North Am 18(1):15, 1991.

11. Myers PM, Larson-Keller JJ, Bergstralh EJ, et al.: Hormonal treatment at time of radical retropubic prostatectomy for stage D1 prostate cancer: results of long-term followup. J Urol 147:910, 1992.

12. Stein A, deKernion JB: Adjuvant endocrine therapy after radical prostatectomy for stage D1 prostate carcinoma. Sem Urol 8(3):184, 1990.

13. van Aubel OG, Hoekstra WJ, Schroder FH: Early orchiectomy for patients with stage D1 prostatic carcinoma. J Urol 134:292, 1985.

14. Zincke H: Combined surgery and immediate adjuvant hormonal treatment for stage D1 adenocarcinoma of the prostate: Mayo Clinic experience. Sem Urol 8(3):175, 1990.

15. Smith JA, Haynes TH, Middleton RG: Impact of external irradiation on local symptoms and survival free of disease in patients with pelvic lymph node metastasis from adenocarcinoma of the prostate. J Urol 131:705, 1984.

16. Lange PH, Reddy PK, Medini E, et al.: Radiation therapy as adjuvant treatment after radical prostatectomy. NCI Monogr 7:141, 1988.

17. Zincke H, Utz DC, Taylor WF: Bilateral pelvic lymphadenectomy and radical prostatectomy for clinical stage C prostatic cancer: role of ad-juvant treatment for residual cancer and in disease progression. J Urol 135:1199, 1986.

18. Zincke H, Utz DC, Thule PM, Taylor WF: Treatment options for patients with stage D1 (T0-3,N1-2,M0) adenocarcinoma of prostate. Urology 30(4):307, 1987.

19. Gervasi LA, Mata J, Easley JD, et al.: Prognostic significance of lymph nodal metastases in prostate cancer. J Urol 142:332, 1989.

20. Stamey TA, Kabalin JN, McNeal JE, et al.: Prostate specific antigen in the diagnosis and treatment of adenocarcinoma of the prostate. II. Radical prostatectomy treated patients. J Urol 141:1076, 1989.

21. Villers AA, McNeal JE, Redwine EA, et al.: Pathogenesis and biological significance of seminal vesicle invasion in prostatic adenocarcinoma. J Urol 143:1183, 1990.

22. Bostwick DG, Graham SD, Napalkov P, et al.: Staging of early prostate cancer: a proposed tumor volume-based prognostic index. Urology 41(5):403, 1993.

23. Andriole GL: New considerations for staging prostate cancer. In Wein AJ, Malkowicz SB (eds): Controversies in the Management of Prostate Cancer, part 8. Philadelphia: CoMed Communications, p 13, 1991.

24. McCarthy P, Pollack HM: Imaging of patients with stage D prostatic carcinoma. Urol Clin North Am 18(1):35, 1991.

25. Terris MK, McNeal JE, Stamey TA: Estimation of prostate cancer volume by transrectal ultrasound imaging. J Urol 147:855, 1992.

26. Rifkin MD, Zerhouni EA, Gatsonis CA, et al.: Comparison of magnetic resonance imaging and ultrasonography in staging early prostate cancer. N Engl J Med 323(10):621, 1990.

27. Ortolano V, Badalament RA, Drago JR: Traditional methods of staging. In Wein AJ, et al. (eds): Controversies in the Management of Prostate Cancer, part 8. Philadelphia: CoMed Communications, p 4, 1991.

28. Paulson DF: Pelvic lymphadenectomy is not essential to staging accuracy in all patients with localized prostate cancer. Sem Urol 1(3):204, 1983.

29. McNeal JE, Villers AA, Redwine et al.: Histologic differentiation, cancer volume, and pelvic lymph node metastasis in adenocarcinoma of the prostate. Cancer 66:1225, 1990.

30. Winkler HZ, Rainwater LM, Meyers RP, et al.: Stage D1 prostatic adenocarcinoma: significance of nuclear DNA ploidy patterns studied by flow cytometry. Mayo Clin Proc 63:103, 1988.

31. deVere White RW, Deitch AD, Tesluk H, et al.: Prognosis in disseminated prostate cancer as related to tumor ploidy and differentiation. World J Urol 8:47, 1990.

32. Heller JE: Prostatic acid phosphatase: its current clinical status. J Urol 137:1091, 1987.

33. Drago JR, Badalament RA, Wientjes MG, et al.: Relative value of prostate-specific antigen and prostatic acid phosphatase in diagnosis and management of adenocarcinoma of prostate. Urology 34(4):187, 1989.

34. Oesterling JE: Prostate specific antigen: a critical assessment of the most useful tumor marker for adenocarcinoma of the prostate. J Urol 145:907, 1991.

35. Burnett AL, Chan DW, Brendler CB, Walsh PC: The value of serum enzymatic acid phosphatase in the staging of localized prostate cancer. J Urol 148:1832, 1992.

36. Partin AW, Carter HB, Chan DW, et al.: Prostate specific antigen in the staging of localized prostate cancer: influence of tumor differentiation, tumor volume and benign hyperplasia. J Urol 143:747, 1990.

37. Parra RO, Andrus C, Boullier J: Staging laparoscopic pelvic lymph node dissection: comparison of results with open pelvic lymphadenectomy. J Urol 147:875, 1992.

38. Huben RP: Pelvic lymphadenectomy. In Fowler, Jr, JE (ed): Urologic Surgery, 1st ed. Boston: Little, Brown, p 595, 1992.

39. deVere White RW: Pelvic lymph node dissection. In Glenn JF (ed): Urologic Surgery, 4th ed. Philadelphia: J.B. Lippincott Co., p 610, 1991, p. 610.

40. Schellhammer PF, Jordan GH, Schlossberg SM: Tumors of the penis. In Walsh PC, et al. (eds): Campbell's Urology, 6th ed. Philadelphia: W.B. Saunders, p 1264, 1992.

41. Prout Jr GR, Heaney JA, Griffin PP, et al.: Nodal involvement as a prognostic indicator in patients with prostatic carcinoma. J Urol 124:226, 1980.

42. Fulgham PF, Feagins BA: Laparoscopic pelvic lymphadenectomy in the staging of adenocarcinoma of the prostate. Infections in Urology 6(2):44, 1993.

43. Rukstalis DB, Gerber GS, Vogelzang NJ, et al.: Laparoscopic pelvic lymph node dissection: a review of 103 consecutive cases. J Urol 1993. Submitted for publication.

44. Schuessler WW, Pharand D, Vancaillie TG: Laparoscopic standard pelvic node dissection for carcinoma of the prostate: is it accurate? J Urol 150:898, 1993.

45. Sosa RE, Poppas DP, Schlegel PN, Lyons JM: Laparoscopic surgery in urology. In Walsh PC, et al. (eds): Campbell's Urology, 6th ed, update 2. Philadelphia: W.B. Saunders, p 1, 1992.

46. Steinberg GD, Epstein JI, Piantadosi S, Walsh PC: Management of stage D1 adenocarcinoma of the prostate: the Johns Hopkins experience 1974 to 1987. J Urol 144:1425, 1990.

47. Brawn P, Kuhl D, Johnson C, et al.: Stage D1 prostate carcinoma: the histologic appearance of nodal metastases and its relationship to survival. Cancer 65:538, 1990.

48. deVere White RW: Radiation and chemotherapy for stage D1 prostate cancer. Sem Urol 1(4):261, 1983.

49. Schmidt JD, Gibbons RP, Bartolucci A, Murphy GP: Prognosis in stage D-1 prostate cancer relative to anatomic sites of nodal metastases. Cancer 64:1743, 1989.

50. Schmidt JD, Gibbons RP, Murphy GP, Bartolucci A: Adjuvant therapy for localized prostate cancer. Cancer 71:1005, 1993.

51. Kramer SA, Cline Jr WA, Farnham R, et al.: Prognosis of patients with stage D1 prostatic adenocarcinoma. J Urol 125:817, 1981.

52. Zincke H: Extended experience with surgical treatment of stage D1 adenocarcinoma of the prostate. Urology 33(5):27, 1989.

53. Catalona WJ: Radical surgery for advanced prostate cancer and for radiation failures (editorial). J Urol 147:916, 1992.

54. Lawton CA, Cox JD, Glisch C, et al.: Is long-term survival possible with external beam irradiation for stage D1 adenocarcinoma of the prostate? Cancer 69:2761, 1992.

55. Bagshaw MA: Potential for radiotherapy alone in prostatic cancer. Cancer 55:2079, 1985.

56. Paulson DF, Cline WA, Koefoot RB, et al.: Extended field radiation therapy versus delayed hormonal therapy in node positive prostatic adenocarcinoma. J Urol 127:935, 1982.

57. Utz DC: Radical excision of adenocarcinoma of prostate with pelvic lymph node involvement: surgical gesture or curative procedure? Urology 24(5):4, 1984.

58. Beland G, Elhilali M, Fradet, et al.: Total androgen ablation: Canadian experience. Urol Clin North Am 18(1):75, 1991.

59. Crawford DE, Eisenberger MA, McLeod DG, et al.: A controlled trial of leuprolide with and without flutamide in prostatic carcinoma. N Engl J Med 321(7):419, 1989.

60. Denis L, Smith P, Carneiro de Moura JL, et al.: Total androgen ablation: European experience. Urol Clin North Am 18(1):65, 1991.

61. Miles BJ, Babiarz J: Maximal androgen ablation: A review. Henry Ford Hosp Med J 40:114, 1992.

62. Blackard CE: The Veterans Administration Cooperative Urological Research Group studies of carcinoma of the prostate: a review. Cancer Chemother Rep 59:225, 1975.

63. Byar DP, Corle DK: Hormone therapy for prostate cancer: results of the Veterans Administration Cooperative Urological Research Group Studies. NCI Monogr 7:165, 1988.

64. Kramolowsky EV: The value of testosterone deprivation in stage D1 carcinoma of the prostate. J Urol 139:1242, 1988.

65. deKernion JB, Neuwerth H, Stein A, et al.: Prognosis of patients with stage D1 prostate carcinoma following radical prostatectomy with and without early endocrine therapy. J Urol 144:700, 1990.

66. Pilepich MV, Krall J, Al-Sarraf, et al.: A phase III trial of androgen suppression before and during radiation therapy (RT) for locally advanced prostatic carcinoma: preliminary report of RTOG Protocol 8610. Proc Am Soc Clin Oncol, Orlando, p 229, 1993.

67. Austenfeld MS, Davis BE: New concepts in the treatment of stage D1 adenocarcinoma of the prostate. Urol Clin North Am 17(4):867, 1990.

68. Carter GE, Lieskovsky G, Skinner DG, Petrovich Z: Results of local and/or systemic adjuvant therapy in the management of pathological stage C or D1 prostate cancer following radical prostatectomy. J Urol 142:1266, 1989.

14

Controversies in the Management of Newly Diagnosed Metastatic Prostate Cancer

Frederick R. Ahmann, M.D., and Bruce L. Dalkin, M.D.

INTRODUCTION

Metastatic prostate cancer remains a major health care problem in the United States and the world. Among men over the age of 60, it rivals lung cancer as being the leading cause of cancer-related mortality. In 1993, it is estimated that 35,000 men will die of prostate cancer,[1] a number that over the last 10 years has continued to rise. Surveillance, Epidemiology and End Results (SEER) data suggest no decline in prostate cancer mortality, primarily reflecting the impact of metastatic disease.[1] This is occurring despite more sensitive and specific modalities for early detection. While this increased mortality may merely reflect the fact that the natural history of cardiovascular disease in men is changing, allowing men to live longer and, hence, allowing a higher number of latent prostate cancers to become clinically significant, prostate cancer and metastatic disease in particular is likely to continue to increase as a major cause of morbidity and mortality among aging men.

It is appropriate to pay tribute to the several historical milestones that mark the development of therapy for metastatic prostate cancer. At a minimum, the important events would include the first description of a useful serum tumor marker for a malignancy, acid phosphatase, in the 1930s.[2] The second event would be the discovery and description in 1941 that endogenous androgens are biologically active in prostate cancer and that reducing androgens results in an antiproliferative effect that benefits a vast majority of patients afflicted with the disease.[3] While the relationship between prostate cancer and androgens may have been suggested as early as 1786,[4] the work of Huggins led directly to a therapeutic benefit for millions of men worldwide and resulted in a Nobel Prize in medicine. And lastly, while not originally targeted toward prostate cancer therapy, the Nobel Prize–winning description by Schally of the pituitary/hypothalamic neuroendocrine control of testicular (and ovarian) endocrine function has also significantly contributed to a lower morbidity from the disease.[5] These accomplishments demonstrate how basic and clinical research, while not curing prostate cancer, has resulted in prolonged survival and improvement in patients' quality of life.

In this chapter, we discuss six different controversies in the initial management of advanced prostate cancer. First, in light of new methods of detecting disease, what is the definition of metastatic prostate can-

Prostate Cancer, pages 215–233 © 1994 Wiley-Liss, Inc.

cer? Second, when metastatic disease is documented, should the timing of therapy initiation be expectant or at diagnosis? Third, what are the known prognostic factors predicting response to and survival with metastatic prostate cancer? Fourth, what are the primary hormonal therapy options and is there an optimal therapy? Fifth, how can a response to therapy be documented and how should patients be followed? And lastly, what therapeutic approach should be taken in patients who present with a consumption coagulopathy, epidural spinal cord compression, or other acute clinical conditions?

A DEFINITION FOR METASTATIC DISEASE

A metastasis is the appearance of cancer at a site distant from the site of origin. The routes of metastases in prostatic cancer are lymphatic, first to regional lymph nodes draining the prostate in the pelvis, and, when more advanced, to periaortic, mediastinal, and supraclavicular nodes. Hematogenous spread of prostate cancer is most commonly represented by sites of disease identified, in descending order of frequency, in bone, liver, lung, and pleura. Hence, the most straightforward definition of metastatic prostate cancer is the documentation of metastatic deposits in any of the above sites. A commonly used modification of the Whitmore-Jewett staging system would classify all distant spread as stage D with two subgroups, stage D-1 (regional lymph node metastases only) and stage D-2 (more distant lymph node metastases or hematogenous metastases).[6]

However, the origin of that simple definition and the commonly used Whitmore-Jewett staging system preceded the development of serum prostate-specific antigen (PSA) measurements. Studies now have demonstrated that patients with micrometastatic disease can be identified with a high degree of accuracy. There are four circumstances in which this is relevant: first,

patients with clinically localized disease who have a markedly elevated serum PSA level[7–10]; second, men after radical prostatectomy in whom the serum PSA level does not become undetectable[7,8,11–14]; third, men after radical prostatectomy who develop a rising serum PSA level[7,8,11–14]; and last, men who after primary radiotherapy for localized prostate cancer develop a rising serum PSA level.[15,16]

After radical prostatectomy, the work of Lange, Stamey, and others has demonstrated that analogous to serum tumor markers in germ cell malignancies, if the serum PSA level does not fall to the lower limits of detection, regardless of the pathologic stage of the resected cancer, prostate cancer persists, albeit clinically undetected. Disease progression over time will occur.[7,8,11–14] It is logical to conclude that such patients had micrometastases at the time of surgery, particularly since postoperative local radiotherapy appears to result in only temporary reductions of persistent or rising PSA levels. There is no staging category for such patients in the Whitmore-Jewett staging system and neither is there an accepted therapeutic approach. We identify these patients as stage D_{PSA}.

In a similar clinical situation are patients who have undergone radical prostatectomy, have had their PSAs fall to the lower limit of detection, and later, develop a rising PSA with no evidence of disease on physical exam or imaging studies.[7,8,11–14] We similarly classify such patients as stage D_{PSA}. Slightly different are patients who have undergone definitive radiotherapy and had their PSAs fall and plateau, but then develop a rising PSA level and have no changes in digital rectal exam or imaging studies. Some of these patients will progress locally and if there is no evidence of disease outside the prostatic bed on physical exam or imaging studies, we label such patients as having recurrent disease. In these men, salvage radical prostatectomy in a select subgroup of these patients is being investigated as an aggressive experimental approach.[17]

Men with clinically localized prostatic carcinoma and moderate elevations in serum PSA (>15 ng/ml) are much less likely to have an optimal surgical outcome (organ-confined cancer on pathologic review) than will men with a lower PSA and similar clinical stage and histologic graded lesions.[7-9] At present, changes in therapeutic intervention, i.e., radical prostatectomy or external beam radiotherapy, cannot be recommended on the basis of serum PSA alone as an outcome determinant. Recently, the investigative use of neoadjuvant medical castration plus radical prostatectomy is being assessed in an effort to improve pathologic stage and eventual survival in this high-risk group. The only diagnostic or therapeutic exception would be to recommend pelvic lymph node dissection, open or laparoscopic, prior to radiotherapy or subsequent (staged) radical prostatectomy, if the decision on proceeding with intervention would be changed by the identification of stage D-1 disease. At present, there is little data to support radiotherapy or radical prostatectomy as potentially curative therapy for stage D-1 prostate cancer.

EARLY VERSUS EXPECTANT THERAPY

A second controversy centers around when to initiate endocrine therapy for metastatic prostate cancer. This issue is a common clinical dilemma and as serum PSA levels enable physicians to identify larger numbers of men with recurrent disease in an asymptomatic state, it will increase with time in significance. It is important to appreciate the historical development of endocrine therapy in order to gain some understanding as to why there is, as yet, no clear best therapeutic approach to this situation.

The work of Huggins in 1941 was received with great enthusiasm and the clinical application of endocrine therapy, either castration or additive estrogen therapy, spread rapidly. Illustrative of this is the retrospective Mayo Clinic Experience reported in 1960 treating prostate cancer during the previous 20 years.[18] One of the objectives was to identify a group of patients not treated with endocrine therapy to serve as a control group in an effort to assess the survival impact of endocrine therapy. However, in this review of over 1,100 patients, less than 10 patients with metastatic disease could be identified in the Mayo Clinic records with prostate cancer who had not been treated with endocrine therapy. This report demonstrates how quickly endocrine therapy was accepted into clinical practice. This fact should not be surprising considering how common the disease was, and how, at the very least, endocrine therapy offered palliation for symptoms.

Hence, the clinical acceptance of Huggins's work left many basic questions about endocrine therapy unanswered. Key among these was the effect of such therapy on overall survival. To date, no definitive answer to this question is known. A study by Nesbit in 1950[19] was the first cooperative urologic study. Nesbit accumulated data from survivals of patients with metastatic prostate cancer, both before and after 1945. A survival advantage for the time period when endocrine therapy was in wide use was demonstrated and seemed to amount to approximately 12 months. The study was retrospective, and during this same time period, other medical developments may have contributed to survival prolongations, including the availability of effective antibiotics. However, these confounding factors seem unlikely to have been the sole explanation for the 12-month difference. Taken together with the common clinical experience of initiating endocrine therapy in a man who is in pain, losing weight, and has a low performance status and then seeing him return, albeit for less than two years on average, to a normal weight and performance status without pain reinforces a conclusion that endocrine therapy appears to contribute to an overall survival benefit.

The Veterans Administration Cooperative Urologic Research Group (VACURG) also tried to address the survival issue in the 1960s. In their first prostate cancer trial studying patients with metastatic disease, the design called for one arm to be a "no treatment" arm. The results of this study did not show an inferior survival for this arm. On initial assessment, this would appear to support a conclusion that endocrine therapy does not significantly prolong survival.[20] However, the study permitted the initiation of endocrine therapy whenever the primary physician felt it was indicated and the study group later reported that, within a year, a majority of patients had had endocrine therapy initiated.[21] Consequently, a more reasonable conclusion in terms of overall survival is that expectant hormonal therapy is equivalent to early endocrine therapy.

Advocates for the early initiation of endocrine therapy would point to the results reported from the Mayo Clinic of their experience in men with pathologic stage D-1 disease.[22] At the Mayo Clinic, careful record has been kept of patients with node-positive disease who immediately underwent bilateral orchiectomy versus those who did not. The time interval to evidence of first progression is prolonged in the patients who undergo early endocrine therapy when compared to delayed endocrine therapy. This result should not be surprising, as there is little debate as to the effectiveness of endocrine therapy in inducing disease regression. However, there is no clear effect on overall disease-specific survival for the entire group and benefit must then return to a discussion of the quality of life resulting with either approach.

More provocative indirect evidence supporting an early initiation of endocrine therapy comes from the Intergroup trial that randomized patients with newly diagnosed metastatic disease to Lupron with or without flutamide.[23] When survival results were analyzed for the subgroup of men with only small numbers of bony metastases, while comprising less than 10% of the study population, a superior survival was found in men treated with "total androgen ablation." The study was not designed to answer this question and the result has not yet been corroborated. The hypothesis is that early, total androgen ablation in patients with low tumor burden results in a superior survival versus testicular suppression/ablation alone. If true, the early initiation of endocrine therapy should be considered in at least some subgroups of patients.

For now, however, we must conclude that there is no definitively proven overall survival benefit for the initiation of endocrine therapy in asymptomatic patients. The decision must then revolve around quality-of-life issues. This topic has been little explored and is multifaceted. Recently, researchers at Memorial Sloan-Kettering Cancer Center in New York have reported a carefully done quality-of-life study in this patient group.[24] Men who were asymptomatic with metastatic prostate cancer either underwent immediate endocrine therapy or were followed. Careful quality-of-life assessments were done prior to endocrine therapy and repeated six months later. There was a measurable decline in quality of life at that time point for the group that underwent early hormonal therapy.

In conclusion, each patient and physician must review the potential advantages as well as the risks of early versus expectant therapy. Neither approach is probably best for all patients. More information regarding this issue is likely to become available in the next five years and clinicians should be alert for new information, particularly as it relates to overall survival effects and quality-of-life issues.

PROGNOSTIC INDICATORS

The wide variability in the natural history of prostate cancer has complicated clinical decision making in the treatment of all stages of prostate cancer. Treatment decisions can and should be influenced by multiple factors in men with metastatic disease. The reported mean and median survivals of men undergoing protocol-directed endocrine therapy for metastatic prostate cancer has slowly increased over the years, possibly due to diagnosing the presence of metastatic disease at earlier time points. Imaging studies have a higher sensitivity for detecting metastatic sites, but the major contributor to this earlier diagnosis is serum PSA levels. Rising serum PSA levels have led to performing imaging studies earlier in asymptomatic patients.

Over the past 10 years, the overall survival of men with metastatic prostate cancer has averaged two to three years.[23,25,26] This survival can be broken down into a period of remission on endocrine therapy lasting on an average between 12 and 24 months and a survival with hormone-resistant disease lasting on average between 6 and 12 months. However, there are wide ranges in these survivals. Ten percent of patients have a rapidly progressive disease course that appears to be minimally influenced by any intervention, and, on the other end of the spectrum, 5% to 10% of treated patients have a prolonged survival with metastatic disease lasting up to 10 years.

An analysis of known prognostic factors can permit a more precise prediction of survival in an individual patient. A knowledge of these prognostic factors is important, both to inform patients as to what

their prognosis is, as well as to aid in the design of a clinical treatment and follow-up plan.

As part of the VACURG studies in prostate cancer, Gleason proposed and subsequently validated the prognostic value of a reproducible histologic grading system for prostate cancer.[27] The Gleason sum score grading of the primary cancer carries with it important prognostic information even for patients with metastatic disease. The prognosis for patients with metastatic disease worsens in direct proportion to the histologic grade sum of the primary and secondary pattern for sum scores 5 to 10. The death rate per year for patients with a Gleason sum score 10 cancer in the VA studies was four times higher than it was for patients with a Gleason sum score 5. At the other end of the spectrum, these studies demonstrated that cancer-related deaths for men with a Gleason sum score 2 prostate cancer were rare in patients with metastatic disease. Other histologic grading systems can be used similarly.

Also of proven prognostic significance are the sites of metastatic disease and the tumor burden.[23,28] While 80% or more of men with metastatic prostate cancer have bony metastases, other sites of disease are not rare. In a series of primary hormone therapy studies of newly diagnosed prostate cancer at the University of Arizona Cancer Center, abdominal and pelvic computed tomography (CT) scans plus chest X-ray and bone scans were performed on all patients. Similar to other studies,[29] the results showed that measurable disease in lymph nodes was present in 33% of all patients found with metastatic disease, with disease in the lung or liver being found in less than 10%. These disease sites do not predict responsiveness to endocrine therapy but do correlate with overall survival. In Tucson, men who had nodal involvement had the same survival as those with bone-only disease. However, those with either liver or lung/pleura involvement had a shorter overall survival.

An analysis of the results of the Intergroup study of Lupron with or without flutamide demonstrated that the amount of bony disease present also correlates with survival.[23] Men who had at diagnosis had three or less bony disease sites had a survival almost double that of men with four or more bony disease sites. In addition, recent analysis of primary hormonal therapy studies have shown that the serum testosterone level prior to the initiation of hormonal therapy predicts both response rate and response duration.[28,30,31] A serum testosterone of less than 200 mg% prior to beginning endocrine therapy results in a significantly shorter survival than does a testosterone level above 200 mg%.[30]

Another multivariant analysis of potential prognostic factors has been carried out on the baseline clinical and laboratory parameters of 240 men with newly diagnosed metastatic prostate cancer who were randomly treated with either a sustained-release luteinizing hormone-releasing hormone (LHRH) agonist (Zoladex) or with castration.[112] Four parameters significantly correlated with a longer survival at two years: the absence of bone pain, a good performance status, a normal serum testosterone level, and a normal serum alkaline phosphatase level. At two years, men in whom all four parameters were favorable had an 82% survival versus only 9% for those patients who had unfavorable values for all four factors. In this study, however, 70% of men had baseline parameters associated with survivals intermediate to the extremes.

And last, serum PSA levels in men with metastatic disease correlate with survival and are clinically useful in several ways.[10] Pretherapy PSA levels correlate with overall tumor burden and hence have been shown to have a general correlation with survival. However, the baseline levels do not predict response rates unless they are less than 10 ng/ml with documented metastases on imaging study. This is a rare circumstance, but in the series in Tucson, such a group of patients have short response durations and overall survivals.

More useful is the prognostic information gained by following serum PSA levels after the initiation of endocrine therapy. The nadir serum PSA level correlates well with response duration and overall survival. Patients with a nadir level less than 4 ng/ml have a mean response duration of 42 months versus 10 months for men whose nadir is above 4 ng/ml.[32]

In summary, there is no definitive multivariant survival formula, but it is possible to classify patients as good, average, or poor prognosis. Table 1 summarizes a simple grading of prognostic factors.

THERAPY OPTIONS

The association of orchiectomy with prostate growth may have been discovered as early as 1786.[4] It was not, however, until the landmark work of Huggins that a rational basis for the successful endocrine therapy of metastatic prostate cancer was established.[3] In Huggins's original description, both castration and additive estrogen therapy were documented as capable of causing reductions in serum levels of acid phosphatase. The exogenous administration of testosterone was shown to reverse these effects. As previously noted, the therapeutic effects were so remarkable that the use of endocrine therapy in men with advanced prostate cancer became widespread before several basic questions were answered. The overall effect of endocrine therapy on survival is not definitively known. And, as we discuss in this section, the relative effectiveness and toxicity of various methods of suppressing or blocking the effects of androgens are still debated.

The effects Huggins described in serum

TABLE 1. Prognostic Factor Grading in Metastatic Prostate Cancer

Prognostic Factor	Favorable	Intermediate	Unfavorable
Gleason histologic score	2 to 4	4 to 7	8 to 10
Number of bony metastases	≤3	—	>3
Liver or lung/pleura metastases	Not present	—	Present
Pretreatment testosterone level	>200 mg%	—	<200 mg%
Pretreatment PSA	10 to 100	100 to 500	<10 or >500
PSA nadir	<10 ng/ml	—	>10 ng/ml
Performance status	ECOG[a] 0 to 1	—	ECOG 2 to 4

[a]ECOG = Eastern Cooperative Oncology Group.

tumor markers, plus improvements in symptoms, can be identified in up to 80% of patients. Little was learned about the overall utility of endocrine therapy until the VACURG sought answers to several questions in men with metastatic prostate cancer. Their first study addressed the question of whether hormonal therapy with 5 mg of diethylstilbestrol (DES) was equally effective as orchiectomy or a combination of 5 mg of DES with orchiectomy, when compared to a placebo arm (delayed endocrine therapy as discussed above). The results in over 800 patients showed that there was no difference in survival seen in any of the four arms, but that there appeared to be excessive cardiovascular deaths in the DES-alone arm. Hence, in the second study, three different doses of DES were compared again with a placebo arm.[33] This much smaller study enrolled a little over 200 patients with metastatic disease and provided results suggesting that 1 mg per day of DES was as effective as 5 mg when overall survival was the endpoint. This lower dose of DES did not appear to have a high cardiovascular complication rate. Because a 1 mg per day dose of DES does not reliably suppress serum testosterone levels to castrate levels, a dose of 3 mg per day is commonly used.[34] The 3 mg/day dose, however, has never been

carefully analyzed for cardiovascular effects.

Generally agreed upon conclusions from the VACURG studies are that the effects of DES and orchiectomy on cancer survival are equivalent and that DES at a dose of 5 mg/day leads to an increase in cardiovascular toxicity.[35] The studies further support a conclusion that delayed or expectant endocrine therapy does not appear to lead to result in inferior disease-specific survival in men with advanced prostate cancer.[21]

The next major development in the endocrine therapy of metastatic prostate cancer was the discovery of a medically reversible castration whose use was not associated with an increase in cardiovascular complications. Schally at Tulane described the endocrine control pathways for testicular androgen secretion through the hypothalamus and pituitary.[5] This led to the isolation of the neurohormone LHRH, a 10 amino acid polypeptide that controls the release of luteinizing hormone/follicle-stimulating hormone (LH/FSH) and hence subsequent testicular testosterone production. Amino acid substitutions at several different positions leads to polypeptides with marked agonist or antagonist activity.[36]

The agonist compounds were initially

hoped to be stimulatory and useful for treating human fertility problems. Clinical trials showed their long-term use to be associated with "receptor down regulation" and with a fall in LH/FSH levels.[37] This medical castration is preceded by a several-day rise in FSH/LH and testosterone levels. The end result, however, was a durable medical castration without significant toxicity other than the effects of androgen withdrawal. Because these small polypeptides cannot be administered orally, clinical trials initially explored an intranasal route of administration.[38] While effective in reducing testosterone levels, this route of administration of LHRH agonists was inconvenient and resulted in unsatisfactory patient compliance.

The practical application of LHRH agonists in prostate cancer was initially accomplished using a daily subcutaneous injection.[41–52] More recently, sustained-release intramuscular or subcutaneous injection formulations have been developed and approved for use by the FDA: Depo Lupron and Zoladex.[39,40] Both compounds in trial appear to be equally effective in chronically suppressing testicular androgen production and both appear to be equally efficacious when compared with bilateral orchiectomy or additive estrogen therapy in controlling prostate cancer.[53] Consequently, the factors physicians and patients must consider in selecting one form of androgen ablative/suppressive therapy include: the requirement for an every-four-week injection by a health care provider for the LHRH agonists, the psychologic concerns some men have associated with surgical removal of the testes, the high cost of LHRH agonist therapy, and the cardiovascular risks of estrogens (Table 2). Efficacy against prostate cancer does not appear to be a factor. Both LHRH agonists and bilateral orchiectomy result in menopausal symptoms, including sweats, hot flashes, loss of libido, weight gain, mild gynecomastia, and skin and hair changes. Additive estrogen therapy has a lower incidence of menopausal symptoms but causes much greater gynecomastia, peripheral edema, and more skin and hair changes.

The most recent controversy in the selection of endocrine therapy for metastatic prostate cancer comes from a hypothesis that adrenal androgens are critically important in the control of androgen-related prostate cancer growth. While the testes are responsible for approximately 90% or more of male androgen production, it has long been recognized that some of the steroids produced by the adrenals are androgens and can be converted peripherally into testosterone and dihydrotestosterone.[40,54,55] When the testes are removed or

TABLE 2. Factors to Consider in Selecting Testicular Suppression/Ablation Therapy for Men with Metastatic Prostate Cancer

Factor	Estrogens	Bilateral Orchiectomy	LHRH Agonist
Convenience	++	+	+++
Psychologic	++	++++	+
Gynecomastia	+++	+	+
Cost	+	++	++++
Skin/hair changes	+++	+	+
Loss of libido	++	++	++
Sweats/hot flashes	+	+++	+++
Cardiovascular risk	+++	−	−
Edema	++	−	−

[a] + indicates the degree of adverse effect.

are medically suppressed, there remain measurable levels of androgens in the body. The significance of these androgens is debated. Some men who have progressive prostate cancer after castration do respond to surgical adrenalectomy and some do respond to inhibitors of adrenal androgen synthesis (aminoglutethimide or ketoconazole) but the probability of a response in that circumstance is low.

Initially, therapy combining LHRH with an antiandrogen was reported to result in response rates approaching 100% with very prolonged response durations.[56] These results spurred a high level of public interest in this approach—"total androgen ablation." It is important to recognize that antiandrogens do not inhibit remaining androgen production but rather block the effects of the androgens at the target cell level. Unfortunately, these initial results have not been duplicated in randomized trials. The results from the randomized trials are nevertheless provocative.

At least eight randomized trials have been conducted comparing different methods of primary testicular suppression/ablation with or without an antiandrogen. Part of the difficulty in interpreting these studies is that there are at least three different options for primary androgen suppression/ablation and several different antiandrogens have been studied. The number of permutations is large and contributes to the difficulty in reaching definitive conclusions.

Among the largest and most significant trials is the Intergroup Trial, which compares Lupron with or without flutamide with a crossover to flutamide at the time of progression in those men who initially did not receive flutamide. This trial is perhaps the best publicized and provides data supporting several conclusions.[54] First, the group of men who initially received LHRH plus flutamide had an overall survival approximately seven months longer (35 versus 28) than the group initially treated

with LHRH alone. Also of interest was the finding that the small subgroup of men with minimal tumor burdens appeared to have most of the overall survival benefit associated with "total androgen ablation." This intriguing observation is being pursued in other trials.

Five other peer-reviewed published analyses of randomized trials have all shown some response benefit for "total androgen ablation" but thus far only one trial, in addition to the Intergroup Trial, has shown statistically significant overall survival benefit. In the Canadian Cooperative Study, 208 men were randomized to either orchiectomy or orchiectomy plus nilutamide.[57] The Danish Cooperative Study randomized 264 patients between orchiectomy or goserelin acetate (Zoladex) plus flutamide, as did the EORTC Trial 30853 (327 men), and the Italian Prostatic Cancer Trial randomized 373 men to either goserelin acetate or goserelin acetate plus flutamide.[55,58,61] The EORTC Trial has recently been updated and now shows a statistically significant overall median survival advantage of approximately seven months for the combination arm.[55] The results of these trials plus the Intergroup Trial and the large Anandron Study Group Trial (published only in abstract form)[62] are displayed in Table 3. Additional follow-up may yet demonstrate significant survival differences between groups in more studies and there are other ongoing studies that are not reviewed here.

Based upon what is published at this time, "total androgen ablation" therapy does appear to result in a higher percent of objective responses and a few trials have shown a slightly longer progression-free survival and overall survival. In the positive trials these differences are measured in terms of months and the effects may be isolated to only some subgroups of patients. A meta-analysis has been organized looking at all randomized trials.[63] This analysis and the results of the ongoing

TABLE 3. "Total Androgen Ablation/Suppression" Trials

Trial (Reference) Rx Arms	No. Enrolled	Relapse-Free Survival Benefit	Overall Survival Benefit
Intergroup[54] LHRH LHRH + Flut.	603	Yes	Yes
Canadian Study[57] Orch Orch + Nilut.	208	No	No
Danish Study[58] Orch LHRH + Flut.	264	No	No
EORTC 30853[55] Orch LHRH + Flut.	327	Yes	Yes
Anandron Study Group[59] Orch Orch + Nilut.	457	No	No
International Prostate Cancer Study Group[60] LHRH LHRH + Flut.	589	No	No
Italian Prostatic Cancer Trial[61] LHRH LHRH + Flut.	373	No	No

Intergroup Trial randomizing patients to orchiectomy with or without flutamide should allow us to reach a more certain consensus in the next few years.

Regardless of what the Intergroup Trial or the meta-analysis shows, many physicians will continue to agonize over this dilemma. On the one hand, some physicians and patients feel passionately about a statistically significant survival difference measured in months, while others consider the down sides of combined androgen ablation. The major limiting factor in the widespread use of this treatment approach is cost. If a patient is treated with "total androgen ablation," the approximate cost for an every-four-week treatment can be over $800, which includes LHRH (approximately $500), flutamide (approximately $300), and an office visit (approximately $35). These costs do not include any routine lab, scans, or X-rays ordered, as they would likely be the same regardless of whatever treatment approach is initiated. For a year encompassing 13 treatments of LHRH plus daily flutamide, the cost can be close to $11,000. Most physicians continue endocrine therapy until death and with an average survival being approximately three years, the cost of total androgen ablation might run as high as $33,000 per patient versus approximately $2,500 for a bilateral orchiectomy. In addition, antiandrogens, while in general being well tolerated, do cause GI toxicity in 10% to 20% of patients.

The decision-making process for physicians and patients is at present not an easy one. In the future, efforts to improve outcome for men in this clinical circumstance are likely to center upon identifying subgroups of patients who may have a large benefit from "total androgen ablation," studying treatment approaches that explore intermittent endocrine therapy, and paying more attention to quality-of-life issues, which will allow physicians and patients to make the most informed and individualized decisions possible.

OTHER PRIMARY HORMONAL THERAPIES

While orchiectomy, additive estrogen therapy, and LHRH agonists are the most commonly utilized primary hormonal manipulations in men with newly diagnosed metastatic prostate cancer, several other endocrine therapies have been evaluated or are in common use in Europe. None of these approaches has been shown in randomized trial to be equivalent to LHRH, orchiectomy, or estrogen therapy and until such trials are completed, all should be considered nonstandard therapies.

Progestational Agents

Megestrol acetate (Megace) and medroxyprogesterone acetate are progestational antiandrogens with demonstrated therapeutic benefit in treating breast cancer. These agents have three effects in men that serve as the basis for their therapeutic potential in prostate cancer: they inhibit LH release; they act as antiandrogens; and they block the 5-alpha-reductase conversion of testosterone to dihydrotestosterone.[64] The most frequently studied dose of Megace is 40 mg four times a day. In previously untreated patients, initial subjective and objective response rates appear approximately equal to that of orchiectomy or LHRH agonists.[65] In EORTC Trial 30761, medroxyprogesterone acetate was compared with DES and the antiandrogen cyproterone in 236 patients.[66] The results demonstrated a shorter progression-free and overall survival for men who received medroxyprogesterone acetate. No other significant randomized comparative trial has been conducted documenting equivalency to standard therapies. Of concern is

the fact that when using megestrol acetate therapy alone, serum testosterone levels after an initial decline tend to return toward normal.[67,68] In response to this, combination trials of megestrol acetate plus low-dose estrogen therapy have been conducted in an attempt to maintain testicular suppression.[69,70] At present, use of these progestational agents as initial therapy should be considered nonstandard.

Estramustine

Estramustine is a chemical combination of the estrogen estradiol phosphate with nitrogen mustard. The drug has combined estrogen effects (suppressing testosterone) with the cytotoxic effects of an alkylator. Of theoretical benefit is the binding of the compound to cells containing the estrogen receptor, thus limiting the alkylator effects to those cells.[71] What importance either or both of these effects have in men with prostate cancer is not clearly determined and the drug's actual mechanism of action is in dispute.[72]

Estramustine therapy in previously untreated patients results in response rates similar to that seen with orchiectomy, LHRH agonists, or DES.[73,74] EORTC Trial 30762 compared estramustine with DES at a dose of 3 mg/day and found no difference in progression-free or overall survival and had toxicity profiles similar for both treatments. At present, no randomized trial supports a conclusion that estramustine is equivalent or superior to DES or other hormonal therapy, and hence the drug is rarely used as initial endocrine therapy for metastatic prostate cancer.

Antiandrogens: Flutamide, Cyproterone Acetate, and Nilutamide

Antiandrogens have as their anticancer mechanism the blockade of the binding of androgens to their receptors.[75] These drugs can be divided based on their chemical structure as steroidal or nonsteroidal compounds. Cyproterone is a progestational agent that has antiandrogen as well as steroid effects. Therapy with cyproterone in patients with previously untreated metastatic prostate cancer appears to have response rates similar to those associated with DES or orchiectomy. However, the toxicity profile includes cardiovascular effects similar to those of estrogens and its long-term therapeutic equivalency is not established.[76]

Both flutamide and nilutamide also bind to androgen receptors but do not have steroid effects.[77–79] In contrast to steroidal antiandrogens, therapy with these drugs has not been associated with any cardiovascular toxicity, fluid retention, or adverse effect on carbohydrate and lipid metabolism.[79–81] However, the drugs do cause gynecomastia and are associated with GI toxicity (diarrhea, nausea, vomiting).[79,82–84] The initial response rates to therapy with either flutamide or nilutamide appear to be similar to those seen with DES, LHRH agonist, or orchiectomy, but no randomized trials have documented survival equivalency. Recently a randomized trial of a new antiandrogen, ICI 176,334 (Casodex), compared this once-a-day antiandrogen as monotherapy with castration or goserelin acetate.[113] Casodex monotherapy at 50 mg orally was inferior to standard therapy in terms of progression-free survival. In conclusion, the use of antiandrogens alone as initial therapy should be regarded as nonstandard.[79,85]

Ketoconazole

Ketoconazole is an antifungal drug that was noted in clinical infectious disease trials to also inhibit steroidal synthesis in both the testes and the adrenals.[86,87] These effects led to its evaluation as a hormonal therapeutic agent in prostate cancer.[88,89] Initial good responses were documented in previously untreated patients, but toxicity and patient compliance limit the

drug's long-term use.[90] No study has documented equivalency with other standard interventions.

Tamoxifen

Additive estrogen therapy in men suppresses pituitary LH secretion and this action is probably the major reason for the beneficial effects seen with such therapy in men with metastatic prostate cancer. However, estrogens have other effects that might also directly affect prostate cancer cell growth. Estrogens increase levels of sex steroid binding globulin, decrease testosterone steroidogenesis in the testis, increase prolactin production, and can decrease DNA synthesis in prostate cells.[114] In addition, prostate cancer cells as well as many other tissues in the body are known to contain estrogen receptors.[115] Because of these varied effects, most of which are modulated via hormone receptors, there exists a theoretical basis for the study of antiestrogens in prostate cancer.

Tamoxifen is a potent antiestrogen with minimal toxicity. Disappointingly, in 13 men with previously untreated metastatic prostate cancer, tamoxifen at a dose of 10 mg orally twice a day resulted in only four tumor responses.[91] Tamoxifen should not be considered an active hormonal agent in prostate cancer.

RESPONSE DETERMINATION AND MONITORING PATIENTS ON ENDOCRINE THERAPY

Over the past 20 years, there has been much debate as to what constitutes a "response" to endocrine or other systemic therapies in men with metastatic prostate cancer. The debate is spurred by a need to compare results from different therapeutic trials. Complex response criteria have been proposed and validated.[92] However, for a patient who is not on an experimental protocol, there are probably only two clinically important parameters to monitor.

The first is relief of cancer-related symptoms such as pain, weight loss, voiding symptoms, lethargy, and fatigue. Monitoring for the relief of cancer-related symptoms is important to determine if additional palliative interventions may be required, such as radiotherapy to a painful bony metastasis or a channel transurethral resection of the prostate (TURP) for significant bladder outlet obstruction. This determination is straightforward and involves serial symptom documentation, serial body weights, quality-of-life assessments, and serial medication use patterns. The control of symptoms is a physician's primary objective with endocrine therapy.

The second group of parameters measured is to assess for disease progression; these are more difficult and of less certain value.[93,95] An individual's prognosis correlates strongly with the onset of disease progression. Progressive disease results in an increased likelihood of worsening symptoms, loss of overall performance status, and a shorter survival. Because at present the systemic therapies available for hormone-resistant disease are of such low efficacy, except for clinical trial objectives, there is no clinically pressing need to document early progression in an asymptomatic patient.[94]

Serial PSA levels appear to provide the most cost-effective and sensitive way of determining hormonal therapy response and response duration. Several studies have shown that the level to which the PSA falls after the initiation of hormonal therapy predicts response duration and overall survival.[32,96,97] Additionally, rising serum PSA levels are usually the first evidence of the emergence of hormone-resistant disease and precede other evidence for disease progression by an average of six months and in some patients by more than a year.[32,96,97]

In conclusion, for patients not on clinical trials, a regular review of a patient's clinical status, including a physical exam, medication use, and a PSA level, are all that is of practical use in monitoring men after the initiation of hormonal therapy. Until such time that effective therapy for hormone-resistant disease becomes available, additional studies done in asymptomatic patients appear to have little practical use.

SPECIAL CLINICAL SITUATIONS

There are several clinical situations with which men with metastatic prostate cancer present that necessitate some alterations in the initial endocrine therapy approach. When aging men present with a consumption coagulopathy, neurologic dysfunction consistent with a lesion in the spinal cord, or with acute renal dysfunction secondary to obstruction, prostate cancer is high on the differential diagnosis list. If the diagnosis is established or highly suspected, then the following should be considered prior to the initiation of endocrine therapy.

Consumption Coagulopathies

The presence of disseminated malignancies can lead to a situation where clotting and coagulation factors are being consumed faster than they can be produced.[98] While not definitely established, it is likely that metastatic prostate cancer in the bone marrow leads to the release/production of a circulation procoagulant that initiates the clotting cascade. There are marked variations in the degree of this consumption. In some patients it can be overwhelming, with clinical bleeding and associated laboratory abnormalities of low platelet counts, high protimes and partial thromboplastin times, low fibrinogens, high fibrin monomers, and high fibrinopeptide A levels. On the other end of the spectrum, patients may have only mild abnormalities of one of these commonly used laboratory tests to document consumption coagulopathies.

The only proven successful long-term therapy for cancer-related consumption coagulopathies is treatment of the underlying malignancy. In prostate cancer, that poses a dilemma.[99–102] Performing an orchiectomy results in an immediate lowering of serum testosterone, a highly desirable result, but entails a surgical procedure. Any surgery, even minor surgery, should be avoided if possible in a patient with a consumptive coagulopathy. The use of LHRH agonists is associated with an initial increase in LH/FSH and testosterone before the onset of testicular suppression.[103] During this time, symptoms can increase and a consumption process could theoretically be exacerbated. Additive estrogen therapy has more rapid onset of action, but estrogens can theoretically adversely alter coagulation and hence their use is probably not ideal.

At present, such clinical situations are probably best handled by the initiation of therapy with ketoconazole.[104,105] Ketoconazole, 400 mg orally every 8 hours, as discussed above, inhibits steroidal synthesis both by the testes and the adrenals and has a rapid onset of action. There is a small published experience with the use of ketoconazole in the presence of a consumptive coagulopathy and hence this drug is probably the treatment of choice.[104,105]

Epidural Spinal Cord Compression

Another clinical scenario is a man with known prostate cancer or with a suspicious digital rectal exam who presents with a neurologic deficit consistent with a spinal cord lesion. If the neurologic deficit is secondary to prostate cancer metastatic to the spine, and causing epidural spinal cord compression, bone radiographs of the spine are usually abnormal, showing collapse and/or blastic/lytic lesions. The diagnosis of spinal cord compression can be confirmed by contrast myelography or magnetic resonance imaging (MRI) of the spine.[106–108] The treatment for epidural spinal cord compression secondary to

prostate cancer is either external beam radiotherapy or decompression laminectomy followed by external beam radiotherapy, both in conjunction with hormonal therapy. In a newly presenting patient, emergent prostate biopsy can establish a diagnosis and endocrine therapy plus radiotherapy or laminectomy can be instituted. There is no need to wait for a serum PSA level, although one should be drawn prior to therapy. When selecting a hormonal therapy for patients presenting with or having an impending epidural spinal cord compression, initial therapy with LHRH because of the initial increase in LH/FSH and testosterone prior to suppression might theoretically either exacerbate or complete a cord compression.[103] Orchiectomy is commonly utilized in this situation or, as an alternative, ketoconazole can be used initially, followed by LHRH once androgen production has been suppressed.

Ureteral and Urethral Obstruction

A majority of men presenting with metastatic prostate cancer have symptomatic urethral obstruction and up to 10% have ureteral obstruction.[109,110] Endocrine therapy has been shown to relieve ureteral obstruction in up to 88% of men and 69% of men requiring catheterization resume voiding within six months of the initiation of endocrine therapy.[109–111] The decision as to whether ureteral stenting should be done in men with obstruction should be based on the degree of obstruction and the need to preserve renal function, as ureteral stents can be quite discomforting to patients. Similarly, in men with urethral obstruction the decision as to whether a channel TURP should be performed is best made on an individual-patient basis with a careful assessment of the risk-benefit ratio. The procedure, in general, is well tolerated. The incidence of urinary incontinence after channel TURP for prostate cancer is somewhat higher than with TURP for benign disease, thought to be secondary to external sphincter involvement from locally aggressive cancer. Before the selection of endocrine therapy in these clinical situations, one needs to consider the possibility that LHRH agonist therapy may temporarily worsen ureteral or urethral obstruction prior to the onset of testosterone suppression. In these circumstances, orchiectomy has the highest reported probability of relieving obstruction in the shortest time period.

CONCLUSION

We have addressed a number of controversies that exist in the treatment of men with either locally advanced or metastatic adenocarcinoma of the prostate. Management of these patients can be optimized through a multispecialty approach including urology, medical oncology, and radiation oncology. There are a number of ongoing clinical studies that will help resolve some of the clinical dilemmas we face so frequently in these men. Hopefully, within the next several years, many of the uncertainties will be clarified by other scientific studies.

REFERENCES

1. Boring CC, Squires TS, Tong T: Cancer Statistics, 1993. CA Cancer J Clin 43:7–26, 1993.
2. Gutman EB, Sproul EE, Gutman AB: Significance of increased phosphatase activity at the cite of osteoplastic metastases secondary to carcinoma of the prostate gland. Am J Cancer 28:485–495, 1936.
3. Huggins C, Hodges CV: Studies on prostatic cancer: the effect of castration, of estrogen and of androgen injection on serum phosphatases in metastatic carcinoma of the prostate. Cancer Res 1:293–297, 1941.
4. Hunter J: Observations on Certain Parts of the Animal Oeconomy, 1st ed. London: Biblioteca Osteriana, p 3839, 1786.
5. Matsuo H, Baba Y, Nair RMG, et al.: Structure of the porcine LH and FSH releasing hormone 1: the proposed amino acid sequence. Biochem Biophys Res Comm 43:1334, 1971.
6. Catalona WG: Staging. In Catalona WJ (ed): Prostate Cancer. Orlando: Grune & Stratton, pp 57–83, 1984.
7. Stamey TA, Yang N, Hay AR, et al.: Prostate-specific antigen as a serum marker for adenocarcinoma of the prostate. N Engl J Med 317:909–916, 1987.
8. Oesterling JE, Cha DW, Epstein JI: Prostate specific antigen in the preoperative and postoperative evaluation of localized prostatic cancer treated with radical prostatectomy. J Urol 139:766–772, 1988.
9. Huber PR, Schnell Y, Hearing F, et al.: Prostate specific antigen. Experimental and clinical observations. Scan J Urol Nephrol 104:33–39, 1987.
10. Oesterling JE: Prostate-specific antigen: a valuable clinical tool. Oncology 5:107–122, 1991.
11. Pontes JD: Biological markers in prostate cancer. J Urol 130:1037–1042, 1983.
12. Kuriyama M, Wang, MC, Lee CL, et al.: Use of human prostate-specific antigen in monitoring prostate cancer. Cancer Res 41:3874–3876, 1981.
13. Ferro MA, Barnes I, Roberts JBM: Tumor markers in prostatic carcinoma. A comparison of prostate-specific antigen with acid phosphatase. Br J Urol 60:69–73, 1987.
14. Lange PH, Ercole CJ, Vessela RL: Tumor markers in the follow-up of initial therapy of prostate cancer. In Lange PH (ed): Tumor Markers in Prostate Cancer. Princeton: Excerpta Medica, pp 16–23, 1986.
15. Russell KJ, Dunatov C, Hafermann MD, et al.: Prostate specific antigen in the management of patients with localized adenocarcinoma of the prostate treated with primary radiation therapy. J Urol 146:1046–1052, 1991.
16. Ritter MA, Messing EM, Shanahan TG, et al.: Prostate-specific antigen as a predictor of radiotherapy response and patterns of failure in localized prostate cancer. J Clin Oncol 10:1208–1217, 1992.
17. Pontes JE, Montie J, Klein E, Huben R: Salvage surgery for radiation failure in prostate cancer. Cancer 71:976–80, 1993.
18. Emmett JL, Greene LF, Papantoniou A: Endocrine therapy in carcinoma of the prostate gland: 10-year survival studies. J Urol 83:471–484, 1960.
19. Nesbit RM, Baum WC: Endocrine control of

prostatic carcinoma. JAMA 143:1317–1320, 1950.

20. Byar DP: The Veterans Administration Cooperative Urological Research Group's studies of cancer of the prostate. Cancer 32:1126–1130, 1973.

21. Hurst KS, Byar DP: An analysis of the effects of changes from the assigned treatment in a clinical trial of treatment for prostatic cancer. J Chron Dis 26:311–324, 1973.

22. Zincke H, Bergstralh EJ, Larson-Keller JL, et al.: Stage D1 prostate cancer treated by radical prostatectomy and adjuvant hormonal treatment. Cancer 70:311–323, 1992.

23. McLeod DG, Crawford ED, Blumenstein BA, et al.: Controversies in the treatment of metastatic prostate cancer. Cancer 70:324–328, 1992.

24. Herr HW, Kornblith AB, Ofman U: A comparison of the quality of life of patients with metastatic prostate cancer who received or did not receive hormonal therapy. Cancer 71:1143–50, 1993.

25. Kozlowski JM, Grayhack JT: Carcinoma of the prostate. In Gillenwater JY, Grayhack JT, Howards SS, et al. (eds): Adult and Pediatric Urology, 2nd ed. Chicago: Year Book Medical Publishers (in press).

26. Schroder FH: Early versus delayed endocrine treatment in metastatic prostatic cancer. In Murphy GP, Khoury S (eds): Therapeutic Progress in Urological Cancers: Proceedings of an International Symposium Held in Paris, France, June 29–July 1, 1988. New York: Alan R. Liss, p 253, 1989.

27. Gleason DF, Mellinger GT: The VACURG: prediction of prognosis for prostate adenocarcinoma by combined histological grading and clinical staging. J Urol 111:58–64, 1974.

28. Soloway MS: The importance of prognostic factors in advanced prostate cancer. Cancer 66:1017–1021, 1990.

29. McCrea LE, Karafin L: Carcinoma of the prostate: metastases, therapy and survival. A statistical analysis of 500 cases. Int Coll Surg J 29:723–728, 1958.

30. Kreis W, Ahmann FR, Lesser M, Scott M, Caplan R, Gau R, Vinciguerra V: Predictive initial parameters for response of stage D prostate cancer to treatment with LHRH agonist goserelin. J Clin Oncol 8:870–874, 1990.

31. Harper ME, Pierrepoint CG, Griffiths K: Carcinoma of the prostate: relationship of pretreatment hormone levels to survival. Eur J Cancer Clin Oncol 20:477–282, 1984.

32. Miller J, Ahmann F, Emerson S, Drach G, Bottauni M: The clinical usefulness of serum PSA following hormonal therapy of stage D-2 prostate cancer. J Urol 147:956–961, 1992.

33. Bailar JC, Byar DP, The Veterans Administration Cooperative Urological Research Group: Estrogen treatment for cancer of the prostate: early results with 3 doses of diethylstilbestrol and placebo. Cancer 26:257–261, 1970.

34. Beck PH, McAninch JW, Goebel JL, Stutzman RE: Plasma testosterone in patients receiving diethylstilbestrol. Urology 11:157–160, 1978.

35. Blackard CE, Doe RP, Mellinger GT, Byar DP: Incidence of cardiovascular disease and death in patients receiving diethylstilbestrol for carcinoma of the prostate. Cancer 26:249–256, 1970.

36. Schally AV, Comaru-Schally AM: Use of luteinizing hormone-releasing hormone analogs in the treatment of hormone-dependent tumors. Sem Reprod Endocrin 5:389–398, 1987.

37. Corbin A: From contraception to cancer: a review of the therapeutic applications of LH-RH analogs as antitumor agents. Yale J Biol Med 55:27–47, 1982.

38. Rajfer J, Handelsman DJ, Crum A, Steiner B, Peterson M, Swerdloff RS: Comparison of the efficacy of subcutaneous and nasal spray Buserlin treatment in suppression of testicular steroidogenesis in men with prostate cancer. Fertil Steril 46:104–110, 1986.

39. Sharifi R, Soloway M, The Leuprolide Study Group: Clinical study of leuprolide depot formulation in the treatment of advanced prostate cancer. J Urol 143:68–71, 1990.

40. Turkes AO, Peeling WB, Griffiths K: Treatment of patients with advanced cancer of the prostate: phase III trial, Zoladex against castration: a study of the British Prostate Group. J Steroid Biochem 27:543–549, 1987.

41. Tolis G, Ackman A, Stellos A, et al.: Tumor growth inhibition in patients with prostatic carcinoma treated with luteinizing hormone-releasing hormone agonists. Proc Natl Acad Sci USA 79:1658–1662, 1982.

42. Labrie F, Dupont A, Belanger A, et al.: New approach in the treatment of prostate cancer: complete instead of only partial removal of androgens. Prostate 4:579–594, 1983.

43. Labrie F, Dupont A, Belanger A, et al.: New hormonal treatment in cancer of the prostate: combined administration of an LHRH agonist and an antiandrogen. J Steroid Biochem 19:999–1007, 1983.

44. Comaru-Schally AM, Ramalho A, Leitao PR,

Schally AV: Clearance of lung metastases of prostate carcinoma after treatment with LH-RH agonist. Lancet 2:281–282, 1984.

45. Borgmann V, Nagel R, Al-Abadi H, Schmidt-Gollwitzer M: Treatment of prostatic cancer with LH-RH analogs. Prostate 99:553–568, 1983.

46. Mathe G, VoVan ML, Duchier J, et al.: An oriented phase-II trial of D-Trp-6-LH-RH in patients with prostatic carcinoma. Med Oncol Tumor Pharmacother 1:119–122, 1984.

47. Waxman JH, Wass JAH, Hendry WF, et al.: Treatment with gonadotrophin releasing hormone analog in advanced prostatic cancer. Br Med J 286:1309–1312, 1983.

48. Walker KJ, Nicholson RI, Turkes AO, et al.: Therapeutic potential of the LHRh agonist, ICI 118630, in the treatment of advanced prostatic carcinoma. Lancet 2:413–415, 1983.

49. Ahmed SR, Brooman PJC, Shalmet SM, et al.: Treatment of advanced prostatic cancer with LHRH analog ICI 118630: clinical response and hormonal mechanisms. Lancet 2:415–418, 1983.

50. Allen JM, O'Shea JP, Mashiter K, et al.: Advanced carcinoma of the prostate: treatment with a gonadotrophin releasing hormone agonist. Br Med J 286:1607–1609, 1983.

51. Gonzalez-Barcena D, Perez-Sanchez P, Ureta-Sanchez S, et al.: Treatment of advanced prostatic carcinoma with D-Trp-6-LH-RH. Prostate 7:21–30, 1985.

52. Koutsilieris M, Tolis G: Gonadotropin releasing hormone agonistic analogs in the treatment of advanced prostatic carcinoma. Prostate 4:569–577, 1983.

53. The Leuprolide Study Group: Leuprolide versus diethylstil-bestrol for metastatic prostate cancer. N Engl J Med 311:1281–1286, 1984.

54. Crawford ED, Blumenstein BA, Goodman PJ, et al.: Leuprolide with and without flutamide in advanced prostate cancer. Cancer 66:1039–1044, 1990.

55. Denis LJ, Whelan P, DeMoura JLC, Newling D, Bono A, DePauw M, Sylvester R: Goserelin acetate and flutamide versus bilateral orchiectomy: a Phase III EORTC Trial (30853). Urology 42:119–129, 1993.

56. Labrie F, Dupont A, Belanger R, et al.: Treatment of prostate cancer with gonadotropin-releasing hormone agonists. Endo Rev 7:67–74, 1986.

57. Beland G, Elhilali M, Fradet, et al.: Total androgen ablation: Canadian experience. Urol Clin North Am 18:75–82, 1991.

58. Iversen P, Christensen MG, Friis E, et al.: A phase III trial of zoladex and flutamide versus orchiectomy in the treatment of patients with advanced carcinoma of the prostate. Cancer 66:1058–1066, 1990.

59. Bertagna C, The International Anandron Study Group: Treatment of metastatic prostate cancer with orchiectomy and Anandron (nilutamide): results of a double-blind study versus orchiectomy and placebo (Abstr). Gynecol Endocrinol 4(Suppl 2):82, 1990.

60. Tyrrell CJ, Altwein JE, Klippel F, Varenhorst E, Lunglmayr G, Boccardo F, Holdaway IM, Haefliger JM, Jordaan JP, Sotarauta M: A multicenter randomized trial comparing the luteinizing hormone-releasing hormone analogue goserelin acetate alone and with flutamide in the treatment of advanced prostate cancer. J Urol 146:1321–1325, 1991.

61. Boccardo F, Pace M, Rubagotti A, Guarneri D, Decensi A, Oneto F, Martorana G, Guiliani L, Selvaggi F, Battaglio M, Delli Ponti U, Petracco S, Cortellini P, Ziveri M, Farraris V, Bruttini GB, Epis R, Comeri G, Gallo G: Goserelin acetate with or without flutamide in the treatment of patients with locally advanced or metastatic prostate cancer. Eur J Cancer 29A:1088–1093, 1993.

62. Boccardo F: Treatment of prostate cancer with LH-RH analogues alone or in combination with pure antiandrogens (Abstr). Gynecol Endocrinol 4(Suppl 2):81, 1990.

63. Denis L, Mettlin C: Conclusions. Cancer 66:1086–1089, 1990.

64. Crombie C, Raghavan D, Page J, et al.: Phase II study of megestrol acetate for metastatic carcinoma of the prostate. Br J Urol 59:443–446, 1987.

65. Geller J, Albert J, Yen SSC: Treatment of advanced cancer of prostate with megestrol acetate. Urology 12:537–541, 1978.

66. Pavone-Macaluso M, de Voogt HJ, Viggiano G, et al.: Comparison of diethylstilbestrol, cyproterone acetate and medroxyprogesterone acetate in the treatment of advanced prostatic cancer: final analysis of a randomized phase III trial of the European organization for research on treatment of cancer urological group. J Urol 136:624–631, 1986.

67. Geller J, Albert J, Yen SSC, et al.: Medical castration of males with megestrol acetate and small doses of diethylstilbestrol. J Clin Endocr Metab 52:576, 1981.

68. Tunn UW, Graff J, Senge TH: Treatment of inoperable prostatic cancer with cyproterone acetate. In Schroder FH (ed): Androgens and

Anti-androgens. Weesp, The Netherlands: Schering Nederland VB, pp 149–159, 1983.

69. Geller J, Albert J, Yen SSC, et al.: Medical castration of males with megestrol acetate and small doses of diethylstilbestrol. J Clin Endocr Metab 52:576–580, 1981.

70. Goldenberg SL, Bruchovsky N, Rennie PS, et al.: The combination of cyproterone acetate and low dose diethylstilbestrol in the treatment of advanced prostatic carcinoma. J Urol 140:1460–1465, 1988.

71. Sinha AA, Blackard CE, Doe RP, Seal US: The in vitro localization of H_3 estradiol in human prostatic carcinoma: an electron microscopic autoradiographic study. Cancer 31:682, 1973.

72. Tew KD, Stearns ME: Hormone-independent, non-alkylating mechanism of cytotoxicity for estramustine. Urol Res 15:155–160, 1987.

73. Fossa SD, Miller A: Treatment of advanced carcinoma of the prostate with estramustine phosphate. J Urol 115:406–408, 1976.

74. Jonsson G, Hogberg K: Treatment of advanced prostatic carcinoma with estracyt: a preliminary report. Scan J Urol Nephrol 5:103, 1971.

75. Ojasoo T, Raynund JP: Unique steroid congeners for receptor studies. Cancer Res 34:4186–4198, 1978.

76. Neumann F, Jacobi GH: Antiandrogens in tumor therapy. Clin Oncol 1:41–66, 1982.

77. Peets E, Henson F, Neri R, Tabachnick I: Effects of nonsteroidal antiandrogen SCH 13521 on testosterone disposition in rats. Fed Proc 32:759, 1973.

78. Varkarakis MJ, Kirdani RY, Yamanaka H, et al.: Prostatic effects of a nonsteroidal antiandrogen. Invest Urol 12:275–284, 1975.

79. Ojasoo T: Nilutamide. Drugs of the Future 12:763–770, 1987.

80. Neri RO, Florance K, Koziol P, VanCleave S: A biological profile of a non-steroidal antiandrogen, SCH-13521 (4'-nitro-3'-trifluoromethyl-isobutyranilde). Endocrinology 91:427–437, 1972.

81. Neri RO, Monahan M: Effects of novel non-steroidal antiandrogen on canine prostatic hyperplasia. Invest Urol 10:123–130, 1972.

82. Crawford ED, Eisenberger MA, McLeod DG, et al.: A controlled trial of leuprolide with and without flutamide in prostatic carcinoma. N Engl J Med 321:419–424, 1989.

83. MacFarlane JR, Tolley DA: Flutamide therapy for advanced prostatic cancer: a phase II study. Br J Urol 57:172–174, 1985.

84. Prout GR, Keating MA, Griffin PP, et al.: Long-term experience with flutamide in patients with prostatic carcinoma. Urology 34(Suppl):37–45, 1989.

85. Sogani PC, Vagaiwala MR, Whitmore WF: Experience with flutamide in patients with advanced prostatic cancer without prior endocrine therapy. Cancer 54:744–750, 1984.

86. Pont A, Williams PL, Azhar S, et al.: Ketoconazole blocks testosterone synthesis. Arch Intern Med 142:2137, 1982.

87. Santen RJ, Van den Bossche H, Symoens J, et al.: Site of action of low dose ketoconazole on androgen biosynthesis in men. J Clin Endocr Metab 57:732, 1983.

88. Pont A: Long-term experience with high dose ketoconazole therapy in patients with stage D2 prostatic carcinoma. J Urol 137:902–904, 1987.

89. Trachtenberg J: Ketoconazole therapy in advanced prostatic cancer. J Urol 132:61–63, 1984.

90. Mahler C, Verhelst J, Denis L: Ketoconazole and liarozole in the treatment of advanced prostatic cancer. Cancer 71:1068–1073, 1993.

91. Glick JH, Wein A, Padavic K, et al.: Phase II trial of tamoxifen in metastatic carcinoma of the prostate. Cancer 49:1367–1372, 1982.

92. Slack NH, Murphy GD, NPCP Participants: Criteria for evaluating patient responses to treatment modalities for prostatic cancer. Urol Clin North Am 11:337–342, 1984.

93. Newling DWW: Criteria of response to treatment in advanced prostatic cancer. In Furr JA, Denis L (eds): Prostatic Cancer: Bailliere's Clinical Oncology, vol 2. London: Bailliere Tindall, pp 505–520, 1988.

94. Yagoda A, Petrylak D: Cytotoxic chemotherapy for advanced hormone-resistant prostate cancer. Cancer 71:1098–1109, 1993.

95. Smith PH, Bono A, da Silva FC, et al.: Some limitations of the radioisotope bone scan in patients with metastatic prostatic cancer: a subanalysis of EORTC Trial 30853. Cancer 66:1009–1016, 1990.

96. Cooper EH, Armitage TG, Robinson MRG, et al.: Prostatic specific antigen and the prediction of prognosis in metastatic prostatic cancer. Cancer 66:1025–1028, 1990.

97. Stamey TA, Kabalin JN, Ferrai M, et al.: Prostate specific antigen in the diagnosis and treatment of adenocarcinoma of the prostate:

IV anti-androgen treated patients. J Urol 141:1088–1090, 1989.

98. Rickles RF, Edwards RL: Activation of blood coagulation in cancer: Trousseau's Syndrome revisited. Blood 62:14–31, 1983.

99. Dobbs RM, Barber JA, Weigel JW, Bergin JE: Clotting predisposition in carcinoma of the prostate. J Urol 123:706–709, 1980.

100. Grignon D, Turnbull DI, Lohmann RC: Carcinoma of the prostate presenting as acute disseminated intravascular coagulation. Can Med Assoc J 135:775–775, 1986.

101. Samaha RJ, Bruns TNC, Ross Jr GJ: Chronic intravascular coagulation in metastatic prostate cancer. Arch Surg 106:295–298, 1973.

102. Ross G, Thompson IM, Samaha RJ: Subacute intravascular coagulation with prostatic carcinoma. Missouri Med 71:177–179, 1974.

103. Waxman J, Man A, Hendry WF, et al.: Short reports: Importance of early tumour exacerbation in patients treated with long acting analogues of gonadotrophin releasing hormone for advanced prostatic cancer. Br Med J 291:1386–1387, 1985.

104. Litt MR, Bell WR, Lepor HA: Disseminated intravascular coagulation in prostatic carcinoma reversed by ketoconazole. JAMA 258:1361–1362, 1987.

105. Lowe FC, Somers WJ: The use of ketoconazole in the emergency management of disseminated intravascular coagulation due to metastatic prostatic cancer. J Urol 137:1000–1002, 1986.

106. Liskow A, Chang CH, DeSanctis P, et al.: Epidural cord compression in association with genitourinary neoplasms. Cancer 58:949–954, 1986.

107. Rodichok LD, Harper GR, Ruckdeschel JC, et al.: Early diagnosis of spinal epidural metastases. Am J Med 70:1181–1188, 1981.

108. Ruff RL, Lanska DJ: Epidural metastases in prospectively evaluated veterans with cancer and back pain. Cancer 63:2234–2241, 1989.

109. Michigan S, Catalona WJ: Ureteral obstruction from prostatic carcinoma: response to endocrine and radiation therapy. J Urol 118:733–738, 1977.

110. Varenhorst E, Alund G: Urethral obstruction secondary to carcinoma of prostate: response to endocrine treatment. Urology 25:354–356, 1985.

111. Fleischmann JD, Catalona WJ: Endocrine therapy for bladder outlet obstruction from carcinoma of the prostate. J Urol 134(3):498–500, 1985.

112. Chodak GW, Vogelzang NJ, Caplan RJ, Soloway M, Smith JA: Independent prognostic factors in patients with metastatic (Stage D-2) prostate cancer. JAMA 265:618–621, 1991.

113. Sharifi R, Chodak G, Venner P, Block S, Callahan-Squire M, Jones J: Casodex versus castration in treatment of Stage D2 prostate cancer: Prostate specific antigen (PSA) as a measure of outcome. Proc ASCO 12:241, 1993.

114. Catalona WG: Endocrine therapy. In Catalona WJ (ed): Prostate Cancer. Orlando: Grune & Stratton, pp 145–171, 1984.

115. Pontes JE, Karr JP, Kirdani RY, Murphy GP, Sandberg AA: Estrogen receptors and clinical correlations with human prostatic disease. Urology 4:399–403, 1982.

15

Recent Therapeutic Advances in "Hormone-Refractory" Metastatic Prostate Cancer: Flutamide Withdrawal, Estramustine Plus Vinblastine, Estramustine Plus Etoposide, and Suramin

Nancy A. Dawson, M.D., Ken Kobayashi, M.D.,
and Nicholas J. Vogelzang, M.D.

INTRODUCTION

Approximately 70% of all men diagnosed with prostate cancer will have metastatic disease at some time in the course of their illness.[1] Standard hormonal therapy for newly diagnosed metastatic disease is reviewed in Chapter 14. Unfortunately, virtually all men will eventually progress, with median time to progression of 12 to 18 months.[2] When metastatic prostate cancer progresses after initial hormonal therapy, it is termed "hormone-refractory." This term may be a misnomer, since many of these patients respond to subsequent hormonal manipulations. A more accurate term may be progressive or failed metastatic prostate cancer, yet "hormone-refractory" is in common use and is retained in this review as well.

Hormone-refractory metastatic prostate cancer is currently not curable. Therapeutic intervention has been predominantly aimed at palliation of symptoms, most commonly bone pain. Subsequent hormonal therapies in common use include high-dose diethylstilbestrol diphosphate, ketoconazole, aminoglutethimide, flutamide, megestrol acetate, prednisone or hydrocortisone, and orchiectomy if the patient has been on diethylstilbestrol or a gonadotropin-releasing hormone (GnRH) analog. These treatments are associated with 15% to 30% response rates, most of which are disease stabilization rather than tumor regression.[3] Single-agent or combination chemotherapy is likewise associated with a low overall objective response rate of 6.5% with 15% disease stabilization. Extensive reviews of the chemotherapy of prostate cancer are available.[4,5] Agents associated with 10% to 15% response rates include low-dose doxorubicin,[6] continuous infusion 5-fluorouracil,[7] daily oral cyclophosphamide,[8] and long-term infusions of mitomycin C[9] and vinblastine.[10] Unfortunately no single chemotherapeutic agent has yet produced a response rate greater than 15%.

In recent years, new therapeutic strategies have emerged that apparently target integral cell structure and function beyond

Prostate Cancer, pages 235–260 © 1994 Wiley-Liss, Inc.

that of the typical chemotherapeutic agent's action on DNA. Three promising new therapeutic interventions that are currently being investigated in progressive metastatic disease are suramin, estramustine combined with vinblastine, and, thirdly, estramustine combined with etoposide. This chapter reviews those therapies. Additionally, the recent observation that withdrawal of flutamide in patients progressing on this hormone may result in tumor regression is initially discussed.

FLUTAMIDE WITHDRAWAL

In response to the recent serendipitous observation that withdrawal of flutamide resulted in a significant prostate-specific antigen (PSA) decline as well as symptomatic improvement,[11] a clinical trial was initiated at Memorial Sloan-Kettering Cancer Center to formally assess this potential therapeutic maneuver.[12] Twenty-five patients who had progressive metastatic prostate cancer on their initial therapy with combined androgen blockade (GnRH analog or orchiectomy plus flutamide) had only the flutamide stopped. Ten of these 25 patients (40%) showed a >50% decline in PSA. In 7 of these 10 patients, the PSA decline was >80%. PSA declines for responders occurred within four weeks of discontinuation of the flutamide and persisted for 2 to 10 or more months (median 5+ months). A reduction in PSA of greater than 50% is correlated with a significant improvement in overall survival compared to those in whom the PSA does not decline by 50%.[13] An additional 11 patients who were initially treated with monohormonal therapy (GnRH analog or orchiectomy followed by flutamide at relapse, flutamide followed by a GnRH analog, or diethylstilbestrol followed by combined androgen blockade) had their flutamide selectively

discontinued at time of tumor progression. None of these patients responded to flutamide withdrawal. Duration of flutamide therapy, extent of disease, and baseline PSA were not significantly different between responders and nonresponders in this cohort of patients.

An independent trial was simultaneously initiated at the National Cancer Institute that combined flutamide withdrawal plus aminoglutethimide and hydrocortisone.[14] This study was also prompted by the dramatic response to this therapeutic maneuver in a single patient. Subsequently 29 men who had progressive metastatic disease were treated with simultaneous withdrawal of flutamide, aminoglutethimide 250 mg orally four times per day, and hydrocortisone 30 mg orally daily. All patients had been heavily pretreated and entered the study on replacement doses of hydrocortisone, which had been prescribed to prevent prior suramin-induced adrenal insufficiency. All patients had castrate levels of testosterone. All patients who had not been surgically castrated were maintained on a GnRH analog. Fourteen of 29 patients (48%) had a >80% decline in PSA that persisted for more than 4 weeks. Predictors of response included a longer duration of flutamide treatment prior to withdrawal (median 26.5 months), a higher initial PSA, and the absence of soft tissue disease. Median response duration was 32 weeks.

In a third clinical trial, Dupont and colleagues at Laval University reported on 40 men with progressive disease following combination therapy in whom flutamide was withdrawn.[15] Twenty-nine of these patients were also being treated with aminoglutethimide and hydrocortisone. Patients were continued on their primary testicular androgen blockade as well as their aminoglutethimide and hydrocortisone. Using the response criteria of the National Prostatic Cancer Project (NPCP),[16] there were one complete, three partial, and 26 stable responses, for an overall response rate of 75%. Using decline in PSA as an endpoint, 32 patients (80%) had a >50% decline, 20 patients (50%) had a >90% decline, and 17 patients (42%) had their PSA return to normal. Three of the patients reported in this study as nonresponders based on NPCP criteria had a PSA decline of >50%. Neither the duration of prior combination therapy nor prior treatment with aminoglutethimide and hydrocortisone impacted on response to flutamide withdrawal. The mean response duration was 14.4 months and the median duration was 11.9 months. Serum concentrations of testosterone-binding globulin increased after flutamide withdrawal. Levels of testicular and adrenal androgens and their main metabolites did not change.

Flutamide is a nonsteroidal antiandrogen. The response to flutamide withdrawal may be explained by the presence of a mutant androgen receptor that recognizes flutamide as an androgen agonist or by the emergence of an androgen-hypersensitive clone of cells or by the unmasking of the agonistic properties of flutamide. In the androgen-responsive human prostate cancer cell line LNCaP, hydroxy-flutamide, the active metabolite of flutamide, demonstrated agonistic properties by stimulating cell growth in vitro.[17] Withdrawal of flutamide may produce secondary tumor regression similar to that reported with tamoxifen withdrawal in patients with breast cancer.[18]

Flutamide withdrawal is a simple, cost-saving, and potentially beneficial therapeutic maneuver and is recommended as a first step in progressive metastatic disease. Previous and future trials in which flutamide is withdrawn simultaneously with initiation of new therapy must be judged cautiously since a flutamide withdrawal response may be misinterpreted as a response to the new treatment.

ESTRAMUSTINE AND VINBLASTINE

Estramustine phosphate (EMP) consists of an estradiol molecule attached to a nor-nitrogen mustard through a carbamate ester linkage. This drug was synthesized in the mid-1960s with the intention of improving the treatment of breast cancer.[19] It was theorized that the steroid component would be taken up by estrogen receptor positive tumors. The cleavage of the carbamate linkage would expose the malignant cells to high intracellular concentrations of cytotoxic nor-nitrogen mustard. However, due to the stability of this linkage, this drug was found to have no significant in vivo alkylating activity.[20] Instead, EMP is rapidly dephosphorylated to its main metabolites, estromustine and estramustine.[21] Only 10% of these metabolites are hydrolyzed to estradiol and estrone, which depress testosterone levels. These steroid metabolites are present in lower concentrations than achieved with standard doses of estrogen used in the treatment of metastatic prostate cancer and are not primarily responsible for the activity of this drug in "hormone-refractory" prostate cancer.[22] EMP cytotoxicity is predominantly attributed to estramustine's ability to bind microtubule-associated proteins (MAP).[23] MAPs are essential to microtubule stability. Estramustine causes microtubules to disassemble as well as prevents their de novo formation, resulting in mitotic arrest during metaphase and cell death. Estramustine preferentially accumulates in prostate cancer apparently due to binding to a "prostatic binding protein" in secretory cells of the ventral prostate.[24] It also binds at the nuclear protein matrix.[25] The relationship between binding to these two sites, to MAP's and tumor response, is presently unknown. In one study, prostate biopsies from men who had been treated chronically with estramustine phosphate showed concentrations of estramustine on an average six times higher than plasma concentrations.[26] In the human prostate cancer cell line DU 145, a relatively hormone-unresponsive cell line, estramustine has been shown to inhibit cell growth and clonogenic survival.[27] In 19 phase II clinical trials (650 patients) assessing EMP as second-line therapy, there was an overall 30% to 35% objective response rate, 15% were in the stable disease category, and 15% to 20% were in the objective response category. The overall subjective response rate was 60%.[28]

Vinblastine is a vinca alkaloid whose cytotoxicity is also attributable to microtubule inhibition, but acts by binding to the beta subunit of the tubulin monomer, a distinctly separate microtubular target. Vinblastine as a single agent has not been extensively evaluated in prostate cancer. In one trial of 39 patients with refractory metastatic prostate cancer, a 21% objective response rate was obtained with continuous infusion vinblastine at a dose of 1.5 mg/m^2 daily for five days, repeated every 3–4 weeks.[10] The median response duration was 28 weeks.

Due to the distinctly unique mechanisms of these two microtubule inhibitors, a potentially synergistic effect was suggested by Tew and Stearns.[23] In vitro studies using the DU 145 human prostatic cell line demonstrated additive (but not synergistic) antimitotic activity for the combination.[29] Additionally, these drugs were demonstrated to have different mechanisms of resistance.[30] In three recent clinical trials involving 82 patients, objective responses (defined as a greater than 50% decline in PSA), were achieved in 35 patients (43%).[31–33] Six of 19 (32%) patients with bidimensionally measurable disease achieved a partial response, defined as a greater than or equal to 50% decrease in the summed products of two or more diameters of all measurable soft tissue lesions. Vinblastine was usually given as a weekly intravenous bolus of 4 mg/m^2 for six consecutive weeks in combination with EMP 10–15 mg/kg/day taken orally on days 1–42. Therapy was repeated after a two-week break if toxicity was acceptable and there was no disease progression. Toxicity was predominantly attributable to the estramustine, which causes cardiovascular toxicity, predominantly arterial and venous thrombosis in 10% of patients. Mild nausea was the most common non-hematologic toxicity reported in 25–50% of patients. The addition of vinblastine did not add significant toxicity. An overall response rate of 43%, based on a greater than 50% PSA decline, probably indicates superior therapeutic benefit for this combination compared to EMP alone. No randomized trials have compared EMP to EMP plus vinblastine.

ESTRAMUSTINE AND ETOPOSIDE

Etoposide is a topoisomerase II inhibitor that inhibits DNA replication selectively at the level of the nuclear matrix.[34] In vitro, etoposide has shown activity against Dunning R3327H prostatic adenocarcinoma[35] and PC-3, a hormone-resistant cell line of prostate cancer.[36] However, in phase II clinical trials, in advanced prostate cancer, results were disappointing with single agent etoposide. Scher reported only one partial response (5%) in 20 adequately treated patients with bidimensionally measurable disease.[36] Treatment consisted of 80–100 mg/M^2 intravenously on days 1, 2, and 3, repeated every 21–28 days. Trump reported similar inactivity using a continuous infusion schedule of 50 mg/M^2 over 24 hours for five days.[37] No responses were seen in 19 adequately treated patients.

Etoposide combined with EMP has been evaluated in vitro and in vivo for synergistic activity. In vitro, etoposide and EMP appear to act synergistically to inhibit cell growth and viability in the human metastatic adenocarcinoma cell line, PC-3, and in metastatic MAT-LyLu (MLL) subline of the Dunning R3327 rat prostatic adenocarcinoma cell line.[38] Using a nascent DNA synthesis assay, in vitro, EMP enhances the ability of etoposide to inhibit DNA synthesis at the level of the nuclear matrix.[38] In vivo, the combination of EMP and etoposide significantly inhibited tumor growth in Copenhagen rats injected subcutaneously with MLL cells compared with etoposide alone treated animals.[38] Etoposide alone inhibited tumor growth by 50% compared to controls ($P < .05$), whereas EMP alone did not significantly inhibit cell growth. These encouraging preclinical results were the basis of a phase I/II clinical trial.[39] Twenty patients with refractory prostate cancer were treated with EMP 15 mg/kg/day and etoposide 50 mg/M²/day, both taken orally for 21 days every 28 days. Fifteen patients were evaluable at time of first report. For the nine patients with measurable disease, six patients achieved a partial response and three patients had stable disease. Of six patients with evaluable only disease, two patients had a partial response, three patients had stable disease, and one patient had progressive disease. Toxicity consisted of mild to moderate nausea, granulocytopenia, and anemia. All patients had alopecia. Median duration of response had not been determined at time of report. No confirmatory trials of this combination have yet been reported.

SURAMIN

Suramin (Moranyl, Bayer 205, Germanin, Fourneau 309 Antrypol, Naganol, Naganin, Naphuride Sodium; Fig. 1) is a polysulfonated naphthylurea analog of trypan blue, synthesized in 1916 by Farbenfabriken Bayer AG as part of an effort to combat the sleeping sickness epidemic in German East Africa. It has been used successfully in the therapy and prophylaxis of trypanosomiasis and onchocercia-

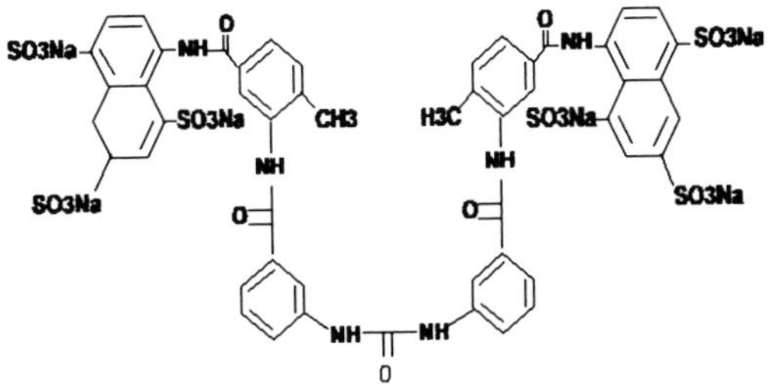

Fig. 1. Chemical structure of suramin.

sis since 1920. In the mid-1980s, it was tested clinically in acquired immunodeficiency syndrome (AIDS) because in vitro activity against reverse transcriptase led to hopes that it would be active against the human immunodeficiency virus. Although no antiretroviral activity of clinical significance was found during these trials, it was noted to cause adrenal insufficiency. A clinical trial in adrenocortical carcinoma was undertaken on the basis of this observation, which demonstrated modest activity. Human cancer clinical trials have since been expanded, with promising activity being noted, most particularly in prostate cancer. Chemically it is the symmetrical 3-urea of the sodium salt of 8-(3-benzamido-4-methyl-benzamido)-naphthalene-1,3,5-trisulfonic acid, is highly sulfonated, and under physiologic conditions carries a high negative charge. These characteristics confer a number of interesting properties on this drug. Although it is postulated to act by interruption of autocrine growth loops, suramin is known to have several cellular effects (Table 1) and the specific mechanism(s) by which suramin exerts its antitumor effects are not known with certainty.

Suramin and Glycosaminoglycan Metabolism

Glycosaminoglycans are polyanionic substances made up of repeating disaccharide units that, like suramin, are polysulfonated and possess a greater negative charge-density than most other molecules

TABLE 1. Biologic Effects and Possible Mechanisms of Action of Suramin

- Interference with glycosaminoglycan metabolism
- Growth factor inhibition
    Transforming growth factor α
    Transforming growth factor β
    Insulin-like growth factor I
    Insulin-like growth factor II
    Bombesin
    Platelet-derived growth factor
    Colorectum-derived growth factor
    Epidermal growth factor
    Basic fibroblast growth factor
    Interleukin 2
- Inhibition of intracellular enzymes
    DNA polymerase α
    Topoisomerase II
- Disruption of cell motility and adhesion
- Disruption of mitochondrial energy balance
- Induction of differentiation
    Human colon adenocarcinoma
    Human promyelocytic leukemia
    Human neuroblastoma
    Rat glioma
- Interference with P_{2x} and P_{2y} purinergic signal transduction
- Immune system effects
    Interference with the delayed-type hypersensitivity reaction
    Impairment of T helper cell function

found in the body. They are covalently bound to proteins in most mammalian tissues, and may occur either attached to cell surfaces or as components of the extracellular matrix. They are involved in cell proliferation, regulation, and cytodifferentiation,[40] and there is evidence that abnormal proteoglycan production by neoplastic cells may alter the extracellular matrix, facilitating tumor growth and/or metastasis.

Suramin damages lysosomal membranes[41] and inhibits several lysosomal enzymes involved in glycosaminoglycan catabolism in vitro.[42,43] At doses equivalent to 10–20 gm/m², it produces hepatic, renal, and smooth muscle changes consistent with mucopolysaccharidosis in animal experiments[44–46] and a sixfold increase in urinary heparan sulfate and dermatan sulfate excretion.[47] This activity has been used to develop preclinical animal models of sphingolipidoses and of lysosomal storage diseases (e.g., Hunter's, Hurler's, and Tay-Sachs diseases), conditions in which abnormal deposition of glycosaminoglycans in various organs and tissues leads to impaired organ function and neurologic abnormalities.

Given the neurotoxicity of suramin (discussed below), it is intriguing that in rat sympathetic neurons and dorsal root ganglion Schwann cells this inhibition of lysosomal enzymes leads to the accumulation of fluorescent inclusion bodies and other pigmented bodies.[48] Tyrosine hydroxylase, an enzyme involved in the synthesis of norepinephrine, also shows decreased immunoreactivity in superior cervical ganglion cells, possibly indicating depletion of these stores.

As is discussed later, the inhibition of glycosaminoglycan metabolism is directly responsible for some of suramin's side effects and may also mediate some of its therapeutic effects. Heparan sulfates isolated from the urine of patients following intravenous administration are cytotoxic to human adrenal and prostate carcinoma cells in vitro and block the stimulatory effects of several growth factors on these cells.[49] It is also possible that heparan sulfate may have a role in regulating nuclear activity; if this hypothesis is correct, then suramin could exert its effect by perturbing glycosaminoglycan metabolism.[50]

Growth Factor Inhibition

The original concept of autocrine growth loops held that malignant transformation occurs by production of endogenous polypeptide growth factors, which in turn act upon the same cells that produced them by interacting with cell surface receptors. For growth factors that are capable of stimulating growth, this series of steps results in a positive feedback loop leading to further cell proliferation,[51] but this hypothesis has recently been modified to allow for negative growth factors (such as TGF-β) that inhibit the growth of malignant cells. Much laboratory evidence has accumulated to show that suramin is capable of interfering with the binding of growth factors to their receptors and thus interrupting the autocrine growth loop.[52–57]

Under the influence of oncogenes, malignant cells may become endogenous producers of polypeptide growth factors, may express more avid growth factor receptors, and/or may have an enhanced postreceptor signal response. The current paradigm of growth factor action holds that after binding to cell surface receptors, the receptor–growth factor complex then alters signal transduction by interacting with GTP-binding proteins, thereby affecting a variety of intracellular events mediated by inositol-1,4,5-triphosphate (ITP), protein kinase C, and phospholipase C. Among the polypeptide growth factors that act in this fashion are transforming growth factors α and β (TGF-α and -β), insulin-like growth factors I and II (IGF-1,2), bombesin, and peptides similar to platelet-derived growth factor (PDGF). Human malignancies with which the autocrine mechanism has been most clearly linked include soft tissue sarcomas,[52–54] astrocytomas, glioma, small-cell lung cancer, head and neck cancer, breast cancer, and squamous carcinoma.

Autocrine growth loop interruption by suramin has been most extensively investigated in systems dependent on PDGF and IGF. Human PDGF is a 30,000 molecular weight serum protein that is a mitogen to connective-tissue-derived cells.[55] The B chain of PDGF is virtually identical to part of the transforming protein v-sis of simian sarcoma virus (SSV), which suggests that a PDGF-like factor mediates transformation. When added to SSV-transformed human fibroblasts, suramin causes a reversible and dose-dependent reversion to the normal phenotype, with complete reversion

at a suramin concentration of 200 μg/ml. Furthermore, although the proliferation of the transformed cells is not inhibited by suramin, their saturation density is reduced to that of nontransformed cells. Suramin can also interfere with the binding of insulin-like growth factor I to its receptor.[52,56] This not only interrupts IGF-I-mediated growth loops but also interrupts an autocrine growth loop involving IGF-I receptor-mediated effects of IGF-II in an embryonal rhabdomyosarcoma line.[57]

The effects of suramin on other growth factors are less well defined. In the non-tumorigenic murine line AKR-2B, suramin interfered with the mitogenic effects and inhibited the binding to these cells of TGF-β, heparin-binding growth factor type-2 (HBGF-2), and epidermal growth factor (EGF).[58] Suramin also inhibits the action of TGF-α on both androgen receptor positive and negative human prostate carcinoma cell lines,[59] and can dissociate colorectum-derived growth factor (CRDGF) from its receptor.[60]

Although suramin is generally considered to be cytostatic, investigators have observed biphasic effects on cell growth in selected instances, with paradoxical stimulation of growth noted in vitro at low concentrations. Individual breast,[61,62] head and neck, bladder, and ovarian carcinoma, large-cell lung cancer, melanoma, osteosarcoma, and glioblastoma cell lines have been observed to exhibit growth in vitro averaging 150% of control when exposed to suramin at concentrations of 50–125 μg/ml.[63,64] Suramin (at 50–500 μg/ml) reversed the activity of the negative growth factor TGF-β in a human renal cell carcinoma model, which in turn allowed cell proliferation,[65] and growth stimulation also occurs in Dunning rat prostate cancer cells at suramin concentrations below 150 μM.[66]

EGF stimulates the growth of many epithelial cells, and the level of expression of its receptor may influence the effects of suramin on any given cell line. This receptor binds both EGF and TGF-α. In an intriguing finding, Cardinali et al. exposed epidermoid squamous carcinoma cells expressing normal amounts of EGF receptor and of TGF-α to suramin under serum-free conditions and observed increased activation of the EGF receptor, increased intracellular tyrosine phosphorylation, and subsequent growth deregulation.[67] However, when they exposed a different epidermoid squamous carcinoma cell line, which constitutively expresses increased amounts of cell surface EGF receptor with normal amounts of TGF-α, to suramin, the cells responded by downregulating the amount of receptor and demonstrating significant growth inhibition. This sequence of events was also accompanied by increased tyrosine phosphorylation, which appears to be the intracellular signal for this event.

Whether or not this growth-stimulatory effect is potentiated by hormonal influences is not clear. In human breast cancer cells, there is no correlation between either estrogen or progesterone receptor status and growth stimulation.[62] However, in primary cultures of cells derived from patients with either normal prostates, benign prostatic hyperplasia, or frank prostate cancer, much lower suramin concentrations (0.14 to 14 μg/ml) are required to stimulate cellular growth than in other cell lines.[68] In the androgen-responsive cell line DDT-1, derived from a Syrian hamster leiomyosarcoma of the ductus deferens, suramin at concentrations of 1.4 to 143 μg/ml stimulated the growth of tumor cells in the presence of testosterone. At higher concentrations or in the absence of testosterone, however, suramin inhibits growth.[69] The implications of these preclinical observations are disquieting, and it is possible that the development of premalignant and malignant skin conditions in patients being treated with suramin (see below) may be a clinical manifestation of this growth-stimulatory phenomenon.

It is clear that suramin has numerous and complex effects on growth regulation. However, doubts regarding the relevance of these effects to suramin's antitumor activity have recently been raised. At in vitro concentrations of albumin approaching that seen in vivo, suramin inhibition of IGF-I-stimulated mitosis was attenuated by 90%, suggesting that this drug may not operate by growth-factor-mediated mechanisms of action in vivo.[70] Furthermore, the autocrine growth factor hypothesis outlined above predicts that inhibition of growth factor binding would lead to decreased tyrosine phosphorylation. However, when certain epidermoid squamous cell and prostate cancer cell lines are exposed to suramin in vitro, an increase in cellular tyrosine phosphorylation is observed.[67,71]

Other Biologic Effects

Although suramin's effects on cell cycle kinetics hold important implications for combined chemoradiotherapy studies, the available information is limited and contradictory. In the androgen-independent prostate cancer cell lines DU 145 and PC-3, suramin increases the fraction of cells in S phase in a dose-dependent fashion up to 300 μg/ml.[72] However, these experiments did not control for the concentration of protein in the ambient medium. When this was done, exposure of PC-3 to similar concentrations of suramin results in redistribution into the G_2/M phases, with no redistribution into the S phase.[73] Exposure of an androgen-responsive cell line, LNCaP, to higher concentrations (1,429 μg/ml) of suramin led to recruitment of cells into the G_0/G_1 phase, with a concomitant decrease in S phase cells.[69] In the human breast cancer cell line MCF-7, exposure to suramin at concentrations ranging from 100 to 5,000 μg/ml in the presence of 10% bovine calf serum led to dose-dependent redistributions in the cell cycle, with accumulation in the G_2/M phase.[74] Human lymphoid tumor[75] and sarcoma cells also accumulate in S phase under the influence of suramin. Flow cytometric analysis of treated osteosarcoma xenografts showed an increase in the S and G_2– M phases following exposure to suramin.[53]

Suramin affects a number of subcellular energy-generating processes, including the H^+-ATPase, oxidative metabolism,[76] and glycolysis.[77] In DU 145, incubation of cells with suramin rapidly uncouples mitochondrial electron transport and ATP generation, resulting in increased oxygen consumption with no increase in ATP generation. This is not reversed by growth factors (including IGF, EGF, and bFGF) and results in loss of the transmembrane potential and progressive toxic mitochondrial changes.[78,79] It is interesting to note that similar pathologic and physiologic parallels exist in the De Toni-Fanconi-Debre syndrome (congenital mitochondrial cytochrome c oxidase deficiency)[80] and in the process of brown fat thermogenesis of hibernating animals and other cold-adapted mammals.[81]

In an interesting series of studies, investigators in France have demonstrated suramin-induced differentiation, as well as growth inhibition, in a human colon adenocarcinoma cell line.[82–84] This probably occurs by blockade of autocrine IGF-I stimulated mechanisms.[85] Similar differentiating effects have been noted in thyroid epithelial cells.[86]

In addition to those enzymes previously discussed, suramin inhibits a variety of enzymes involved in the complement cascade, the coagulation cascade, and DNA synthesis. These include urease, hexokinase, fumarase, succinic dehydrogenase, kallikrein, thrombin, plasmin, and chymotrypsin.[87,88] It both inhibits the binding of low-density lipoprotein (LDL) to its receptor, and dissociates bound LDL,[89–91] and can block iron uptake by interfering with

its binding to transferrin and inhibiting receptor-mediated endocytosis.[92] Inhibition of the mammalian enzymes DNA primase and DNA polymerase-α[93] or of DNA topoisomerase II[94] may be responsible for inhibition of DNA synthesis in human osteogenic sarcoma and rhabdomyosarcoma lines.[95]

Suramin and the Immune System

Suramin appears to produce a clinically significant impairment of the immune response to gram-positive infection, and several instances of gram-positive sepsis in association with indwelling central venous catheters have been observed in the clinical trials reported to date. However, the effects of suramin in vitro on various components of the immune system are contradictory. Suramin has been reported to be selectively lymphocytotoxic[96] and interferes with cell-mediated immunity, as shown by a poor response to *Listeria monocytogenes* and to *Mycobacterium bovis*[97] in a rat model, and by impaired delayed-type hypersensitivity reactions in mice treated with sheep erythrocytes.[98] Such impairment of cell-mediated immunity can be due to either increased suppressor T cell activity[99] or to impaired helper T cell activity. Suramin reversibly decreases the cell surface expression of the CD4 (T helper) antigen, possibly by tyrosine kinase-mediated pathways,[100] and it may also interfere with the binding of interleukin-2 to its receptor.[101] In contrast, other investigators have reported an increase in phagocytic activity of human monocytes in vitro.[102] With regard to effects on neutrophil function, suramin induced a dose-dependent defect in bactericidal activity of polymorphonuclear leukocytes obtained from healthy volunteers against *Staph. aureus*, with some impairment noted at 100 μg/ml and complete disappearance of activity at a concentration of 500 μg/ml. This defect was somewhat overcome by the addition of granulocyte colony-stimulating factor at lower concentration of suramin. No effects on fungicidal activity were noted. Phagocytic activity, but not the oxidative metabolic burst and intracellular killing activity, was also impaired.[103] These findings may reflect impaired binding to the leukocyte cell surface Fc and complement receptors.

Preclinical Antitumor Activity

Suramin is active in vitro against a variety of other growth factor- and/or hormone-responsive malignant human cell lines, including osteogenic sarcoma, rhabdomyosarcoma, rat glioma,[104] a variety of lung cancer and mesothelioma cell lines,[64,105] ovarian and endometrial cancer,[106] and human breast cancer,[107] both estrogen-responsive and -unresponsive.[61,108] In the estrogen receptor-positive line MCF-7, the cytostatic effect occurs by a dose-dependent inhibition of IGF-I and -II, EGF, and E_2-stimulated pathways.[61] Results from work with endoglycosidases produced by both human and murine melanoma cells[109] also suggest that suramin may inhibit these enzymes and reduce the potential for invasiveness and metastasis.

In fresh specimens obtained from 135 patients undergoing initial surgery for ovarian cancer, the median IC-50 of suramin alone in the human tumor cloning assay (HTCA)[110] was 50 µg/ml; 85% of cell lines tested were sensitive at 200 µg/ml, and 57% at 50 µg/ml. Endometrial cancer was the most sensitive, with an extrapolated IC_{50} of 0.625 µg/ml; non-small-cell lung and ovarian cancer lines were also easily inhibited, and a clear dose-response effect was noted. Based on their data, these investigators proposed that clinical trials using suramin should strive to maintain plasma levels in excess of 50 µg/ml. Hepatoma, myeloma, Burkitt's lymphoma, and the HL-60 human leukemia cell lines also exhibit growth inhibition in vitro,[111] and growth of human osteosarcoma,[53] hepatoma,[111] and sarcomatoid renal cell cancer[112] xenografts in nude mice is inhibited when suramin is injected intraperitoneally.

Preclinical Studies of Suramin in Prostate Cancer

Suramin alone is cytostatic for prostate cancer cells, as demonstrated by in vitro culture of cells derived from specimens obtained at the time of radical or open prostatectomy for prostate cancer.[113] In these cells, the IC_{50} was found to be 10 µg/ml, which was not appreciably altered by addition of EGF, insulin, hydrocortisone, pituitary extract, or cholera toxin.

The effect of suramin on prostate cancer cells may be modulated by other hormonal influences. LaRocca et al.[114] evaluated the morphologic and growth-inhibitory effects of suramin both alone and in combination with various growth factors, including testosterone, on LNCaP, DU 145, and PC-3 in vitro. The androgen-sensitive line LNCaP-FGC was more sensitive to suramin alone in the colony formation assay than the androgen-independent lines PC-3 and DU 145, with IC_{50} levels of 230.3, 335.3, and >600 µg/ml, respectively. Suramin inhibits bFGF-stimulated cellular proliferation in both DU 145 and in LNCaP, but at a concentration of 300 µg/ml only partially opposes the growth-stimulatory effects of testosterone on LNCaP cells in steroid-depleted serum, and this effect wanes with time.

Some of the confusion regarding the sensitivities of various prostate cancer cell lines to suramin may be explained by considering the amounts of growth factor receptor that are produced by cells. LNCaP is known to respond to EGF, the synthetic hormone R1881, and androgens, while the cell line DDT-1, mentioned previously, responds to PDGF and bFGF. In the LNCaP line, suramin alone at concentrations of

1,429 µg/ml completely blocks not only cell proliferation but also the stimulatory effects of EGF and R1881. However, in the line DDT-1, suramin alone at one-tenth the dose (143 µg/ml) effectively blocks tumor growth, blocks the effect of testosterone, and significantly inhibits the effects of PDGF and bFGF.[69] This wide variation in sensitivity to suramin may be reflected clinically as well. In another study, suramin mitigated the growth-stimulatory effects of EGF on LNCaP cells by interfering with I^{125}-EGF binding to its receptor in a concentration-dependent fashion, while androgen stimulation of LNCaP cell growth was only incompletely opposed by suramin.[59]

Preclinical Studies of Combination Chemotherapy with Suramin

Synergistic activity has been reported for suramin plus dexamethasone in dexamethasone-sensitive human T-cell lymphoma and myeloma[75] and for suramin with doxorubicin in breast cancer.[115] Suramin does not appear to be synergistic with genistein in human colon cancer.[116] In prostate cancer, synergistic activity of suramin with tumor necrosis factor and doxorubicin has been described,[117] as has synergy between tumor necrosis factor, interferon γ, and suramin.[118]

Early Phase I and II Trials of Suramin

Although by far the greatest activity has been noted in patients with prostate cancer (vide infra), encouraging results have also been observed in patients with adrenocortical cancer,[119,120] non-Hodgkin's lymphoma,[121] renal cell carcinoma, and adult T-cell leukemia/lymphoma. These therapeutic results are not further discussed here, although the toxicity and pharmacokinetic data is reviewed in the following sections.

On the basis of encouraging preclinical data, clinical trials of suramin were eagerly anticipated, yet the selection of the optimal dose and schedule of suramin has been difficult. Early clinical trials used doses and schedules that were adapted from those used in AIDS trials and in the treatment of patients with trypanosomiasis and onchocerciasis. However, early observations of a severe demyelinating polyneuropathy at the National Cancer Institute[122] generated substantial concern, since it appeared to be related to sustained plasma levels of over 300 µg/ml. At the same time, the preclinical data reviewed above suggested that a threshold level of about 200 µg/ml was required in order to obtain therapeutic activity. Thus, suramin was postulated to have a very narrow therapeutic window, and most studies conducted to date have utilized highly sophisticated adaptive control methods to maintain plasma concentrations within this range. Such methods utilize real-time pharmacokinetic drug monitoring with continuous dosage adjustments to maintain plasma levels within the specified limits, and have been successfully applied to the dosing of digoxin, aminoglycoside antibiotics, phenytoin, and methotrexate. However, for a drug with a long elimination half-life and delayed toxic effects such as suramin, adaptive control strategies are very demanding, labor-intensive, and costly for patients. Furthermore, they require expertise that is currently available only in a limited number of centers, thus restricting the availability of treatment with this drug to a selected segment of the population. In general, such effort is best justified when an agent is known to have a narrow therapeutic index, when either the interpatient or intrapatient variability is wide, and when a pharmacodynamic relationship exists between plasma levels and either toxicity or therapeutic benefit.[123] Critical reexamination of suramin's clinical characteristics has shown that these preconditions do not necessarily hold and has led to the conclusion that such efforts are probably unnecessary. Since suramin is expected to be widely administered in the community, it is important to establish the safety and efficacy of alternative schedules for administering this agent, and fixed-dose intermittent infusion schedules are currently being developed.

The first study of suramin administered as a chemotherapeutic agent to patients with cancer began with a dose of 850–1,400 mg/m^2 given as a weekly IV bolus, repeated until a plasma suramin level of 250–300 µg/ml was achieved. After eight patients were entered, the schedule of administration was modified to 350 mg/m^2/d, given by continuous IV infusion until the target serum concentration was reached. Hydrocortisone support (40 mg/d) was initiated following the first trial to overcome the effects of suramin-induced adrenal insufficiency.

Myers et al.[124] reported a 40% partial-response rate among 15 patients with measurable soft tissue disease; of these, three had complete disappearance of all measurable soft tissue disease and three had significant improvement in PSA level. Among 20 other patients with "bone-only" involvement, 75% had either normalization or significant improvement in PSA levels and more than 70% had significant pain relief following treatment. Similar response rates were reported by Armand et al.[125] This experience is typical of the reported studies of suramin in treating hormone-refractory metastatic prostate cancer, with impressive response rates being observed when PSA level and pain level are used to measure outcome.

Eisenberger et al.[126] treated 33 patients with metastatic hormone-refractory prostate cancer using intermittent doses of suramin. Doses were adjusted to achieve steady-state plasma levels of between 150 and 300 mcg/ml. Seventy-seven percent achieved a reduction in PSA level of 50% or more, while 55% achieved a reduction of 75% or more. An overall response rate of 50% in patients with measurable disease

was reported, including one complete and five partial responses. Toxicity was substantial, with seven patients developing neurotoxicity within 3–6 months following termination of treatment, seven patients developing adrenal insufficiency, and a syndrome of malaise, fatigue, and lethargy being the main dose-limiting toxicity in most patients. As in previous reports, a high incidence of skin rash was noted. All patients experienced some reduction in creatinine clearance, although this was usually reversible. Although no pharmacokinetic data was reported, the authors of this study noted that the adaptive control strategy entailed a substantial institutional commitment of time and effort, and recommended a critical evaluation of the need for this methodology. These investigators have published preliminary results of a follow-up trial evaluating a fixed, empiric dosing scheme[127] designed to maintain suramin plasma concentrations between 100 and 300 µg/ml. This schedule employs an initial test dose on day 1, followed by a loading dose and daily infusions for the next five days in decrementally decreasing doses. Subsequent doses are given at gradually increasing time intervals. In the 15 patients treated, the mean peak suramin concentrations were 260 µg/ml, with pretreatment trough levels of 158 µg/ml. No dose-limiting neurotoxicity has been noted, and approximately 36% of patients have experienced a ≥75% decrease in the PSA. Kelly et al.[128] have also derived an empiric dosing schedule in which fixed doses of 750 mg/m^2 are administered on days 1 and 4, with doses of 500 mg/m^2 then being administered subsequently at gradually increasing time intervals. Suramin concentrations were maintained between 150 and 300 µg/ml without neurotoxicity in eight patients. Response data in this group of patients was limited, but encouraging. A contrasting view of suramin's utility is provided by Van Oosterom et al.,[129] who reported on nine patients treated with periodic prolonged infusions of suramin targeted to maintain plasma levels between 130 and 200 μg/ml. Four patients achieved PSA reductions of greater than 50%, and the remaining five were nonresponders. The duration of response was short, lasting only a few weeks, and seven of the nine patients had died of malignancy in a mean follow-up period of nine weeks. Van Rijswijk et al.[130] recently reported their experience with adaptive control regimens for suramin, and concluded that an initial loading dose followed by intermittent weekly infusions could maintain mean serum concentrations between 150 and 300 μg/ml. However, despite their efforts, patients still encountered neurotoxicity. No response data was reported.

In the particular case of suramin, the studies to rigorously demonstrate the relationship between peak plasma levels and neurotoxicity that have been proposed by others have not yet been published, and the presumption of a narrow therapeutic index has yet to be proven. Investigators at the University of Chicago began conducting a phase I dose escalation trial in January 1992 using a fixed-dose scheme without adaptive control to test the hypothesis that a pharmacokinetically based empiric dosing scheme is both feasible and safe.[131] The dosing schedule was simulated using prior estimates for the population pharmacokinetic parameters supplied by investigators at the University of Maryland, and is based on delivering intermittent doses of suramin by a one-hour infusion on days 1, 2, 8, and 9 of a 28-day cycle, which will provide a smooth approach to the steady state. Given the long elimination half-life of suramin, doses are decrementally decreased throughout the course of therapy, following a day 1 loading dose, in order to avoid progressively rising peak plasma concentrations in later cycles.

We have treated 59 patients, including 51 patients with prostate cancer, two with renal cell cancer, two with colon cancer, one with lymphoma, one with breast cancer, one with non-small cell lung cancer, and one with a malignant schwannoma, with a median of two cycles per patient. Three patients have experienced neurotoxicity, one developed a steroid-related myopathy, and two developed impotence. Other dose-limiting nonhematologic toxicity has been extremely heterogeneous, including four (reversible) episodes of nephrotoxicity, two instances of neutropenia, two instances of thrombocytopenia, one episode of pancreatitis, one episode of disseminated intravascular coagulopathy, one episode of adrenal insufficiency, and one pericardial effusion. It is worth remarking that the pattern of toxicity is not clearly dose related. Similar to the reported experience of other investigators, we have also noted common, but not dose-limiting, toxicities of a diffuse macular skin rash, lower extremity paresthesias, and fever with rigors. As is discussed later, several new skin lesions have also appeared in patients while being treated.

PSA levels have fallen by >50% in 37% of the prostate cancer patients and by >75% in 19% of these patients. Two patients (one with breast cancer and one with nodular lymphoma) maintained stable disease while on protocol treatment but ultimately progressed. Of the responding prostate cancer patients, two patients normalized their PSA levels and maintained this response for 14 and 11 months, respectively.

Despite the encouraging results of these trials in prostate cancer, and despite the wealth of information gained from developing Bayesian adaptive control methods in suramin clinical trials, these trials uniformly suffer from several drawbacks. First, it is known that hydrocortisone alone is able to elicit a response rate of about 10%,[132] and glucocorticoids have been shown to interrupt autocrine growth loops in human mammary adenocarcinoma lines in vitro.[133] Since hydrocortisone was routinely administered concurrently with suramin in most reported trials to date, it is unclear whether the reported objective and subjective responses are due to suramin, to hydrocortisone, or to the combination of the two agents. Second, many patients in these trials had their flutamide discontinued either shortly before or during suramin therapy, and the evidence reviewed previously suggests that discontinuation of flutamide has a therapeutic benefit in and of itself.[11,12,14,15] Third, although there is increasing evidence of the value of PSA monitoring in early prostate cancer, its use in advanced disease is still being questioned.[13] In particular, defining the relationship of changes in PSA levels with changes in actual disease extent is problematic at best. In view of the myriad unwanted clinical effects and the unique pharmacokinetic profile of suramin, it is important to address the issue of suramin's intrinsic activity with carefully designed clinical trials that control for flutamide withdrawal, the use of hydrocortisone, and that include other response assessments besides PSA measurements during the further development of this agent.

Pharmacokinetics

Suramin plasma concentrations as low as 0.5 μg/ml can be reliably quantitated by reverse-phase ion-paired high-performance liquid chromatography (HPLC).[134,135] More rapid HPLC assays that require only small volumes of plasma have recently been described.[136-138]

Suramin is not well absorbed when given by mouth, and causes intense local irritation when administered subcutaneously or intramuscularly. It is 99.7% bound to many different proteins, including serum globulins, albumin, casein, fibrinogen, gelatin, and histones.[87,139,140] Protein binding by albumin is saturable, and at plasma concentrations beyond 500 μg/ml the free fraction rises sharply.[141] The interaction with albumin is pH dependent[140,142] and alters its secondary structure, thereby affecting the binding of other drugs such as digoxin.[143]

Suramin accumulates principally in the kidneys and adrenal glands, the lung, liver, spleen, and large bowel, but not in muscle, red blood cells, or cerebrospinal fluid.[144-146] It is not metabolized to any significant extent, and it is principally cleared through the kidney, with renal clearance accounting for approximately 80% of total drug removal. It has an initial half-life of about two days and an elimination half-life of 40–50 days.[147,148] Total body clearance is correspondingly slow, being less than 0.5 ml/min.

In addition to the dose–toxicity relationship alluded to above, an issue of crucial importance in designing dosing regimens for suramin is the extent of inter- and of intrapatient variability. If there is wide variability, then it may not be possible to predict the appropriate doses for achieving tight control without plasma level monitoring. However, if administration of a given dose of the drug can be reliably expected to result in a given plasma concentration, regardless of differences in pharmacokinetic parameters either between patients or within the same patient over time, then there is little need for adaptive control.

The U.S. AIDS trials[147,148] reported relatively little interpatient variability in suramin pharmacokinetic behavior. In cancer clinical trials conducted at the NCI, Cooper et al.[149] and Lieberman et al.[150] found that a continuous infusion of 350 mg/m²/day resulted in blood levels ranging from 75–300 μg/ml at one week. In a three-compartment model, the population mean clearance was 0.33 ml/hr/kg (32% coefficient of variation), central volume of distribution 0.052 L/kg, volume of distribution at steady state 32.7 liters, and elimination

TABLE 2. Bayesian Estimates of Two-Compartment Kinetic Parameters for Suramin

Study	N	Volume of the Central Compartment (V_c) (L/m²)	Volume of the Peripheral Compartment (V_p) (L/m²)	Distributional Clearance (CL_d) (L/hr/m²)	Total Clearance (CL_t) (L/hr/m²)
Chicago, in progress[a]	27	6.17	15.75	0.102	0.03
MSKCC renal, 1992[a]	25	5.6	10.1	Not reported	0.001
MSKCC prostate, 1992[a]	7	4.38	10.3	0.083	0.017
Maryland, 1991[a]		3.8	9.4	97	15
NCI, 1992[b]	36	0.018 L/kg			0.34 ml/hr/kg

[a] ADAPT II estimates.
[b] NONMEM estimates.

half-life 1,205 hours (40% coefficient of variation). These investigators also noted a correlation between tumor bulk and suramin blood level, with lower blood concentrations achieved in patients with greater tumor burden.[149] This suggestion of a pharmacodynamic relationship with response is supported by a subset analysis of heavily pretreated patients with ovarian carcinoma treated with suramin. Patients with disease stabilization following treatment with suramin were found to have significantly lower rates of total body drug clearance and longer elimination half-lives than those patients who continued to progress.[151] No patient achieved tumor reduction. Kilbourn et al.,[152] administering suramin by IV bolus twice weekly at doses ranging from 250 to 750 mg/m², observed peak drug levels as high as 600 μg/ml, which decreased to 60% of peak within 24 hours with highly variable plasma half-lives.

Scher et al.[153] and Iversen et al.[154] evaluated the impact of individualized pharmacokinetic dosing on outcome in patients with prostate cancer and renal cell carcinoma. Suramin was administered by continuous infusion of 350 mg/m²/day to target a plasma concentration of 280 μg/ml. The average peak concentration was 287 ± 30 μg/ml. Site-specific differences for total time of suramin concentration >100 μg/ml, total systemic exposure, and elimination rate were found, suggesting pharmacokinetic differences between prostate and renal cell cancer. In a phase II study of suramin in patients with advanced renal cell carcinoma[155] using a continuous infusion with dose rates individualized to target a plasma level of 280–300 μg/m² with a nomogram developed at the NCI, wide interpatient variability in all pharmacokinetic parameters was noted. Again, subset analysis revealed that patients with either stable disease or partial responses had slower median elimination half-lives, although this difference could not be explained on the basis of alterations in either clearance or volume of distribution.

In a preliminary communication of data from an ongoing phase I trial of an intermittent infusion schedule, Hutson et al.[156] have suggested the possibility that suramin may recirculate during its distribution phase and have observed a dose-dependent change in the area under the concentration × time curve. A summary of suramin pharmacokinetic data evaluated using a two-compartmental model is given in Table 2.

The clinical results of the University of Chicago phase I trial of intermittent infusion without adaptive control have already been discussed. Using the mean peak plasma levels (excluding day 1) over the first two cycles as a measure of the peak concentrations being attained over time, mean peak levels of 385 mcg/ml are being achieved at the current dose level, with a median administered dose of 9,325 mg per patient at that cohort. Overall inter- and intrapatient variability has been low, with median coefficients of variation of 12% and 21% at the second and sixth cohorts (600 mg/m^2 and 1,440 mg/m^2), respectively.[131] Thus, in our trial, there appears to be little interpatient variability in plasma levels, and the neurotoxicity of suramin does not appear to be related to peak plasma levels.

Toxicity

In cancer patients, formal dose-finding studies have not yet been performed and no single dose-limiting toxicity has been defined. However, a number of interesting reactions have been reported, and it is clear that patients receiving suramin regularly experience a variety of significant side effects.

In patients treated with suramin, decreased activities of factors V, VII, X, XI, and XII leads to prolongations of the prothrombin time (PT) and the activated partial thromboplastin time (PTT).[157] Standard mixing tests with aliquots of plasma from normal patients correct these abnormalities with the exception of that reported with factor V, indicating the presence of an inhibitor, thought to be suramin itself. The loss of factor V activity is irreversible, suggesting that suramin somehow interacts directly with this procoagulant, and it is possible that the presence of albumin protects the other factors from similar irreversible inhibition. The increased amounts of circulating heparan sulfate and dermatan sulfate in the plasma of these patients interferes with the action of thrombin upon fibrinogen, thus prolonging the thrombin time.[158] Although these coagulation abnormalities are frequently asymptomatic, they can predispose patients to

hemorrhage, particularly during periods of hepatic injury, when large amounts of glycosaminoglycans are suddenly released into the circulation.[158] The idea that glycosaminoglycans may play a role in suramin's antitumor activity is supported by the observation of a tight temporal correlation between the development of anticoagulation and tumor shrinkage in patients treated with suramin.[159]

Suramin-related keratopathy has been reported by Teich et al.,[160] by Holland et al.,[161] and by the U.S. Suramin Working Group trial.[162] Bilateral vortex keratopathy was documented in six adrenocortical carcinoma patients. In two patients, the changes were symptomatic with complaints of mild pain and photophobia. Histopathologic findings included deposits similar to those seen in lipid storage diseases, and this condition appears to result from the deposition of excess glycosaminoglycans in the cornea. It appears to be related to both the total dose of suramin and to the rate of drug delivery. Treatment with topical lubricants improved the symptoms; the underlying lesions improved or resolved with the discontinuation of therapy.

Neuromuscular toxicity has been the most feared complication of suramin therapy, and initial observations of its occurrence led to the adoption of adaptive control methods for dosing suramin, as discussed above. In the original report describing this peripheral neuropathy, two patients developed a severe, progressive, polyradiculopathy resembling Guillain-Barré syndrome,[122] while two others developed a nonprogressive peripheral neuropathy. Electrical nerve testing revealed severe demyelinating neuropathy with conduction block; an elevated cerebrospinal fluid protein level was also noted. Plasmapheresis and high-dose steroid therapy were of little value; however, these patients all improved within 6 to 12 weeks of the onset of their symptoms. The risk of developing neurotoxicity appeared to be correlated with peak blood suramin levels, approaching 100% at 400 μg/ml, although the sample size on which this conclusion was based is small. The etiology of the neurotoxicity is unclear; hypotheses include an immune mechanism and direct or indirect damage to the nerve sheath. In addition, a recent report describes the presence of a mitochondrial myopathy resembling that seen with congenital cytochrome c oxidase deficiency,[163] characterized by hypophosphatemia, further emphasizing the clinical significance of suramin's effects on cellular metabolism.

In addition to a commonly occurring diffuse macular erythematous rash, a variety of interesting cutaneous reactions to suramin have been described, including lethal toxic epidermal necrolysis,[164,165] disseminated superficial actinic porokeratosis, and keratoacanthoma.[166] In our currently ongoing phase I trial of suramin administered by fixed-dose intermittent infusion, one patient developed six basal cell and two squamous cell cancers of the skin while on treatment with suramin, and two other patients developed keratoacanthomas.[167]

Other common side effects[168] have included proteinuria (up to 2 g/day), with a decline in creatinine clearance (20–40%), and occasional episodes of hematuria. These generally resolve with discontinuation of therapy. Thrombocytopenia and leukopenia may occur but are rarely severe; an immune-mediated phenomenon may account for some instances of thrombocytopenia.[169] Glycosaminoglycans commonly accumulate in the liver and spleen, causing hepatosplenomegaly, and drug-related hepatic injury has been reported. Most patients report paresthesias involving the lower extremities, and a syndrome of fever, chills, and a skin rash often occurs following completion of the infusion during the first cycle. The severity of this last syndrome usually decreases with time,

and its occurrence is not due to the presence of infection. Other, more global disturbances of mood, vision, and hearing occur, as does a severe flu-like syndrome. A number of endocrinologic and electrolyte abnormalities have been noted, including both hypo- and hyperglycemia (possibly related to concurrent steroid administration), hypocalcemia, hypomagnesemia, and hyperamylasemia.

The issue of whether, and to what extent, suramin causes end-organ adrenal dysfunction is an interesting and important one given the questions raised by the current standard of concurrent hydrocortisone replacement. Instances of Addisonian crisis developing in patients being treated with suramin for pemphigus have been reported,[170,171] with pathologic examination at autopsy showing the presence of adrenal cortical necrosis in two patients. Humphreys and Donaldson at the University of Chicago found zonal degeneration of the adrenal cortex[172] in the adrenal glands of guinea pigs, rats, and dogs treated with suramin, and in 1986, Stein et al. described a patient with AIDS and Kaposi's sarcoma who became hypoadrenal while receiving treatment with suramin.[173] These observations are historically important, for they led to the initial investigations of suramin's utility in cancer therapy.

Suramin may exert its adrenolytic actions at the level of the adrenal gland, and the finding that cynomolgus monkeys treated with suramin show biochemical evidence of end-organ hyporesponsiveness to adrenocorticotropic hormone (ACTH) stimulation and adrenal cortical necrosis[174] is consistent with the hypothesis that suramin-induced adrenal cortical necrosis is responsible for the adrenal insufficiency observed clinically. However, exposure to 75–400 μg/mL of suramin results in a concentration- and time-dependent inhibition of steroid hormone production by cultured adrenal gland carcinoma cell lines,[175–177] suggesting that suramin may inhibit adrenal steroidogenesis by a direct cellular effect. This is supported by the observation that suramin causes a concentration-dependent decrease in activity of the microsomal enzymes 17-β- and 21-hydroxylase, 17,20-desmolase, and mitochondrial 11β-hydroxylase in normal human adrenal tissue in vitro.[178] When dispersed adrenal cortical cells are exposed to ACTH, suramin, and other stimulants of adrenal steroidogenesis,[179] suramin exhibits a dose-dependent inhibition of ACTH-stimulated corticosterone release, once a threshold dose of 10^{-5} M was exceeded. Furthermore, this inhibition was either reversible or preventable when the cells were coincubated with agents that stimulate steroid biosynthesis by mechanisms independent of ACTH receptor binding. Chromatographic elution studies using ^{125}I-labeled ACTH and suramin on a column containing a molecule that is structurally similar to suramin showed that ACTH binds strongly to suramin-like molecules. This evidence suggests that the adrenal inhibitory effect is due to interference with ACTH binding to its receptor, in a mechanism analogous to its postulated effects on growth factor receptors, rather than by destruction of functional adrenal tissue.

The observed adrenal insufficiency may be only a manifestation of a more generalized endocrine defect, but few clinical studies conducted to date have addressed the possibility of higher-level interference with the hypothalamic–pituitary–end organ axes. Suramin inhibits both basal and secretagogue-stimulated ACTH release in cultured rat anterior pituitary cells[180] in isolation; however, this effect is abrogated by the addition of bovine serum albumin or of fetal calf serum. When patients were treated with a 10-day continuous infusion of suramin at a dose of 350 mg/m²/day,[181] decreases in both T4 and the thyroid-stimulating hormone (TSH) response to the hypothalamic hormone thyroid-releasing hormone (TRH) were noted, as well as an increase in both plasma ACTH and bas-

al cortisol levels. However, no impairment in pituitary–adrenal axis function was noted on ACTH stimulation testing. Of interest in this regard is the finding that adrenal cortical cells treated with suramin followed by removal of the suramin and washing did not show any impairment of steroidogenesis when compared with untreated cells, suggesting that the inhibition of adrenal cellular function may be reversible.[176] Since the largest experience with suramin has been in patients with prostate cancer, obvious clinical signs of other endocrine deficiencies such as impotence may have been obscured by the effects of hormonal therapy for their illness. Suramin reversibly suppresses testosterone production by rat Leydig cells, as well as estradiol production by Sertoli cells, by noncompetitive inhibition of follicle-stimulating hormone (FSH) and luteinizing hormone (LH) at the receptor level.[182] LaRocca et al.[114] found that the levels of dehydroepiandrosterone sulfate, dehydroepiandrosterone, and androstenedione decreased in patients with hormone-refractory prostate cancer treated with suramin. These effects on androgen production may also contribute to suramin's activity in advanced prostate cancer.

To ameliorate the expected adrenal insufficiency, current guidelines call for the simultaneous initiation of hydrocortisone (30–40 mg per day) with the beginning of suramin therapy. However, although cogent evidence exists to show that adrenal insufficiency is an important toxicity of suramin therapy, the response issues and data reviewed earlier indicate a need for carefully designed trials to examine the role of routine steroid replacement therapy and its contribution to the overall response rates in patients undergoing treatment with suramin.[183,184]

CONCLUSION

There remains a need for continuing studies to improve conventional cytotoxic chemotherapy for patients with hormone-refractory metastatic prostate cancer. The most promising new agent, suramin, may act by a novel mechanism of growth factor inhibition. However, issues of the optimal dose, schedule, and of the need for ancillary supportive therapy remain as yet unsettled. Furthermore, given the frequency of side effects encountered with this drug, it is crucial that further studies to define the extent of its activity be conducted. Despite this, the simplest and least harmful maneuver in appropriate patients who develop evidence of progressive prostate cancer is the withdrawal of flutamide with careful observation of the response.

REFERENCES

1. Klein LA: Prostatic carcinoma. N Engl J Med 300:824–833, 1979.

2. The Veterans Administration Co-operative Urological Research Group: Treatment and survival of patients with cancer of the prostate. Surg Gynecol Obstet 124:1011–1017, 1967.

3. Dawson NA: Treatment of progressive metastatic prostate cancer. Oncology 7:17–27, 1993.

4. Eisenberger MA, Abrams JS: Chemotherapy for prostatic carcinoma. Sem Urol 6:303–310, 1988.

5. Yagoda A, Petrylak D: Cytotoxic chemotherapy for advanced hormone-resistant prostate cancer. Cancer Suppl 71:1098–1109, 1993.

6. Rangel C, Matzkin H, Soloway MS: Experience with weekly doxorubicin (Adriamycin) in hormone-refractory stage D2 prostate cancer. Urology 39:577–582, 1992.

7. Hansen R, Moynihan T, Beatty P, et al.: Continuous systemic 5-FU infusion in refractory prostatic cancer. Urology 37:358–361, 1991.

8. von Roemeling R, Fisher HAG, Horton J: Daily oral cyclophosphamide is effective in hormone refractory prostate cancer. A ph-I/II pilot trial. Proc Am Soc Clin Oncol 11:213, 1992.

9. Becker H, Otto U, Hoffmann B, et al.: Phase 2 study of longterm infusion with MMC in patients with progressive prostate cancer (Abstr 825). J Urol 147:419A, 1992.

10. Dexeus F, Logothetis CJ, Samuels ML, et al.: Continuous infusion of vinblastine for advanced hormone-refractory prostate cancer. Cancer Treat Rep 69:885–886, 1985.

11. Kelly WK, Scher HI: Prostate specific antigen decline after antiandrogen withdrawal: the flutamide withdrawal syndrome. J Urol 149:607–609, 1993.

12. Scher H, Kelly WK: Flutamide withdrawal syndrome: its impact on clinical trials in hormone-refractory prostate cancer. J Clin Oncol 11:1566–1572, 1993.

13. Kelly WK, Scher HI, Mazumdar M, et al.: Prostate-specific antigen as a measure of disease outcome in metastatic hormone-refractory prostate cancer. J Clin Oncol 11:607–615, 1993.

14. Sartor O, Cooper M, Weinberger D, et al.: Surprising activity of flutamide withdrawal when combined with aminoglutethimide in treatment of "hormone-refractory" prostate cancer. J Natl Cancer Inst 86:222–227, 1994.

15. Dupont A, Gomez J, Cusan L, et al.: Response to flutamide withdrawal in advanced prostate cancer in progression under combination therapy. J Urol 150:908–913, 1993.

16. Murphy GP, Slack NH: Response criteria for the prostate of the USA National Prostatic Cancer Project. Prostate 1:375–382, 1980.

17. Wilding G, Chen M, Gelmann EP: Aberrant response in vitro of hormone responsive prostate cancer cells to antiandrogens. The Prostate 14:103–115, 1989.

18. Howell A, Dodwell DJ, Anderson H, et al.: Response after withdrawal of tamoxifen and progestogens in advanced breast cancer. Ann Oncol 3:611–617, 1992.

19. Fex HJ, Hogberg KB, Konyves I, et al.: Certain steroid N-bis-(halo-ethyl)-carbamates. U.S. Patent No. 3 299 104, 17.1.

20. Tew KD, Erickson LC, White G, et al.: Cytotoxicity of estramustine, a steroid-nitrogen mustard derivative, through non-DNA targets. Mol Pharmac 24:324–328, 1983.

21. Gunnarsson PO, Forshell GP, Fritjofsson A, et al.: Plasma concentrations of estramustine phosphate and its major metabolites in patients with prostatic carcinoma treated with different doses of estramustine phosphate (Estracyt). Scand J Urol Nephrol 15:201–205, 1981.

22. Van Poppel H, Baert L: The present role of estramustine phosphate in advanced prostate cancer. EORTC Genito-urinary Group Monograph, 10:323–341, 1991.

23. Tew KD, Stearns ME: Estramustine—a nitrogen mustard/steroid with antimicrotubule activity. Pharmac Ther 43:299–319, 1989.

24. Aumuller G, Seitz J, Heyns W: Intracellular

localization of prostatic binding protein (PBP) in rat prostate by light and electron microscopic immunocytochemistry. Histochemistry 76:496–516, 1982.

25. Hartley-Asp B, Kruse E: Nuclear protein matrix as a target for estramustine-induced cell death. Prostate 9:387–395, 1986.

26. Norlen BJ, Andersson SB, Bjork P, et al.: Uptake of estramustine phosphate (estracyt) metabolites in prostatic cancer. J Urol 140:1058–1062, 1988.

27. Hartley-Asp B, Gunnarsson PO: Growth and cell survival following treatment with estramustine, nor-nitrogen mustard, estradiol and testosterone of a human prostatic cancer cell line (DU 145). J Urol 127:818–822, 1982.

28. Janknegt RA: Estramustine phosphate and other cytotoxic drugs in the treatment of poor prognostic advanced prostate cancer. The Prostate Suppl 4:105–110, 1992.

29. Mareel MM, Storma GA, Dragonett CH, et al.: Anti-invasive activity of estramustine on malignant MO4 cells and on DU145 human prostate carcinoma cells in vitro. Cancer Res 48:1842–1849, 1986.

30. Speicher LA, Sheridan VR, Godwin AK, et al.: Resistance to the antimitotic drug estramustine is distinct from the multidrug resistant phenotype. Br J Cancer 64:267–273, 1991.

31. Amato RJ, Logothetis CJ, Dexeus FH, et al.: Preliminary results of phase II trial of estramustine and vinblastine for patients with progressive hormone refractory prostate carcinoma. Proc Am Assoc Cancer Res 32:186, 1991.

32. Seidman AD, Scher HI, Petrylak D, et al.: Estramustine and vinblastine: use of prostate specific antigen as a clinical trial end point for hormone refractory prostatic cancer. J Urol 147:931–934, 1993.

33. Hudas GR, Greenberg R, Krigel RL, et al.: Phase II study of estramustine and vinblastine, two microtubule inhibitors, in hormone-refractory prostate cancer. J Clin Oncol 10:1754–1761, 1992.

34. Kaufman SH, Shaper JH: Association of topoisomerase II with the hepatoma cell nuclear matrix: the role of intermolecular disulfide bond formation. Exp Cell Res 192:511–523, 1991.

35. Mador D, Ritchie B, Meeker B, et al.: Response of the Dunning R3327H prostatic adenocarcinoma to radiation and various chemotherapeutic drugs. Cancer Treat Rep 66:1837–1843, 1982.

36. Scher HI, Sternberg C, Heston WDW, et al.: Etoposide in prostatic cancer: experimental studies and phase II trial in patients with bi-dimensionally measurable disease. Cancer Chemother Pharmacol 18:24–26, 1986.

37. Trump DL, Loprinzi CL: Phase II trial of etoposide in advanced prostatic cancer. Cancer Treat Rep 68:1195–1196, 1984.

38. Pienta KJ, Lehr JE: Inhibition of prostate cancer growth by estramustine and etoposide: evidence for interactions at the nuclear matrix. J Urol 149:1622–1625, 1993.

39. Pienta KJ, Redman BG, Hussain M, et al.: A combination of estramustine and etoposide orally may be an effective regimen in the treatment of hormone refractory prostate cancer. Proc Am Soc Clin Oncol 12:246, 1993.

40. Iozzo RV: Biology of disease proteoglycans: structure, function, and role in neoplasia. Lab Invest 53:373–396, 1985.

41. Akanji MA: Labilising effect of suramin on rat kidney lysosomes in vivo. Toxicol Lett 23:273–277, 1984.

42. Constantopoulos G, Rees S, Barranger JA: Suramin-induced storage disease. Am J Pathol 113:266–268, 1983.

43. Skoglund G, Ahren B, Lundquist I: Insulin secretion and islet lysosomal enzyme activities in the mouse. Int J Pancreatol 4:29–40, 1989.

44. Marjomäki V, Salminen A: Morphological and enzymatic heterogeneity of suramin-induced lysosomal storage disease in some tissues of mice and rats. Exp Mol Pathol 45:76–83, 1986.

45. Rees S, Constantopoulos G, Brady R: The suramin-treated rat as a model of mucopolysaccharidosis: reversibility of biochemical and morphological changes in the liver. Virchows Arch [Cell Pathol] 51:235–245, 1986.

46. Sjölund M, Thyberg J: Suramin inhibits binding and degradation of platelet-derived growth factor in arterial smooth muscle cells but does not interfere with autocrine stimulation of DNA synthesis. Cell Tissue Res 256:35–43, 1989.

47. Constantopoulos G, Rees S, Cragg BG, et al.: Experimental animal model for mucopolysaccharidosis: suramin-induced glycosaminoglycan and sphingolipid accumulation in the rat. Proc Natl Acad Sci USA 77:3700–3704, 1980.

48. Koistinaho J: Suramin-induced changes in sympathetic neurons: correlation between catecholamine fluorescence, tyrosine hydroxylase immunoreactivity and accumula-

tion of pigment bodies. Neurosci Lett 112:19–24, 1990.

49. Cooper M, Danesi R, LaRocca R, et al.: Suramin induces the production of antiproliferative heparan sulfate in patients with malignancies. Proc Am Assoc Cancer Res 31:200, 1990.

50. Ishihara M, Fedarko NS, Conrad HE: Transport of heparan sulfate into the nuclei of hepatocytes. J Biol Chem 261:13575–13580, 1986.

51. Sporn MG, Roberts AB: Autocrine growth factors and cancer. Nature 313:745–747, 1985.

52. Pollak M, Richard M: Suramin blockade of insulinlike growth factor I-stimulated proliferation of human osteosarcoma cells. J Natl Cancer Inst 82:1349–1352, 1990.

53. Walz TM, Abdiu A, Wingren S, et al.: Suramin inhibits growth of human osteosarcoma xenografts in nude mice. Cancer Res 51:3585–3589, 1991.

54. Fleming TP, Matsui T, Heidaran MA, et al.: Demonstration of an activated platelet-derived growth factor autocrine pathway and its role in human tumor cell proliferation in vitro. Oncogene 7:1355–1359, 1992.

55. Westermark B, Heldin CH: Platelet-derived growth factor as a mediator of normal and neoplastic cell proliferation. Med Oncol Tumor Pharmacother 3:177–183, 1986.

56. Pollak M, Polychronakos C, Richard M: Suramin interferes with the binding of insulin-like growth factor I (IGF-I) to IGF-I receptors. Proc Am Assoc Cancer Res 31:47 (279), 1990.

57. Minniti C, Maggi M, Helman L: Suramin inhibits the growth of human rhabdomyosarcoma by interrupting the insulin-like growth factor II autocrine growth loop. Cancer Res 52:1830–1835, 1992.

58. Coffey RJ Jr, Leof EB, Shipley GD, et al.: Suramin inhibition of growth factor receptor binding and mitogenicity in AKR-2B cells. J Cell Physiol 132:143–148, 1987.

59. Knabbe C, Kellner U, Schmahl M, et al.: Suramin inhibits growth of human prostate carcinoma cells by inactivation of growth factor action. Proc Am Assoc Cancer Res 30:295 (1172), 1989.

60. Culouscou JM, Garrouste F, Remacle-Bonnet M, et al.: Autocrine secretion of a colorectum-derived growth factor by HT-29 human colon carcinoma cell line. Int J Cancer 42:895–901, 1988.

61. Vignon F, Prebois C, Rochefort H: Inhibition of breast cancer growth by suramin. J Natl Cancer Inst 84:38–42, 1992.

62. Foekens JA, Sieuwerts AM, Stuurman-Smeets EMJ, et al.: Pleiotropic actions of suramin on the proliferation of human breast cancer cells in vitro. Int J Cancer 51:439–444, 1992.

63. Olivier S, Formento P, Fischel JL, et al.: Epidermal growth factor receptor expression and suramin cytotoxicity in vitro. Eur J Cancer 26:867–871, 1990.

64. Mórocz IÁ, Lauber B, Schmitter D, Stahel RA: In vitro effect of suramin on lung tumour cells. Eur J Cancer Clin Oncol 29A:245–247, 1993.

65. Wade TP, Kasid A, Stein CA, et al.: Suramin interferes with TGF-beta induced inhibition of human renal cell carcinoma. Proc Am Assoc Cancer Res 30:70n (276), 1989.

66. Pienta K, Isaacs W, Vindivich D, et al.: The effects of basic fibroblast growth factor and suramin on cell motility and growth of rat prostate cancer cells. J Urol 145:199–202, 1991.

67. Cardinali M, Sartor O, Robbins K: Suramin, an experimental chemotherapeutic drug, activates the receptor for epidermal growth factor and promotes growth of certain malignant cells. J Clin Invest 89:1242–1247, 1992.

68. Mitchen J, Rago R, Wilding G: Effects of suramin on the proliferation of primary epithelial cell cultures derived from normal, benign hyperplastic and cancerous human prostates. Prostate 22:75–89, 1993.

69. Berns EMJJ, Schuurmans ALG, Bolt J, et al.: Antiproliferative effects of suramin on androgen-responsive tumour cells. Eur J Cancer Clin Oncol 26:470–474, 1990.

70. Richard M, Pollak R: Protein binding of suramin affects bioactivity as well as pharmacokinetics: loss of activity of suramin as an inhibitor of peptide growth factor binding in the presence of albumin (Abstr). Proc Am Soc Clin Oncol 12:157, 1993.

71. Sartor O, McLellan CA, Myers CE, et al.: Suramin rapidly alters cellular tyrosine phosphorylation in prostate cancer cell lines. J Clin Invest 90:2166–2174, 1992.

72. Kim JH, Sherwood ER, Sutkowski DM, et al.: Inhibition of prostatic tumor cell proliferation by suramin: alterations in TGF alpha-mediated autocrine growth regulation and cell cycle distribution. J Urol 146:171–176, 1991.

73. Ewing MW, Liu SC, Gnarra JR, et al.: Effect of suramin on the mitogenic response of the human prostate carcinoma cell line PC-3. Cancer 71:1151–1158, 1993.

74. Foekens JA, Sieuwerts AM, Stuurman-Smeetss EMJ, et al.: Effects of suramin on cell-cycle kinetics of MCF-7 human breast cancer cells *in vitro*. Br J Cancer 67:232–236, 1993.

75. Freter C, Wolfson A, Brown A, et al.: Dexamethasone and suramin block lymphoid tumor cells in different phases of the cell cycle. Proc Am Assoc Cancer Res 31:345 (2041), 1990.

76. Calcaterra N, Vicario L, Roveri O: Inhibition by suramin of mitochondrial ATP synthesis. Biochem Pharmacol 37:13575–13580, 1986.

77. Fantini J, Rognoni JB, Roccabianca M, et al.: Suramin inhibits cell growth and glycolytic activity and triggers differentiation of human colic adenocarcinoma cell clone HT29-D4. J Biol Chem 264:10282–10286, 1989.

78. Rago R, Mitchen J, Cheng AL, et al.: Disruption of cellular energy balance by suramin in intact human prostate carcinoma cells, a likely antiproliferative mechanism. Cancer Res 51:6629–6635, 1991.

79. Rago RP, Brazy PC, Wilding G: Disruption of mitochondrial function by suramin measured by rhodamine 123 retention and oxygen consumption in intact DU145 prostate carcinoma cells. Cancer Res 52:6953–6956, 1992.

80. Brooke MH: A Clinician's Guide to Neuromuscular Diseases, 2nd ed. Baltimore: Williams and Wilkins, p 306, 1986.

81. Stryer L: Biochemistry, San Francisco: W.H. Freeman, p 346, 1975.

82. Baghdiguain S, Verrier B, Marvaldi J, et al.: Short-term suramin treatment followed by the removal of the drug induces terminal differntation of HT29-D4 cells. J Cell Physiol 150:168–174, 1992.

83. Baghdiguain S, Verrier B, Marvaldi J, et al.: Kinetics of biochemical, electrophysiological, and morphological events (including lysosomal disorder) during the course of suramin-induced differentiation of the human colon cancer cell clone HT29-D4. Int J Cancer 49:608–615, 1991.

84. Fantini J, Verrier B, Robert C, et al.: Suramin-induced differentiation of the human colonic adenocarcinoma cell clone HT29-D4 in serum-free medium. Exp Cell Res 189:109–117, 1990.

85. Baghdiguian S, Verrier B, Gerard C, et al.: Insulin like growth factor I is an autocrine regulator of human colon cancer cell differentiation and growth. Cancer Lett 62:23–33, 1992.

86. Trieb K, Dorfinger K, Neuhold N, et al.: Suramin affects differentiated and undifferentiated human thyroid epithelial cells *in vitro*. J Endocrinol 134(3):505–511, 1992.

87. Hawking F: Suramin: with special reference to onchocerciasis. Adv Pharmacol Chemother 15:289–322, 1978.

88. Eisen V, Loveday C: Effects of suramin on complement, blood clotting, fibrinolysis and kinin formation. Br J Pharmac 49:678–687, 1973.

89. Schneider WJ, Beisiegel U, Goldstein JL, et al.: Purification of the low density lipoprotein receptor, an acidic glycoprotein of 164,000 molecular weight. J Biol Chem 257:2664–2673, 1982.

90. Chiang CP, Caulfield JP: The binding of human low-density lipoproteins to the surface of schistosomula of *Schistosoma mansoni* is inhibited by polyanions and reduces the binding of anti-schistosomal antibodies. Am Pathol 134:1007–1018, 1989.

91. Tamai T, Patsch W, Lock D, et al.: Receptors for homologous plasma lipoproteins on a rat hepatoma cell line. J Lipid Res 24:1568–1577, 1983.

92. Forsbeck K, Bjelkenkrantz K, Nilsson K: Role of iron in the proliferation of the established human tumor cell lines U-937 and K-562. Effects of suramin and a lipophilic iron chelator (PIH). Scand J Haematol 37:429–437, 1986.

93. Ono K, Nakane H, Fukushima M: Differential inhibition of various deoxyribonucleic and ribonucleic acid polymerases by suramin. Eur J Biochem 172:349–353, 1988.

94. Bojanowski K, Lelievre S, Markovits J, et al.: Suramin is an inhibitor of DNA topoisomerase II in vitro and in Chinese hamster fibrosarcoma cells. Proc Natl Acad Sci USA 89:3025–3029, 1992.

95. Hargis JB, Danesi R, Myers C, et al.: Suramin activity in human sarcoma cell lines. Proc Am Assoc Cancer Res 31:410 (2433), 1990.

96. Spigelman Z, Dowers A, Kennedy S, et al.: Antiproliferative effects of suramin on lymphoid cells. Cancer Res 47:4694–4698, 1987.

97. Brandely M, LaGrange P, Hurtrel G: Effects of suramin on the *in vivo* antimicrobial resistance against Listeria monocytogenes and Mycobaterium bovis (BCG) in mice. Clin Exp Immunol 63:118–126, 1986.

98. Brandely M, LaGrange P, Hurtrel B, et al.: Effects of suramin on the immune responses to sheep red blood cells in mice. I. *In vivo* studies. Cell Immunol 93:280–291, 1985.

99. Motta I, Brandely M, Truffa-Bach I, et al.: Effects of suramin on the immune responses to sheep red blood cells in mice. II. *In vitro* studies. Cell Immunol 93:292–302, 1985.

100. Allen PD, Johnston DH, Macey MG, et al.: Modulation of CD4 by suramin. Clin Exp Immunol 91:141–146, 1993.

101. Mills GB, Zhang N, May C, et al.: Suramin prevents binding of interleukin 2 to its cell surface receptor: a possible mechanism for immunosuppression. Cancer Res 50:3036–3042, 1990.

102. Sipka S, Danko K, Nagy P, et al.: Effects of suramin on phagocytes in vitro. Ann Hematol 63:45–48, 1991.

103. Roilides E, Paschalides P, Freifeld A, et al.: Suppression of polymorphonuclear leukocyte bactericidal activity by suramin. Antimicrob Agents Chemother 37:495–500, 1993.

104. Danesi R, LaRocca R, Stein C, et al.: Effect of suramin on the human glioma cell line U706T. Proc Am Assoc Cancer Res 30:578 (2300), 1989.

105. Bergh J: Suramin is a potent inhibitor of the cell proliferation in human non-small cell lung cancer cell lines. Proc Am Assoc Cancer Res 30:77, 1989.

106. Crickard U, Abu-Sitta M, Crickard K: Suramin and growth factor effects on proliferation of human gynecologic cancer cells *in vitro*. Proc Am Assoc Cancer Res 31:58 (345), 1990.

107. Foekens JA, Stuurman-Smeets EMJ, Groenenboom-De Munter IK, et al.: Reversible proliferative and antiproliferative effects of suramin on human breast cancer cells *in vitro*. Proc Am Assoc Cancer Res 31:50 (298), 1990.

108. Berthois Y, Martin P, Dong XF, et al.: Suramin EGF-mediated reversible inhibition of hormone dependent growth in the MCF-7 cell line. Proc Am Assoc Cancer Res 31:57, 1990.

109. Nakajima M, Dechavigny A, Johnson, et al.: Suramin: a potent inhibitor of melanoma heparanase and invasion. J Biol Chem 266:9661–9666, 1991.

110. Alberts D, Miranda E, Dorr R, et al.: Phase II and pharmacokinetic and human tumor cloning assay study of suramin in advanced ovarian cancer. Proc Am Soc Clin Oncol 10:187,1991.

111. Bai L, Naomoto Y, Miyazaki M, et al.: Antiproliferative effects of suramin on human cancer cells in vitro and in vivo. Acta Med Okayama 46:457–463, 1992.

112. Chang SY, Yu DS, Sherwood E, et al.: Inhibitory effects of suramin on a human renal cell carcinoma line causing nephrogenic hepatic dysfunction. J Urol 147:1147–1150, 1992.

113. Peehl D, Wong S, Stamey T: Cytostatic effects of suramin on prostate cancer cells cultured from primary tumors. J Urol 145:624–630, 1991.

114. LaRocca R, Danesi R, Cooper M, et al.: Effect of suramin on human prostate cancer cells *in vitro*. J Urol 145:393–398, 1991.

115. Favoni RE, Rosso R, Pirani P, Repetto L, Nicolin A, Miglietta L: Synergistic activity of suramin and doxorubicin on human breast cancer cell lines. Proc Am Assoc Cancer Res 32:384 (2282), 1991.

116. Clark J, Chu M, Calabresi P: Growth inhibition of colon cancer cells by genistein and suramin. Proc Am Assoc Cancer Res 30:557 (2218), 1989.

117. Fruehauf JP, Myers CE, Sinha BK: Synergistic activity of suramin with tumor necrosis factor α and doxorubicin on human prostate cancer cell lines. J Natl Cancer Inst 82:1206–1209, 1990.

118. Liu S, Ewing M, Anglard P, et al.: The effect of suramin, tumor necrosis factor, and interferon γ on human prostate carcinoma. J Urol 145:389–392, 1991.

119. Allolio B, Reincke M, Arlt W, et al.: Suramin for treatment of adrenocortical carcinoma. Lancet 2:277, 1989.

120. Vierhapper H, Nowotny P, Mostbeck G, et al.: Effect of suramin in a patient with adrenocortical carcinoma. Lancet 1:1207, 1989.

121. LaRocca RV, Cooper MR, Stein CA, et al.: A pilot study of suramin in the treatment of progressive refractory follicular lymphomas. Ann Oncol 3:571–573, 1992.

122. LaRocca R, Meer J, Gilliatt R, et al.: Suramin-induced polyneuropathy. Neurology 40:954–960, 1990.

123. Kobayashi K, Jodrell DI, Ratain MJ: Pharmacodynamic-pharmacokinetic relationships and therapeutic drug monitoring. Cancer Surveys (in press).

124. Myers C, Cooper M, Stein C, et al.: Suramin: a novel growth factor antagonist with activity in hormone-refractory metastatic prostate cancer. J Clin Oncol 10:881–889, 1992.

125. Armand JP, Bonnay M, Gandia D, et al.: Phase I–II suramin (SRM) study in advanced cancer patients (pts). Proc Am Assoc Cancer Res 32:175 (1042), 1991.

126. Eisenberger MA, Reyno LM, Jodrell DI, et al.: Suramin, an active drug for prostate cancer: interim observations in a phase I trial. J Natl Cancer Inst 85:611–621, 1993.

127. Reyno LM, Egorin MJ, Eisenberger MA, et al.: Development and validation of a pharmacokinetically (PK) based fixed dosing scheme for suramin (Abstr). Proc Am Soc Clin Oncol 12:135, 1993.

128. Kelly WK, Scher H, Bajorin D, et al.: Empiric dosing of suramin therapy in hormone refractory prostate cancer (Abstr). Proc Am Soc Clin Oncol 12:139, 1993.

129. Van Oosterom AT, De Smedt E, Denis L, et al.: Suramin for prostatic cancer: a phase I/II study in advanced extensively pretreated disease. Eur J Cancer 26:411, 1990.

130. van Rijswijk REN, van Loenen AC, Wagstaff J, et al.: Suramin: rapid loading and weekly maintenance regimens for cancer patients. J Clin Oncol 10:1788–1794, 1992.

131. Kobayashi K, Vokes EE, Janisch L, et al.: A phase I cohort study of suramin (SUR) in patients with advanced cancer (CA) (Abstr). Proc Am Soc Clin Oncol 12:161, 1993.

132. Tannock I, Gospodorowicz M, Meckin W, et al.: Treatment of metastatic prostate cancer with low-dose prednisone: evaluation of pain and quality of life as pragmatic indices of response. J Clin Oncol 7:597, 1989.

133. Alexander DB, Goya L, Webster MK, et al.: Glucocorticoids coordinately disrupt a transforming growth factor alpha autocrine loop and suppress the growth of 13762NF-derived Con8 rat mammary adenocarcinoma cells. Cancer Res 53:1808–1815, 1993.

134. Klecker RW Jr, Collins JM: Quantification of suramin by reverse-phase ion-pairing high-performance liquid chromatography. J Liquid Chrom 8:1685–1696, 1985.

135. Teirlynck O, Bogaert MG, Demedts P, et al.: Rapid high-performance liquid chromatographic determination of suramin in plasma of patients with acquired immune deficiency syndrome (AIDS) or AIDS-related complex (ARC). J Pharm Biomed Anal 7:123–126, 1989.

136. Supko JG, Malspeis L: A rapid isocratic HPLC assay of suramin (NSC 34936) in human plasma. J Liquid Chrom 13:727–741, 1990.

137. Tong WP, Scher HI, Petrylak DP, et al.: A rapid HPLC assay for suramin in plasma. J Liquid Chrom 13:2269–2284, 1990.

138. Tjaden U, Reeuwijk H, van der Greef J, et al.: Bioanalysis of suramin in human plasma by ion-pair high-performance liquid chromatography. J Chromatogr 525:141–149, 1990.

139. De Clercq E: Suramin in the treatment of AIDS: mechanism of action. Antiviral Res 7:1–10, 1987.

140. Vansterkenburg ELM, Wilting J, Janssen LMH: Influence of pH on the binding of suramin to human serum albumin. Biochem Pharmacol 38:3029–3035, 1989.

141. de Bruijn EA, Pattyn G, Denis L, et al.: Therapeutic drug monitoring of suramin and protein binding. J Liquid Chrom 14:3719–3733, 1991.

142. Bos OJM, Vansterkenburg ELM, Boon JP, et al.: Location and characterization of the suramin binding sites of human serum albumin. Biochem Pharmacol 40:1595–1599, 1990.

143. Müller WE, Wollert U: Spectroscopic studies on the complex formation of suramin with bovine and human serum albumin. Biochimica Biophysica Acta 427:465–480, 1976.

144. Cooper M, Jamis-Dow C, Weiss G, et al.: Suramin: a clinically relevant physiologic pharmacokinetic model. Proc Am Soc Clin Oncol 9:81 (314), 1990.

145. Jamis-Dow CA, Weiss GH, Cooper MR, et al.: Pharmacokinetics and biodistribution of suramin. Proc Am Assoc Cancer Res 31:385 (2285), 1990.

146. Edwards G, Rodick CL, Ward SA, et al.: Disposition of suramin in patients with onchocerciasis (Abstr). Acta Pharmacol Toxicl 59(Suppl V);222, 1986.

147. Broder S, Collins JM, Markham PD, et al.: Effects of suramin on HTLV-III/LAV infection presenting as Kaposi's sarcoma or AIDS-related complex: clinical pharmacology and suppression of virus replication in vivo. Lancet 2(8456):627–630, 1985.

148. Collins JM, Klecker RW, Yarchoan R, et al.: Clinical pharmacokinetics of suramin in patients with HTLV-III/LAV infection. J Clin Pharmacol 26:22–26, 1986.

149. Cooper M, Lieberman R, LaRocca R, Gernt PR, Weinberger MS, Headlee DJ, Kohler DR, Goldspiel BR, Peck CC, Myers CE: Adaptive control with feedback strategies for suramin dosing. Clin Pharmacol Ther 52:11–12, 1992.

150. Lieberman R, Katzper M, Cooper M, et al.: Nonmem (NM) population (POP) pharmacokinetic (PK) analysis and Bayesian forecasting (FOR) during suramin (SUR) therapy in

prostate cancer: one-versus two-compartment models. Proc Am Soc Clin Oncol 9:68 (262), 1990.

151. Reed E, Cooper MR, LaRocca RV, et al.: Suramin in advanced platinum-resistant ovarian cancer. Eur J Cancer 28A:864–866, 1992.

152. Kilbourn R, Dexeus F, Amato R, Sella A, Bui C, Logethetis C, Trevino M, Newman RA: Clinical pharmacology of suramin administered by IV bolus injection in patients with refractory prostate cancer. Proc Am Soc Clin Oncol 10:112 (319), 1991.

153. Scher H, Jodrell D, Iversen J, et al.: Use of adaptive control feedback to individualize suramin dosing. Cancer Res 52:64–70, 1992.

154. Iversen J, Scher H, Motzer R, Forrest A, Curley T, Tong W, Niedzwiecki D: Suramin (sur): impact of individualized pharmacokinetic (PK) dosing on outcome in patients with prostatic cancer (PC) and renal cell carcinoma (RCC). Proc Am Soc Clin Oncol 10:103 (283), 1991.

155. Motzer RJ, Nanus DM, O'Moore P, et al.: Phase II trial of suramin in patients with advanced renal cell carcinoma: treatment results, pharmacokinetics, and tumor growth factor expression. Cancer Res 52:5775–5779, 1992.

156. Hutson PR, Tutsch K, Spriggs D, et al.: Evidence of an absorption phase after short intravenous suramin infusions. Cancer Chemother Pharmacol 31:495–499, 1993.

157. Horne III MK, Wilson O, Cooper M, et al.: The effect of suramin on laboratory tests of coagulation. Thrombosis Hemostasis 67:434–439, 1992.

158. Horne MK III, Stein CA, LaRocca RV, et al.: Circulating glycosaminoglycan anticoagulants associated with suramin treatment. Blood 71:273–279, 1988.

159. Stein CA, LaRocca RV, Thomas R, et al.: Suramin: an anticancer drug with a unique mechanism of action. J Clin Oncol 7:499–508, 1989.

160. Teich SA, Handwerger S, Mathur-Wagh U, et al.: Toxic keratopathy associated with suramin treatment. N Engl J Med 314:1455–1456, 1986.

161. Holland EJ, Stein CA, Palestine AG, et al.: Suramin keratopathy. Am J Ophthalmol 106:216–220, 1988.

162. Cheson BD, Levine AM, Mildvan D, et al.: Suramin therapy in AIDS and related disorders. JAMA 258:1347–1352, 1987.

163. Rago R, Suffitt R, Miles J, et al.: Suramin (SUR) weakness due to Fanconi's syndrome and mitochondrial myopathy supports disruption of mitochondria or energy balance as mechanism of activity (Abstr). Proc Am Soc Clin Oncol 11:114, 1992.

164. Falkson G, Rapoport BL: Lethal toxic epidermal necrolysis during suramin treatment. Eur J Cancer 28:1294, 1992.

165. May E, Allolio B: Fatal toxic epidermal necrolysis during suramin therapy. Eur J Cancer 27:1338, 1991.

166. O'Donnell B, Dawson N, Weiss R, et al.: Suramin-induced skin reactions. Arch Dermatol 128:75–79, 1992.

167. Kobayashi K, Vogelzang N, Pezen D, et al.: Suramin and skin neoplasms, submitted.

168. NCI investigators brochure.

169. Seidman AD, Schwartz M, Reich L, et al.: Immune-mediated thrombocytopenia secondary to suramin. Cancer 71:851–854, 1993.

170. Mahoney LJ, Barrie HJ: Adrenal insufficiency after suramin treatment of pemphigus (letter). Br Med J 2:655–656, 1950.

171. Wells HG, Humphreys EM, Work EG: Significance of the increased frequency of selective cortical necrosis of adrenal as a cause of Addison's disease. JAMA 109:490–493, 1937.

172. Humphreys EM, Donaldson L: Degeneration of the adrenal cortex produced by germanin. Am J Pathol 14:767–775, 1941.

173. Stein CA, Saville W, Yarchoan R, et al.: Suramin and function of the adrenal cortex. Ann Intern Med 104:286–287, 1986.

174. Feuillan P, Raffeld M, Stein CA, et al.: Effects of suramin on the function and structure of the adrenal cortex in the cynomolgus monkey. J Clin Endocrinol Metab 65:153–158, 1987.

175. LaRocca RV, Stein CA, Danes R, et al.: Suramin in adrenal cancer: modulation of steroid hormone production, cytotoxicity *in vitro*, and clinical antitumor effect. J Clin Endocrinol Metab 71:497–504, 1990.

176. Dorfinger K, Vierhapper H, Wilfing A, et al.: The effects of suramin on human adrenocortical cells *in vitro*: suramin inhibits cortisol secretion and adrenocortical cell growth. Metabolism 40:1020–1024, 1991.

177. Dorfinger K, Niederle B, Vierhapper H, et al.: Suramin and the human adrenal cortex: results of experimental and clinical studies. Surgery 110:1100–1105, 1991.

178. Ashby H, DiMattina M, Linehan WM, et al.: The inhibition of human adrenal steroidogenic enzyme activities by suramin. J Clin Endocrinol Metab 68:505–508, 1989.

179. Marzouk H, Zuyderwijk J, Uitterlinden P, et al.: Suramin prevents ACTH-stimulated corticosterone release by dispersed adrenocortical cells. Endocrinology 126:666–668, 1990.

180. Marzouk H, Hofland LJ, den Holder FH, et al.: Effects of suramin on hormone release by cultured rat anterior pituitary cells. Mol Cell Endocrinol 72:95–102, 1990.

181. Klijn JGM, Setyono-Han B, Bakker GH, et al.: Growth factor-receptor pathway interfering treatment by somatostatin analogs and suramin: preclinical and clinical studies. J Steroid Biochem Mol Biol 37:1089–1095, 1990.

182. Daugherty R, Cockett A, Schoen S, et al.: Suramin inhibits gonadotropin action in rat testis: implications for treatment of advanced prostate cancer. J Urol 147:727–732, 1992.

183. Pinedo HM, van Rijswijk RE: Suramin awakes? J Clin Oncol 10:875–877, 1992.

184. Harland SJ, Duschesne GM: Suramin and prostate cancer: the role of hydrocortisone (letter). Eur J Cancer 28:1295, 1992.

16

Radiopharmaceutical Therapy of Cancer Pain from Bone Metastases

Edward B. Silberstein, M.D.

INTRODUCTION

Of the 970,000 patients who will have cancer diagnosed in 1993, up to 75% of them will eventually develop osseous metastases. Bone pain from metastatic cancer is estimated to occur in 75–85% of the 120,000 patients in the United States annually who have osseous metastatic disease. The spine accounts for over 40% of marrow/bone metastases, pelvis about 25%, skull 12%, and ribs 6%. Many of these patients require an analgesic, usually a narcotic, and a third or more of the total have a diminished quality of life due to both pain and opioid treatment.[1,2]

Besides the reduction or relief of such pain, other goals of therapy in these patients include the prevention of pathologic fracture, improvement in patient mobility and function, reduction in the number of new metastases, and, of course, increasing survival. Radiopharmaceuticals with high skeletal affinity that have achieved many of these goals are now available.

MECHANISMS OF PAIN RELIEF FROM RADIATION

Pathologic fracture, impending or actual, and epidural tumor are sources of bone pain in these patients that must be quickly recognized and treated. The mechanism of bone pain in most patients is, however, not entirely clear. Marrow, bone, and periosteum are innervated with neural fibers that carry pressure and pain impulses to the central nervous system, and compression of these endosteal, periosteal and marrow nerves by tumor invasion does occur.

Intramedullary pressure in excess of 50 torr is also painful. However, it is of more than theoretical interest that pain relief may occur within days of the delivery of a single dose of 400–800 rads (4–8 Gy) of external beam radiotherapy before any reduction in tumor mass would be expected to occur. Just after radiotherapy there may well be increase in blood flow and edema to the tumor site, factors that would increase tumor volume. A variety of local humoral mechanisms for pain modulation have therefore been invoked, including several interleukins and prostaglandins. Low levels of radiotherapy could have an early lethal effect on highly radiosensitive cells such as lymphocytes producing these cytokines, thus explaining, at least theoretically, the prompt reduction in pain following radiation under 1,000 rads (10 Gy). Of course pathologic fracture, which occurs in 16–30% of bone metastases, will also be painful, and, if there is no displacement of bone around the fracture, radiographs may miss it.

Prostate Cancer, pages 261–268 © 1994 Wiley-Liss, Inc.

TABLE 1. Measures of Pain Relief

1. Changes in mobility and activity levels (Karnofsky or Eastern Cooperative Oncology Group [ECOG] Scales)
2. Hours of sleep
3. Semiquantitative pain scales
4. Radiation Therapy Oncology Group (RTOG) pain score (pain severity related to pain frequency)
5. Radiation Therapy Oncology Group narcotic score (medication type and frequency)

EVALUATIVE TOOLS

The evaluation of pain relief is a difficult process and one must be careful to use the proper tools. There are few experimental models for pain reduction. Table 1 indicates some of the measures of pain reduction which have been employed in the literature.

TELETHERAPY

External beam radiotherapy for focal painful metastatic disease has been employed for many years. The probability of pain relief is 70–90% when radiotherapy is given either as an 800-rad (8 Gy) single dose, as 2,000 rads (20 Gy) over two weeks (10 days of therapy), or as 3,000 rads (30 Gy) over three weeks (15 days of therapy). When there are multiple areas of pain, however, attempting to control all of these with focal radiation becomes extremely difficult, and a larger volume of normal tissue may be irradiated than is desirable.

Wide-field radiation is then a treatment option. A major collaborative study employed single-dose hemibody radiation to treat multiple areas of painful osseous metastases.[3] Six hundred rads (6 Gy) to the upper hemibody or 800 rads (8 Gy) to the lower hemibody were employed. Thirty percent of those treated became pain free, 50% had a partial response, and 20% were unchanged.

Eighty percent of responses occurred in one week and 95% within two weeks. The mean duration of pain relief was three months. Nausea, vomiting, or diarrhea was mild or moderate in 35% of the patients, with 15% of the total having severe or life-threatening diarrhea. Twenty-four percent of patients had mild to moderate hematologic effects and 9% of the hematologic effects were classified as life-threatening.[3]

INTERNAL BETA-EMITTERS

Ideal Characteristics

The administration of radiopharmaceuticals with a high affinity for the skeleton could lead to pain reduction or relief if there were selective targeting of osteoblastic metastases. An ideal radiopharmaceutical would have a sufficiently long half-life and sufficiently energetic beta emission to delivery a therapeutically significant radiation dose selectively to intraosseous tumor. Such a radiopharmaceutical should have no toxic effects requiring hospitalization.

It is difficult *a priori* to predict the optimum half-life for these therapeutic radiopharmaceuticals. A higher dose rate from a radiopharmaceutical with a shorter half-life might, on theoretical grounds, cause greater cell killing and resultant reduction in tumor volume. This is being tested with rhenium-188 etidronate, with a half-life of 0.7 days. On the other hand, a radiopharmaceutical with a more extended half-life might remain on or in bone long enough to decrease the appearance of new metastatic disease. The reactive bone-to-marrow uptake ratio for any radiopharmaceutical employed for therapy must be high. Excretion from sites other than tumor must be prompt so as to reduce irradiation of the marrow, kidneys, bladder, and intestine.

Difficulties with the Data

In reviewing the available data for the most widely used radiopharmaceuticals, one must be aware that the study of pain

TABLE 2. Patient Exclusions in Studies Evaluating Radiopharmaceutical Efficacy for Pain Relief

1. Pathologic fractures
2. Epidural metastatic disease
3. Short life expectancy (less than 1–2 mos.)
4. Significant leukopenia and thrombocytopenia
5. Negative bone scan
6. Change in hormone therapy within three months
7. Use of chemotherapy or external beam radiotherapy within the previous 4–6 weeks
8. Pretreatment bone scan shows deposition of the radiopharmaceutical in extraskeletal sites (except kidneys and bladder)
9. Known allergy to the radiopharmaceutical

requires a rigorous evaluative system in order to be reproducible, and such systems have not always been employed in the data we discuss here. Furthermore, in order to properly study pain relief in patients receiving radiopharmaceuticals, there are certain important patient exclusions that should occur in any such study. These are summarized in Table 2. One cannot determine in each of the studies of phosphorus-32, strontium-89, rhenium-186 etidronate, and samarium-153 ethylenediaminetetramethyl phosphonate (EDTMP) that these exclusions have been rigorously applied, although, in general, the more recent the data, the more documentation has been provided to determine the quality of the study, and the flaws in recent studies are few.

The radiopharmaceuticals currently in use for which extensive data are available include phosphorus-32 as orthophosphate, strontium-89 as the cation (strontium chloride), and two phosphonate chelates, [186]Re-etidronate and [153]Sm-ethylenediaminetetramethylenephosphonate (EDTMP) (Table 3). The two labeled phosphonates are chemically absorbed to the surfaces of metabolically active bone. Orthophosphate easily enters the hydroxyapatite crystal structure, and strontium-89, a member of the same periodic table group II as calcium, substitutes for it in hydroxyapatite. All these radiopharmaceuticals have high bone affinity, with ratios of uptake by metastatic to normal bone measured at 3–5 to 1, occasionally as high as 15 to 1 employing external scintigraphic quantitative techniques.

The two radionuclides chelated to phosphonates (Re-186, Sm-153) have sufficient gamma abundance, as noted in Table 3, to permit imaging of osteoblastic lesions. Comparison of images obtained with these agents with those from commercially available diphosphonates such as ^{99m}Tc-MDP has shown identical distribution, but slightly better spatial resolution of metastases with the latter.

There are now adequate data on the four beta-emitting bone-seeking radiopharmaceuticals listed in Table 3 to demonstrate successful relief of pain from bone metastases by each, when the reactive bone around the metastatic tumor has concentrated the administered material to a greater extent than normal bone.

TABLE 3. Radiopharmaceutical Characteristics of Therapeutic Compounds for Painful Osseous Metastases

Radiopharmaceutical	Physical Half-life (days)	Gamma Energy (keV) (% of Decay Events Yielding a Gamma Emission)	Avg. Beta Energy (keV)	Mean Beta Range in Tissue (mm)
[32]P-orthophosphate	14.3	—	690	3.0
[186]Re(Sn)HEDP	3.8	137 (9)	346	1.1
[153]Sm-EDTMP	1.9	103 (28)	290	0.8
[89]Sr-chloride	50.5	910 (0.01)	583	2.4

PHOSPHORUS-32

Phosphorus-32 (P-32) as sodium ortho-phosphate has been used in the treatment of intractable bone pain secondary to skeletal metastases since the 1940s.[4,5] This material may be administered orally or intravenously. Since oral phosphate absorption ranges between 40–80%, the intravenous route appears preferable in most instances. However, if P-32 is given under standardized conditions orally, it is effective and is far less expensive than if administered parenterally, since it does not have to be sterile or pyrogen-free under these circumstances. The P-32 bone-to-muscle ratio peaks at 6–10 by 72 hours. Dosimetry employing phosphorus-32 is complicated by the fact that some phosphate is also taken up by marrow cells, appearing in a variety of structural and metabolically active compounds, including ATP, DNA, and RNA. The radiation dose to normal bone has been estimated at 20–63 rads per mCi depending on the assumptions employed. There have been many treatment schedules for administration of phosphorus-32. Single or multiple intermittent doses have all been administered, with or without pretreatment with testosterone and/or parathyroid hormone to increase osseous uptake. Single doses have ranged from 4–12 mCi with total activity for multiple treatments totaling 5–20 mCi. There are no comparative data using two treatment schedules in the same study to indicate the optimum schedule. About 30 studies have documented the efficacy of phosphorus-32 in relieving intractable bone pain, with an overall response for breast cancer of 84% and for prostate carcinoma 77%, independent of total activity and type of pretreatment given, as long as about 8 mCi or more were administered.[5] No careful dose-escalation study has ever been performed.

We have noted that the methodology of measuring pain is a difficult problem, and,

of all the radiopharmaceuticals, the P-32 data, which are generally older, most frequently demonstrate this. A therapeutic effect was typically defined as substantial or complete alleviation of pain, a decrease in or complete elimination of analgesic requirements, and/or partial or complete improvement in functional capabilities. The duration of response to P-32 has ranged from 1.5–28 months. Radiographs have shown healing of lesions in 11–80%, depending on the series. Mild marrow suppression occurs in the majority of P-32-treated cases, occurring between three and eight weeks of initiation of therapy. Only one, and possibly a second, death have been related to myelosuppression by phosphorus-32, in both cases after multiple doses totaling 20 mCi. An agent such as P-32 that suppresses bone marrow not only from beta-irradiation coming out of adjacent bone but also from intracellular marrow (localization and subsequent marrow self-radiation) could theoretically show a greater degree of myelosuppression than agents that are deposited only on the surface of metabolically active (largely trabecular) bone. Also P-32 decays to sulfur, which would alter the structure of DNA molecules containing the radionuclide, probably with lethal or sublethal results.

All skeletal-seeking beta-emitters cause some degree of myelosuppression. With these agents it is wise to require an adequate leukocyte and platelet count, in the range of 4,000–5,000/μl and 100,000/μl, respectively. Also chemotherapy or radiotherapy given within 4–8 weeks of the administration of these radiopharmaceuticals can lead to impressive myelosuppression.

Polyphosphates and chelating phosphonates (e.g., etidronate, EDTMP) are strongly chemisorbed (absorbed by chemical bonds) to the surface of hydroxyapatite. These moieties have also been labeled with phosphorus-32. Polyphosphates are hydrolyzed in vivo to the orthophosphate and thus have the same efficacy. While

P-32–HEDP (hydroxethylidene diphosphonate) was found to have a high bone tumor-to-marrow ratio, at an administered activity of only 3 mCi marked bone marrow despression was observed, and only one of five patients who received 3 or 9 mCi of P-32-HEDP had relief of bone pain.[6]

STRONTIUM-89

Strontium-89 was first suggested as having a possible therapeutic role in the palliation of bone pain associated with metastatic bone disease in 1942, even preceding the earliest reports of phosphorus-32 for this purpose (although P-32 had been used for therapy of hematologic diseases since 1936). Total skeletal uptake of strontium has been found to range from 11–88% depending on the degree of osteoblastic response, the extent of metastatic skeletal involvement, and renal function.[7] Metastatic bone has been shown to retain strontium (and the phosphonate chelates of Re-186 and Sm-153) longer than normal bone, but the mechanism is unknown.[7] The average dose to tumor in bone from a 4-mCi injection of strontium-89 appears to be 3,000–3,500 rads (30–35 Gy) with tumor doses as high as 13,000 rads (130 Gy) noted, compared with about 150–300 rads (1.5–3 Gy) delivered to the bone marrow. Responses, defined as reduction in pain and analgesic consumption, and improvement in performance scores, have been reported in 55–80% of patients. Complete relief of pain has been documented in 5–20% after a single infusion. Time to response is 1–4 weeks, with a median duration of benefit of 3–6 months. Treatment has been possible at approximately three-month intervals, with pain relief after the second injection possible about 50% of the time. As with all of the radiopharmaceuticals under discussion, myelosuppression is the only toxic effect (besides a brief flare noted in some series), with the platelet and leukocyte counts falling to 30–70% of pretreatment levels within 3–7 weeks.[7-12] Myelosuppression is more severe in patients with extensive osseous neoplastic involvement and those with previous large-field radiotherapy or intensive chemotherapy. Most researchers do not find a direct relation between the total activity of strontium administered and the degree of pain relief from the agent, or between pain relief and reduction in serum acid phosphatase levels,[7-9,11,12] although a recent study did demonstrate a statistically significant ($P <$ .01) descrease in both acid phosphatase and prostate-specific antigen (PSA) levels in strontium-89-treated patients compared to controls treated with placebo.[10] Response to strontium-89 is independent of narcotic requirements, tumor type, and performance status.[8] One recent study has found a reduction in new painful sites in patients given local external beam therapy followed by strontium-89,[10] but there are no data yet published that show improved survival in responders.

The reporting of response rates in the published data on strontium-89 must be analyzed carefully. For example, some investigators report only responses of those who survive for three or more months. We have found approximately 55% response in uncensored patients when response was defined as either an increase of two steps in the 10-step Karnofsky scale or reduction in analgesic medication by 25%.[8] Some nonresponders died within 3–4 weeks of injection, however, before evaluation could be completed. With removal of patients having characteristics listed in Table 2, Sr-89 efficacy rises to 70%. In contrast, Schmidt et al., giving doses of 1–3 mCi, reported a complete response rate of 59%, a partial response rate of 28%, with only 14% showing no response.[9] The definitions and measurements of responses, severity of pain, and extent of tumor vary widely in these different series. Strontium-89 appears to be efficacious in almost all reports, with response rates as high as those reported for hemibody radiation and similar to those from phosphorus-32 for prostate and breast cancer.[12] A review of 18 articles covering treatment of 715 patients with strontium-89 showed 467, and 65%, had a complete or partial response.

Recently strontium-89 chloride injection (trade name: Metastron) was approved by the Food and Drug Administration (FDA) for the relief of bone pain in patients with painful skeletal metastases. The recommended dose is 4 mCi (10 ml) over 1–2 minutes and repeated doses are not recommended at intervals of less than 90 days. The nadir of platelet depression occurs 5–8 weeks after Sr-89 administration with a slow recovery, typically reaching preadministration levels 10–16 weeks after treatment in most investigators' experience, although the package insert states this could take six months.

RHENIUM-186 DIPHOSPHONATE

The stable bone-seeking diphosphonates were labeled with Tc-99m for diagnostic uses in 1971. The chemical properties of rhenium and technetium are very similar, as both are in group VIIA of the periodic table. In 1979 Mathieu et al. labeled HEDP with rhenium-186 and described its distribution in rats.[13] Like technetium-99m diphosphonate, therapeutic rhenium-186 diphosphonate agents are not pure chemical species but include rather complex, time-dependent mixtures of polymers of various sizes. These mixtures can be separated by high-performance liquid chromatography (HPLC) and the separated components have been shown to have significantly different biodistributions and in vivo kinetics. Employing HPLC and then a simple gravity-flow chromatographic procedure, therapeutically useful bone-seeking rhenium-186 HEDP was purified,[14] and clinical trials have been performed.[15] The distribution of ^{99m}Tc-

medronate, a widely used bone-imaging agent, and ^{186}Re-etidronate was found to be virtually identical, with very similar kinetics to ^{99m}Tc-etidronate, also a bone-imaging radiopharmaceutical. The mean marrow dose from an average of 33.5 mCi given intravenously has been calculated at 118 cGy with a tumor dose about 3,500 cGy,[15] although the dosimetry models employed are being reexamined by these workers. Maxon et al. found clinically significant pain relief in 79% of patients by 2–3 weeks. A flare response occurred in 10%. The average therapeutic response lasted for five weeks, although follow-up was limited to eight weeks.[15] A double-blind crossover study of ^{186}Re-HEDP and ^{99m}Tc-MDP has also been completed by this group, showing that rhenium-186, and not the diphosphonate moiety, causes pain relief. About 50% of patients who responded to a first treatment responded to a second or even a third injection of ^{186}Re-HEDP.

SAMARIUM-153 EDTMP

Samarium-153 is another beta-emitting radionuclide with physical properties useful in the formulation of radiotherapeutic agents. It has a short half-life (46.3 hours) not too different from that of rhenium-186 (90.6 hours). The University of Missouri group examined several multidentate (moieties capable of multiple chelations) aminophosphates to chelate samarium and found the best combination of high bone uptake with low nonosseous uptake and rapid blood clearance to be a samarium complex with EDTMP. ^{153}Sm-EDTMP was found to clear more rapidly from blood than ^{99m}Tc-MDP, to provide very similar scintigraphic images and bone to marrow ratios,[16-19] and to be excreted more rapidly in the urine than rhenium-186 HEDP.

In cancer patients, myelotoxicity has been seen in doses between 0.6 and 1.0 mCi/kg, generally when the marrow dose exceeded 200 rads. A phase I study of [153]Sm-EDTMP indicated a wide range of retained skeletal activity (40–95%) similar to that noted with strontium-89.[20] Any prior chemotherapy where a marrow-toxic agent has been employed enhanced the myelotoxicity of this and all beta-emitting radiopharmaceuticals. Several research teams have found that pain has been fully or partially relieved in about 65% of evaluable patients for periods ranging from 1–11 months following a single or multiple intravenous administrations. Pain recurrence responded to retreatment in 5 of 9 patients in Australia, with dose-limiting toxicity predictably being thrombocytopenia. Platelet counts returned to pretreatment levels within 10 weeks of therapy. Responders noted improvement within 14 days with no obvious dose–response relationship (i.e., increasing response with increasing activity given) noted for this radiopharmaceutical,[19,20] similar to the data for P-32 and Sr-89. There was also no correlation of the clinical response to [153]Sm-EDTMP with acid or alkaline phosphatase or with skeletal radiographic changes. PSA was not measured.

CONCLUSIONS

The currently available and widely studied internally administered radiopharmaceuticals (P-32, Sr-89, Re-186-HEDP, Sm-153-EDTMP) for skeletal metastases can reduce pain due to metastases positive on bone scan in 65–80% of patients. Prior to treatment, patients who will respond cannot be distinguished from nonresponders, except perhaps by performing complex dosimetry of individual lesions with a tracer dose, although this has never been shown for these beta-emitters given to relieve bone pain. All of these radiopharmaceuticals have the advantage of toxicity limited to mild or rarely moderate hematopoietic depression, and about a 10% prevalence of a flare response (brief local

pain increase). In contrast, hemibody radiation leads not infrequently to nausea, vomiting, diarrhea, or cystitis. The response to hemibody radiation may be several days more rapid than that to the internal emitters.

Controlled comparative trials of the available bone-seeking radiopharmaceuticals must be instituted to determine the radiolabeled compound combining greatest efficacy with least toxicity. Since all of these beta-emitters can be myelosuppressive, combining these with chemotherapy must be done cautiously. There are no problems with concurrent hormone therapy. The cost of strontium-89 alone exceeds $1,700 U.S. dollars for a single dose. Phosphorus-32 currently costs $750 for 10 mCi.

Thus, of the therapeutic goals listed in the introduction to this review, pain reduction, improvement in patient mobility and function, and reduction in the number of new painful metastases are now all possible with the use of beta-emitting bone-seeking radiopharmaceuticals.

REFERENCES

Treatment with Teletherapy

1. Poulson HS, Nielsen OS, Klee M, et al.: Palliative irradiation of bone metastases. Cancer Treat Rev 16:41–48, 1989.
2. Tong D, Gillick L, Hendrickson FR: Palliation of symptomatic osseous metastases. Cancer 50:893–899, 1982.
3. Salazar OM, Rubin P, Hendrickson FR, et al.: Single dose half-body irradiation for palliation of multiple bone metastases from solid tumors. Final Radiation Therapy Oncology Group report. Cancer 58:29–36, 1986.

Phosphorus-32

4. Van Nostrand D, Silberstein EB: Therapeutic uses of [32]P. In Freeman LM, Weissman HS (eds.): Nuclear Medicine Annual 1985. New York: Raven Press, pp 285–344, 1985.
5. Silberstein EB: Phosphorus-32 radiopharmaceuticals for the treatment of painful osseous metastases. Sem Nucl Med 22:17–27, 1992.

6. Potsaid MS, Irwin RJ Jr, Castronovo FP, et al.: ^{32}P-diphosphonate dose determination in patients with bone metastases from prostatic carcinoma. J Nucl Med 19:98–104, 1978.

Strontium-89

7. Blake GM, Zivanovic MA, McEwan AJ, et al.: Sr-89 therapy: strontium kinetics in disseminated carcinoma of the prostate. Eur J Nucl Med 12:447–454, 1986.

8. Silberstein EB, Williams C: Strontium-89 therapy for the pain of osseous metastases. J Nucl Med 26:345–348, 1985.

9. Schmidt CG, Firusian N: ^{89}Sr for the treatment of incurable pain in patients with neoplastic osseous infiltrations. Int J Clin Pharmacol 9:199–205, 1974.

10. Porter AT, McEwan AJB, Powe JE, et al.: Results of a randomized phase-III trial to evaluate the efficacy of strontium-89 adjuvant to local field external beam irradiation in the management of endocrine resistant metastatic prostate cancer. Int J Rad Oncol Biol Phys 25:805–813, 1993.

11. Kloiber R, Molnar CP, Barnes M: Sr-89 therapy for metastatic bone disease: scintigraphic and radiographic follow-up. Radiology 163:719–723, 1987.

12. Robinson RG, Preston DF, Spicer JA, et al.: Radionuclide therapy of intractable bone pain: emphasis on strontium-89. Sem Nucl Med 22:28–32, 1992.

Rhenium-186 HEDP

13. Mathieu L, Chevalier P, Galy G, et al.: Preparation of rhenium-186 labeled HEDP and its possible use in the treatment of osseous neoplasms. Int J Appl Rad Isotopes 30:725–727, 1979.

14. Deutsch E, Libson K, Vanderheyden JL, et al.: The chemistry of rhenium and technetium as related to the use of isotopes of these elements in therapeutic and diagnostic nuclear medicine. Nucl Med Biol 13:465–477, 1986.

15. Maxon HR, Thomas SR, Hertzberg VS, et al.: Rhenium-186 hydroxethylidene diphosphonate for the treatment of painful osseous metastases. Sem Nucl Med 22:33–40, 1992.

Samarium-153-EDTMP

16. Goeckeler WF, Troutner DE, Volkert WA, et al.: ^{153}Sm radiotherapeutic bone agents. Nucl Med Biol 13:479–482, 1986.

17. Ketring AR: ^{153}Sm-EDTMP and ^{186}Re-HEDP as bone therapeutic radiopharmaceuticals. Nucl Med Biol 14:223–232, 1987.

18. Logan KW, Volkert WA, Holmes RA: Radiation dose calculations in persons receiving injections of samarium-153 EDTMP. J Nucl Med 28:505–509, 1987.

19. Holmes RA: [^{153}Sm] EDTMP: a potential therapy for bone cancer pain. Sem Nucl Med 22:41–45, 1992.

20. Turner JH, Claringbold PG, Hetherington EL, et al.: Phase I study of samarium-153 ethylenediaminetetramethylene phosphate therapy for disseminated skeletal metastases. J Clin Oncol 7:1926–1931, 1989.

Index

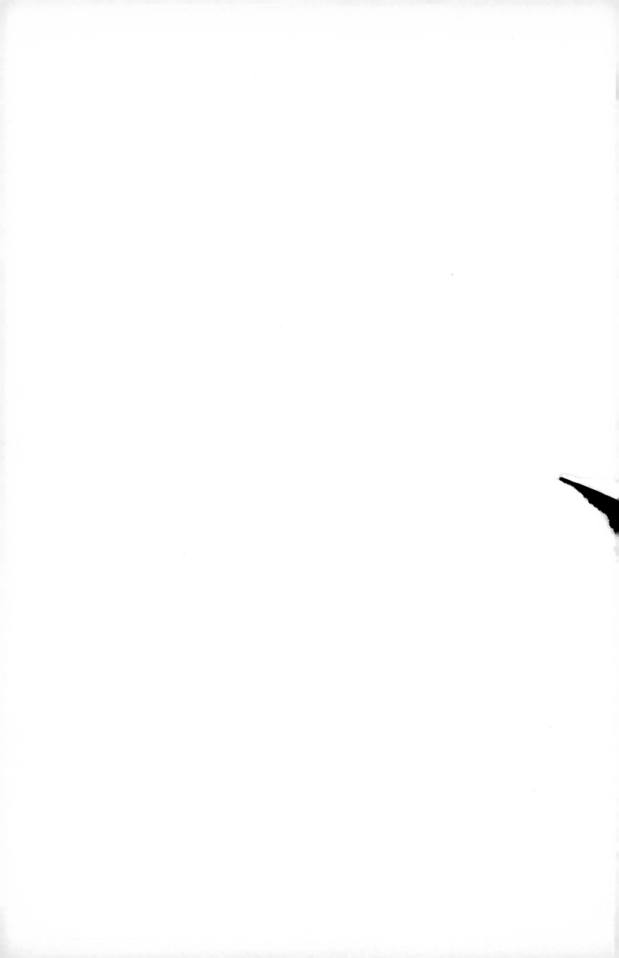